NOT
SO
FAST

NOT
SO
FAST

The Smarter, More Gradual Approach to
Intermittent Fasting Benefits That Last

MARISA MOON, NBC-HWC

ISBN: 979-8-89109-589-2 - paperback

ISBN: 979-8-89109-590-8 - ebook

ISBN: 979-8-89109-591-5 - hardcover

Medical Disclaimer

This book provides general information about the potential benefits of intermittent fasting, a reduced carbohydrate diet, and sufficient intake of animal protein and nutrient-dense foods. The information and recommendations do not constitute medical advice. Consult your physician before making major dietary changes, especially if you have medical conditions or take prescription medications. The author specifically disclaims any and all liability arising directly or indirectly from the use of any information in this book.

Marisa Moon is a Certified Master Primal Health Coach and National Board-Certified Health and Wellness Coach.

Health/Wellness coaching is not a substitute for the advice, treatment, and/or diagnosis of a qualified licensed medical professional or registered dietitian.

References and products mentioned in this book are provided for informational purposes only and do not constitute an endorsement.

Download the
Not So Fast Action Guide

To get the best experience with this book, readers who download the PDF Action Guide are able to implement with more clarity and take the next steps needed to start intermittent fasting for results that last.

Scan This QR Code to Download Your Guide:

In the Action Guide you will find:

- Bulleted key teaching points for parts 1-7 of this book
- At-a-glance action step summaries for each part 1-7
- FAQs and how to work with Marisa

Save time with the Action Guide so the action steps are at your fingertips.

Get your free Action Guide
by scanning the QR code above or visit:
Marisamoon.com/notsofast/resources

Table of Contents

PART 3: EAT NOURISHING FOODS

PART 4: EXTEND YOUR FASTS

PART 5: THOUGHTFULLY ADAPT

PART 6: SLEEP: A CRITICAL PIECE OF THE PUZZLE

PART 7: CRAFTING YOUR UNIQUE FASTING LIFESTYLE

Introduction

It's quite ironic that I'm sitting here writing a book about fasting when I love food more than anything in life. Food is my greatest hobby—reading food magazines, shopping for food, preparing and cooking food in my free time, trying new foods any chance I get. I love learning about food, sharing food with others, and eating it, too, of course!

I first learned about intermittent fasting (IF) in 2012 when I was introduced to the Paleo Diet. Though the ideas behind fasting made perfect sense, it didn't appeal to me whatsoever. At this point, I was pretty darn healthy. I was only twenty-nine years old and had just fixed my terrible IBS (irritable bowel syndrome) by ditching gluten and eating a more Paleo-ish diet. Those felt like massive changes in my life, like I was already sacrificing a lot.

My interest only grew once I came across the concept of Bulletproof fasting—coined by famous biohacker Dave Asprey, who's behind the wildly trendy coffee recipe known as Bulletproof coffee. I was already drinking Bulletproof coffee at this point because I'd learned the healthy fats would provide my brain with clean-burning ketone energy that could assist me in my battle with inattentive-type ADHD.

I struggled massively with time management, initiating tasks, switching tasks, and bringing tasks to completion. I found it nearly impossible to force my brain to do something it didn't feel like doing. And since I got into the Paleo Diet and living more naturally, I resisted using ADHD medication as the sole solution to my brain-chemistry troubles. I wanted to boost my brainpower naturally instead.

In comes that idea of Bulletproof fasting. Mornings were a struggle for my hazy, disorganized brain. I had a lot of shit to think about and manage at the start of each day, so I loved the idea of drinking only my Bulletproof coffee and foregoing breakfast as 'the most important meal of the day'. If I could still be healthy and skip breakfast, I thought, it would save me a lot of thinking, time, and effort in the mornings.

Welp! That was easy.

Making breakfast, or even thinking about breakfast, was a pain in the ass. This, however, came naturally to me. Drink my fatty coffee and wait to eat until I get some shit done. I did that a few days in a row, and I noticed immediate benefits! It wasn't just the time-saving, effort-saving effects of my morning fasts that paid off big time. By noon, my concentration and mental energy were on a level I'd never experienced before.

Fasting helped free up so much energy inside me. I felt more alive. I felt more *with it*. More capable. More awake. On mornings when I ate instead, I'd feel so lazy and checked out afterward. My energy went way down—not just in my body, but in my brain.

That's where it became so obvious to me. If I want to be productive and I want my brain to have the energy it needs to get shit done, I need to prioritize my brain over my love of eating. I need to give my body a break from digestion so it can focus on sending blood flow, oxygen, and life-giving energy to my brain, where I desperately need and want it.

On days I fasted, I was better able to manage my lazy-yet-scattered brain and had more energy to tackle the day ahead. I'd finally found a natural way to boost my brain and follow my dreams in a way I never before thought was possible for me.

Maybe what surprised me most about intermittent fasting was that I felt less obsessed with food. It wasn't on my mind every hour of the friggin' day. When I fasted, I could focus my attention on things I needed to accomplish instead of, *What else should I eat?*

Before fasting came into my life, my hunger and fullness meters were all out of whack. Like, crazy-messed-up. I could eat anytime, anywhere, and there still seemed to be no end to my appetite. I'm pretty confident in saying your hunger-fullness meters are probably out of whack, too.

The American diet, and pretty much every diet out there besides lower-carb, messes up your hunger and fullness signals. It makes your appetite more and more voracious over time. Our human brains are wired to see food as something highly rewarding. This was extremely beneficial back in the most ancient of times. Seeing food as a reward helped us survive harsh conditions because we'd prioritize food above almost any other thing that needed our time, energy, and effort to accomplish. Without that relentless drive to eat or acquire food, humans never would've survived as a species.

Fast forward to modern society, and we don't face those harsh conditions. Where we live, food scarcity is rare. Food, whether it be junk food or real food, is ridiculously accessible. Things get more complicated with the advertisements that practically surround us—like that little video player on the gas station pump, those familiar golden arches, or the burger-and-fry billboards we drive past in the city.

Edible food-like stuff is available literally everywhere. We're taunted when we least expect it—like the candy bowl at the bank, the free granola bars in the waiting room at the auto shop, the onslaught of snacks within arms reach while waiting to checkout at Walgreens, and the 24-hour drive-thrus that tease our subconscious with that familiar junk food craving that's locked into our stored memories. If only they taunted us with blueberries, salads, and braised beef, we might be alright.

What makes things worse is that food manufacturers know we fall prey to the drug-like allure of processed, highly-palatable foods. We can't resist the tastes, textures, and rewarding experiences we get from eating their scienced-up imposter food. We're hooked. Our stores, streets, and pantry shelves are filled with items far more rewarding than their natural counter-parts—real food. It's downright trickery we're being fooled with, and we're so enraptured we don't even realize the spell we're under until it's broken.

I'll teach you how to break that spell. Whenever you want to experience the freedom, you can improve your relationship with food and shield yourself from the trickery of modern processed foods. I almost called this book Intermittent Fasting Freedom. That's the name of my online program in which hundreds of others have learned my approach to flexible fasting and real-food living. I'll teach you how to put an end to dieting that sucks and experience more food freedom that's so rewarding you want to keep doing it.

It's not just our food system that's messed up or the hunger-fullness signals in our brains. If you ask our DNA, we live in pretty messed up times. Stress is chronically high, and the body can't contain it or sustain it. Maybe that's because our sleep is so low in quality or quantity, and the body can't function like that for much longer. Activity levels are low—we're sitting all friggin' day and night—and we're emotionally and intellectually exhausted.

We're exposed to mad toxins in our food, our medications, our supplements, the air we breathe, the water we drink, the soap-like chemicals we wash our clothes with, and the fragrance-laced products we freshen our homes with. Soil quality and farming methods are disgraceful, misinformation is flooding our digital landscapes, mental health disorders are at an all-time high, the state of our gut health is continuously threatened and declining, and chronic disease and dependence on pharmaceuticals are also at all-time highs. And all these things work against our ability to fight disease, feel healthy, and lose excess weight (even with fasting).

You know you can't keep going at the rate you're going and still be there for your grandkids. You know something's gotta change, and this something must be out there. You know you need to eat more healthy foods, but you want something you can stick with. You want something you can enjoy if you're out with friends or want a glass of wine. You want something that feels so good you *don't want to* get off that wagon. *Right?*

You're in the right place. It's time to play a more active role in your own health and well-being. Your health can no longer take last place compared to all the other priorities in your life. As keto coach Ben Azadi said, "I believe that when you treat your health casually, you will end up a casualty."

This will require some drastic, yet, rewarding changes. It will require you to be curious and venture outside of your comfort zone. It'll require you to believe in yourself. To reinvent yourself. You *are* a healthy person. You are someone who prioritizes healthy living. You are already an action-taker because you're reading this book. Nice work!

This is the most comprehensive walkthrough I've ever created to help guide you through the change, how to make healthy eating a priority in your life, how to free yourself from the grips of your appetite, and how to experience energy and confidence with your health like never before.

If you're not already intermittent fasting, you will be once you're through with the next few chapters because I'll lay out a simple foundation for you. And it is missing in your life. I'm a firm believer that pretty much every adult should be doing 12-hour overnight fasts, at minimum, on a daily basis. It's like basic maintenance, so your metabolic hormones don't go haywire, and your body can focus on other important jobs besides digesting food and combatting unnecessary food toxins.

I'm not writing a book about the science of fasting or the fastest road to weight loss. It doesn't sit right with me to label this a diet book. This book is about making your health your hobby and improving your relationship with food. This book is about the way we humans are designed to consume food, and how to do it at a pace our bodies respond favorably to.

I realize it's quite likely that what you want most is to lose some excess weight in the hopes it will result in you being healthier, more energized, and happier in your day-to-day life. That's what most people expect: to lose weight and *then* get healthy (mind and body) *as a result*. That's what your doctor made it sound like, too, when he suggested you lose some excess weight to help with your high blood pressure and arthritis. But what they don't acknowledge, and what I hope you'll soon accept, is that you must first step into a version of yourself that's *healthy*. You make more choices that a healthy *you* would make, because then the weight can finally come off and stay off for good. I can help you get healthy, and that will inevitably lead to weight loss, but I can't help you lose weight in order to get healthy. It's going to work the other way around, and I can promise you that (*especially* if you're a woman over forty. *Hey girl!*).

I'll show you my RESET method to start or restart with intermittent fasting and healthy-*ish* eating so your body has what it needs to be health-*ier* and shed stubborn pounds. I'll give you lists and tricks and tools to make healthy eating more enjoyable, more effective, and more doable. I'll challenge you with mindset shifts that are essential if you want to overcome self-sabotaging patterns that have been holding you back from experiencing significant changes in your health and in your life.

I'll give you the 'go' on some rule-breaking, and I'll give you just enough of the science so you know why and how things are working for you or against you. I'm going to address some absolutely critical things, like stress and sleep, that cannot be ignored any longer if you want to see changes in your body and become the healthy version of yourself you've been fantasizing about for a decade now.

You will get answers, and you will get solutions. Are you ready to receive them?

I've seen hundreds of clients who are facing the same self-limiting obstacle: *How can I get what I want without sacrificing the other things I want to keep doing?* You need to really want this. You need to be willing to change things in your life that are holding you back. You'll need to sacrifice things that are only getting in the way of what you truly want. You'll need to be imaginative and optimistic and adopt a new sense of determination. There's a new life for you, one you can mold and create for yourself. No one can make that happen for you, so it's your turn to show up for yourself big time.

I won't ask you to exercise like a maniac or fast like hell. Nope. Oftentimes, I'll ask you to slow down. It was months into writing this book that I realized the title it truly needed. *Not so fast.* People want to jump in and speed things along because they're desperate for change, but a certain degree of consideration and patience is absolutely required. I'm sure you're busy—like crazy busy these days, and you feel you need results, like, *yesterday.* You're tired of trying new diets and want one that works for daily life. You know you need to stick to healthier habits, but you haven't found anything that's realistic to stick with. Well, I've got thousands of clients and followers who've willingly chosen to stick with this, and it's quite reasonable to assume that you will, too. Patience and persistence are the only two things you really need if you want to succeed.

I always tell my new clients that everyone succeeds as long as they don't give up. It's quite likely your journey will be longer than you expect. Do yourself a favor and stop comparing yourself or your journey with someone else's situation. Thousands of variables make your situation unique, your body unique. And that's what makes comparison a deceitful, treacherous road to travel.

It's time to celebrate your uniqueness and become so familiar with it that you become a student of your own life. A lifelong student of your own body and mind. How does that sound? You're a fascinating subject, to be sure.

CHAPTER 1

In Case You Don't Read
Further Than This

I t astounded me to learn that fewer than 10 percent of people finish an online course they've purchased. We're not as bad with books, but still, we never get around to reading about 40 percent of the books we've purchased. On the bright side, that means around 60 percent of the books we've purchased will reach their destination. And you're here. You're reading this, so you're on the advantageous side of that statistic.

What Lies Ahead

What beliefs do you have about your willingness to finish this book? Some serious FOMO might kick in once I finish telling you what lies ahead. This book consists of seven parts. I named most of them after certain phases of my proven RESET method for intermittent fasting. Thousands of people have used the RESET method to train their bodies for enjoyable fasting that's more likely to become a healthy lifestyle.

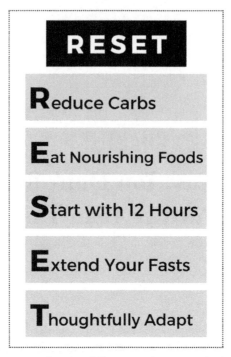

RESET is an acronym for the following phases, and it's designed to help anyone start—or restart—with intermittent fasting for long-term success:

Reduce Your Carbs

Eat Nourishing Foods

Start With 12 Hours

Extend Your Fasts

Thoughtfully Adapt

I've compiled the RESET method into a free PDF manual for my followers to learn this simple method and start with confidence. You can download my RESET manual now at *marisamoon.com/iffreedom*. Along with the digital manual, for 12 days, you'll get my coaching emails, which provide plenty of advice to help you with the process. Join the thousands of people who've successfully implemented this proven framework and see what your body is truly capable of.

Assuming you're ready for a deeper dive into the incredible world of intermittent fasting and healthy, doable eating, get ready for what's ahead:

In *Part 1: Start With 12 Hours*, I'll teach you why I refer to 12 hours as your home base (a majority of which will occur while you sleep). I'll bust the myth that breakfast is the most important meal of the day, and we'll review the importance of your biological clock, known as the circadian rhythm. I'll give you extensive guidelines on how coffee can be an enjoyable part of your daily fast, and you'll get my *What Breaks a Fast* lists. The action steps in Part 1 will guide you to put this info into action and train for intermittent fasting right away.

In *Part 2: Reduce Your Carbs*, you'll learn about the difference between burning carbs and sugar for energy and burning fat. You want to burn body fat, right? That's where your relationship with carbohydrates becomes critical to face and rectify. I'll give you action steps on how to do a gradual 21-day carbohydrate reduction so your life isn't turned upside down by these changes, so you're not too uncomfortable or inconvenienced, and so you start feeling way better than you have in years.

In *Part 3: Eat Nourishing Foods*, I'll give you some real talk regarding why you can't go on without giving a crap about the nutrition in your diet. You'll learn about two key terms: metabolic flexibility and mitochondria (where energy is created inside your cells). I'll help you make nutritious eating more practical, and I'll squash nonsense dogma that's left you wondering: *Which foods are actually healthy?* Part 3 ends with action steps that show you how to build a nutrient-dense plate because the more nutritious your diet, the more progress you'll make, and the more incredible you'll feel. Did I mention that fasting comes easier when you eat this way, too? Way easier.

In *Part 4: Extend Your Fasts*, you'll really get clear on why I named this book *Not So Fast*. You'll learn about hormesis, a beneficial adaptation to stress you're tapping into whenever you fast or exercise for better health. I'll teach you about stress so you can see what your current living situation is doing to your health and how likely you are to succeed under those circumstances. I'll introduce you to what I call fasting safeguards, the things you can do to prevent backslides, and barriers that inhibit progress with fasting. Finally, you'll see the most common mistakes and mindset tricks people get caught up in at this stage. I'll give you clear action steps to put this info to good use while you work on extending your fasting window the *not-so-fast* way.

In *Part 5: Thoughtfully Adapt*, I'll teach you the difference between fasting as a lifestyle versus fasting as a diet. You'll learn about the most important fasting safeguards that I call *3-Meal Days* and how to thoughtfully adapt for flexibility and results. This book would be insufficient if I didn't address the differences between female and male bodies in response to fasting and how women can tweak their practice to work in concert with their hormones to prevent those dreaded plateaus. The action steps help you prioritize what's next so you can play a more active role in your success.

In *Part 6: Sleep. A Critical Piece of The Puzzle*, I bet you can guess what we'll be covering. You can't hide from it any longer if you want results. Sorry, but sleep matters. If you want to lose significant weight, improve your health, and sustain results, it's time to get smart about your sleep. And I've got plenty of tips, tricks, and lists to help you do just that.

In *Part 7: Crafting Your Fasting Lifestyle*, I'll introduce you to the importance of gut health and how to improve your gut so your efforts make the greatest impact. We'll review the many types of fasting schedules to consider, and I'll even talk about fasts that involve food. With the *5 Types of Hunger*, you'll uncover the distinct triggers that prompt your urge to eat, ranging from physical hunger to various emotional and situational cues. Some of the most important lessons you'll learn are how to revise your self-image so self-sabotage doesn't screw you in this process, and how self-reflection and experimentation are key to your long-term success.

In Case You Only Read This Chapter

Your time is valuable, and it's good that you dedicated some time and—actually—sat down to start this book. If you don't read beyond this chapter, start with the following steps right now to see significant changes in the way you feel and how your body responds to the way you eat.

Step 1: Start with 12 hours

If you're not currently fasting at all, you want to start with 12-hour overnight fasts. That means that if your last bite of food (or gummy vitamin or sip of wine) occurs at 9 p.m., for example, you're not eating or consuming any carbohydrates or protein until 9 a.m. the next day.

Just by doing that, you'll begin to improve your metabolism, burn through superfluous energy stores, sleep better (especially if you allow ≥ 3 hours of fasting before bed), and achieve more efficient detox and recovery. Just so you know, Part 1 of this book focuses entirely on this topic. If you have questions, it's likely you'll find the answer in Part 1. What if a 12-hour fast is difficult for you? That's a sign your metabolism is sorely out of shape, and it really needs you to take this seriously—so your health and energy improve for life.

Step 2: Improve Your Diet by Cutting Out The Following Crap

- Ditch the fried foods, partially-hydrogenated oils (Crisco, margarines, powdered creamer), and strictly limit vegetable seed oils (canola oil, rapeseed oil, soybean oil, sunflower seed oil, cottonseed oil, safflower oil, grape seed oil, peanut oil).

  o Replace inflammatory seed oils with pourable healthy oils like 100 percent avocado oil, extra virgin olive oil, or cultured oil (like the new one by Zero Acre Farms); and safe saturated fats, like unrefined coconut oil; unrefined, sustainable palm oil; butter, ghee (clarified butter), and clean-sourced animal fats like tallow, duck fat, and lard.

- Drastically reduce added sugar.

  o A good rule of thumb: keep total sugar per sitting under 10 g if fat-loss is your goal.

  o Cut out excuses for daily desserts. Dessert shouldn't be a daily occurrence unless it's like a square of ≥ 70 percent dark chocolate, a handful of organic berries, or one serving of seasonal fruit. Dessert is, otherwise, best saved for times of celebration.

- Say no to sweetened drinks and sweetened coffee creamers (exceptions are limited to pure stevia, pure monk fruit extract, allulose, xylitol, or erythritol).

- Drastically reduce simple carbohydrates—especially flour-based foods.

  o Aim to cut down on your consumption of flour-based foods by limiting them to one meal per day or less (limit to once per week for faster results).

- Conquer your nighttime eating habits.

  o Aim to stop calorie intake at least 3 hours before bed. Night eating is extremely habit-forming, so it's important to try and overcome it. When you stop eating at least 3 hours before bed, you facilitate deeper sleep and increased fat-burning abilities.

  o This habit is easier to change when you work your way up to it. If you currently eat before bed, start by trying to stop eating one hour before bed. Then, once that's locked in, increase it to ninety minutes before bed, and so on.

If you just do the above steps along with Step 3 listed below, you can make some massive improvements in your health. Massive!

Step 3: Patiently increase your fasting window.

Once 12 hours feels comfortable for you, try 12.5 hours. Take your time here. Little by little, over weeks at a time, you'll increase the length of your routine fasts. If, or whenever, you abandon fasting entirely for three weeks or longer, to avoid further setbacks, I always suggest you return to 12-hour fasts to help retrain your body.

5 Reasons You'll Want to Keep Reading

1. Two years from now, you'll wish you had. Think about what you were doing two years ago—doesn't that seem like eons ago? Yet here you are, still feeling the same way about your body, your diet, your health. It's time to take life by the horns and get serious about changing your health for the long run. You absolutely can do it!

2. If you stopped reading, what would you do with the time instead? It's likely your time would be used up by doing whatever you usually do, and nothing will change. Keep reading; do something different.

3. Think of all you'll learn about the body, about health, about yourself. Learning expands what's possible for you, it prevents age-related brain decline, and it empowers you to believe you're capable of more—because you are!

4. Unlike most diet books, the concepts I'll present to you aren't based on trends or ideas that will soon be outdated. These concepts have been time-tested throughout human existence, but they've recently been left behind due to rapid changes in the ways we eat and live in modern society. These concepts deserve your attention and will change your life for the better, starting now. Be a trailblazer! Others will see what you've accomplished and feel so inspired to improve their health, too.

5. Your body is an incredible thing, and it's capable of abundant health and reform. Don't you deserve to experience what that feels like?

7 Key Factors That Make or Break Your Progress with Fasting

As you work your way through this book, you'll see frequent mention of the many factors that (strongly) influence your fasting results. Some of them might be obvious to you, such as the length of your fasting window or your activity level, but there's far more nuance to consider.

First, take a glance at the list that follows. Then, continue reading to find an overview for each factor so you're primed for what we'll cover in the rest of this book. Keep in mind how some of the nuance shared here is relevant to your own circumstances.

7 Key Factors That Make or Break Your Progress with Fasting

1. **Fasting Window** (timing, length, and consistency)

2. **Diet & Dieting History** (carbohydrate content, nutrient density, and offensive foods)

3. **Sleep**

4. **Stress** (psychological, emotional, physical, and physiological)

5. **Activity Level**

6. **Hormonal & Metabolic Health**

7. **Mindset**

From personally coaching hundreds of individuals through a fasting lifestyle since 2018, I can confidently say your progress will, at some point, be hindered by one or more of these 7 factors.

1. Fasting Window

As you know, the length of your "fasting window' can have one of the most significant impacts on your ability to achieve results. That much is obvious. But what isn't so obvious is that the length of your fast must work in harmony with your current circumstances.

Circumstances to consider when determining the most fitting fasting length:

- Are you just starting out with fasting?

- Are you just returning to fasting after a hiatus?

- Have you been sleeping fewer than 6 hours a night, or are you frequently awakened throughout the night?

- Are you dealing with sudden compounding stressors in your life?

- Women, are you menstruating, pregnant, or nursing?

- Has your activity level recently changed?

- Does your current fasting window feel effortless or arduous?

- Are you extremely routine with your fasting window?

- Do you binge eat when your eating window opens?

That list could've been 50 questions long, but the following six factors will help inform the other variables to consider when adjusting your fasting window more appropriately.

2. Diet

No matter which method of fasting you follow, diet has a major influence on your abilities to:

- Sustain a fasting habit

- Achieve results

- Maintain any results you accomplish.

Although some people do succeed at fasting without changing their diet, the odds are greatly stacked against you. The crappier your diet is, the longer you'd need to fast to counter the effects of the poor diet. Should you read a fasting book that encourages this type of fasting, such as *Delay Don't Deny*, you might find it alluring to still eat at the McDonald's drive-thru, order pizza, and have dessert as long as you fast 20–36 hours at a time—but, it won't be long before you realize that such a yo-yo dieting pattern leaves you at war with your body and brain. Your body will be starved of critical nutrients and the consequences will compound, dangerously, over time.

Although a handful of clients I've worked with chose to fast longer rather than improve their diet, I can't think of a single one who ultimately reached their fasting goals that way. Why? Because they eventually quit or change the plan after suffering long enough through the tug-of-war that happens between a junky diet and aggressive fasting (and the voices in their head).

What you eat has undeniable effects on your:

- Appetite and hunger levels
- Thoughts about food
- Fasting stamina
- Ability to turn this into a lifestyle
- Mindset about what's possible (self-efficacy)
- Mood
- Brainpower
- Physical energy
- Stress tolerance
- Pain, inflammation, and healing
- Immunity
- Fat-burning abilities

From where I stand, diet must be considered in the equation. This could be the one thing standing in your way of adopting a healthier lifestyle—one you truly want to stick with. Once you're habitually opting for nutritious foods, it transforms the way you think about your health and the way your body functions. You won't know what's possible until you experiment openly and figure out what's sustainable for you through different phases of your life.

This isn't just about eating healthy foods. It's also about discovering which foods are inflammatory for you. Which foods disagree with *your* gut? Which foods spin *your* appetite out of control? This is where the freedom really begins because once you can make the connection between specific foods and your personal reactions to them, you're finally in control of how comfortable or energized you feel (physically, mentally, and emotionally) in response to the food choices you make.

The exploration doesn't stop there. What was your diet like in your twenties, thirties, forties, and so on? How often have you been on a diet? Do you have a history of extreme dieting and dynamic weight loss and regain? When it comes to your expectations about how your body will respond to intermittent fasting and a new diet, those are important facts that must be considered.

3. Sleep

Are you getting enough quality sleep? The duration and quality of sleep you get on a daily and weekly basis have an incredible influence on your fasting results and your appetite. Your metabolism can slow down when your body lacks sufficient sleep. Your body and brain become too stressed from the concurrent demands of your lifestyle, and the consequences are obvious.

Shorter sleep times plateau your waistline.

When you're short on quality sleep, you also experience undesirable symptoms caused by increased hunger hormones and decreased satiety hormones. You want more even though you just ate.

Yup, that's right. *Lack of sleep makes you eat.*

More concerning effects include an increase in the stress hormone known as cortisol (which, at the very least, equals more belly fat) and increased insulin levels (which equals more fat storage). The body senses sleep deprivation as a chronic stressor.

No one who's sleep-deprived enjoys having the sleep discussion with me. Just the very nature of the conversation probably brings up feelings from adolescence when our parents demanded, "Lights out by 10 p.m.!" And since sleep-time generally occurs in the evening when our willpower is tanked and our *f*ck it!* attitude takes over, bedtime for adults feeds into a never-ending cycle of rebellious behavior and grumbling *shoulds. I should go to bed earlier, I should get more sleep, I should watch less TV, etc.*

I'd say that at least half of my clients struggle to prioritize sleep and achieve quality sleep. Most of those clients have a great reason to be short on sleep (like a new baby or poorly managed anxiety), and many are caught in an exhausting trap of family demands or work pressure that makes sleep seem impossible to prioritize. Even if I help them to see it is possible, many will feel unmotivated to make this improvement because nighttime is when they finally get some alone time and indulge in mindless activities, which are tough habits to break, regardless of how unfulfilling they are.

If only they could see the bigger picture. If only they knew how much their life would improve from this shift in priorities. Collectively, this gives you an idea of why deep sleep and sleep tracking are on my list of *Fasting Safeguards* (which you'll learn about in Chapter 38), and why an entire section of this book, Part 6, is dedicated to the topic of Sleep.

4. Stress

It helps to categorize stress into two types:

1. Psychological/emotional stress
2. Physical/physiological stress

Psychological/emotional stress is the mental stuff—your kid gets bullied at school, and you feel helpless to make it stop, or your normal state is to feel anxious at work all day, every day. Physical stress can be from an injury, arthritis, or an inflamed gastrointestinal tract from unknown food intolerances. Stress can also be physiological, like stressing your cells and immune system. For example, the hormonal stress of a woman's period approaching, your body's efforts to fight off a lingering cold, too much exercise without adequate recovery time, or the chemical cascade of stressors that results from being chronically under-slept.

Stress plays a massive role in your ability to achieve results with intermittent fasting. You could say stress plays the largest role because fasting *is* a stressor. That's why fasting works (or *doesn't* work). It's a hormetic stressor, and you'll learn all about that in Part 4. Stress comes up in nearly every chapter because your ability to apply what you've learned and benefit from it is greatly influenced by stressors in your life that might be overwhelming your system at the time.

If you try to fast too long for your body or mind's current threshold of stress tolerance, you can see it backfire in the form of:

- Binge eating
- Stalled weight loss
- Increased hunger
- Forgetfulness
- Rebellion
- Apathy towards self-improvement
- Self-sabotage
- Feelings of defeat or failure
- Exhaustion
- Recurring or frequent infections or injuries
- Chronic pain and inflammation
- Hormonal dysfunction (spotty periods, terrible PMS, thyroid dysfunction, infertility, etc.).

To ignore the stress component is to ignore your ultimate goal of sustainable weight loss.

5. Activity Level

Many variables related to your exercise regime will have a big influence on your fasting abilities. The following questions give you an idea of how many factors you may need to consider at different times in your life.

- How hard do you exercise?
- What time do you exercise?
- How often do you exercise?
- What type of exercise is it, and how long is it?
- How do you fuel your exercise and recover from it?
- Have you recently changed up your exercise habit?
- How much do you move around during the day?
- How much do you enjoy or look forward to the exercise?

My clients who are exercise enthusiasts tend to exercise too much, too often, or too hard to see continued results with fasting—especially in comparison to their fasting window, sleep habits, and the quality of their diet. These variables must be considered if you want to reach your fasting goals and continue a dedicated regime that includes both exercise and fasting. Exercise and fasting don't always work in a complimentary way. This is a place where a fasting coach or informed trainer really pays off.

6. Hormonal & Metabolic Health

This one's a doozy. Boy, let me tell you, with each one of these seven factors I'm writing, I'm like, "Oooo, this one's really important. No, *this* one's really important. No, *this one's* really important." And here we are at hormonal health, which is probably the most misunderstood, under-emphasized set of factors controlling your likelihood of success with *any* diet or intermittent fasting.

As you'll learn in this book, weight gain is essentially a hormonal problem with a hormonally-centered solution. By the time someone comes to me, it's not a problem related to how many calories they're taking in or how much exercise they're *not* getting. It's a problem with their hormones.

When someone says the word *hormones*, you probably think about sex hormones like estrogen and testosterone. But hundreds of hormones exist, and far more than sex hormones are at play here. Hormones influence every single function in your body. To address the more common hormonal imbalances I see as a coach, we'll cover stress hormones, satiety, and hunger hormones, metabolic hormones (like insulin!), anti-aging hormones, inflammatory hormones, sex hormones, and neurotransmitters (hormones that send messages between your brain cells!).

Questions related to hormonal dysfunction or metabolic impairment:

- Is your thyroid function impaired?

- How adequately do your adrenal glands handle stress? Are you on the verge of burnout?

- Do you suffer from insulin resistance like most Americans do today?

- Have you been diagnosed with pre-diabetes, type 2 diabetes, or metabolic syndrome?

- Is your waistline larger than your chest or hip circumference?

- Do you struggle with leptin resistance and have trouble stopping eating once you're full?

- Are you pregnant or breastfeeding?

- Are you going through perimenopause (or those early stages of perimenopause where you're not even sure that's what's going on)?

- Is your period approaching within the next week?

- Are you doing any hormone replacement therapy?

Any of these circumstances may suggest that your metabolism is highly impaired, which means you want to approach intermittent fasting the *not-so-fast* way. Start slow, give your body a chance to correct your systems and adapt over time. Hormones are key to explore and understand, specifically, where you're at right now, because this will have a major impact on your ability to seek better health with the help of fasting and/or any sort of dieting.

7. Mindset

Anytime you're trying to make a new habit, break an old habit, do something to better yourself, or step outside of your comfort zone, your mindset can make or break you. That's why, naturally, when it comes to fasting, the mind plays so many tricks.

Mindset work is sort of messy. Most of the time, we're not consciously aware of our thoughts or patterns of thought. If you don't get something out of your head, you can't logically analyze or improve it. Some ways to become more consciously aware are to speak your thoughts out loud, either in conversation or to yourself, by journaling or tracking in another written form, or by meditating and observing through mindfulness training. Yet the work doesn't stop there. Noticing is a huge piece, but what comes next is an active effort to reflect on those patterns, practice self-compassion, and experiment with new, supportive self-talk or 'reframes' that help tweak your perspective.

This isn't easy to do on your own or in the day-to-day hustle of life. That's why most people don't do it until they hit rock bottom or when they're up against incredible odds, which leads them to seek support from a licensed therapist, a business coach, a life or health coach. Some may even take a sabbatical to recover from burnout and focus more deeply on their self-care as a result.

The three most common mindset tricks I see people get tripped up with on their health journey:

1. Viewing a diet as temporary

2. The mindset: if *some* is good, *more is better*

3. All-or-nothing thinking

Through the chapters ahead, we'll visit these mindset tricks time and time again. Soon, you'll be more aware of the hold they have on you and can patiently strive to overcome them as you transform your health.

PART 1

Start With 12 Hours

RESET

R	Reduce Carbs
E	Eat Nourishing Foods
S	Start with 12 Hours
E	Extend Your Fasts
T	Thoughtfully Adapt

CHAPTER 3

12 Hours is Home Base

This is home base for you, for me, for everyone. This is where you start and where you return to any time you've given up on fasting and slipped back into an eat-all-day, eat-all-night lifestyle.

It may require some trust in me to consider this an essential starting place if you're inspired to jump head-first into fasting. It requires some patience with yourself as you start or *restart* with 12 hours. After reading this, you'll understand why it's often the best way to go.

Other intermittent fasting methods skip this essential starting line. I consider it essential for dozens of reasons you'll see below. A general explanation is that you must give your body and mind time to adapt to the changes so you're not discouraged by the negative effects experienced from starting out too aggressively.

Not so fast....

When you rush into a new fasting routine without training for it, you might experience one or more of these consequences:

- Moodiness and irritability
- Brain fog and being easily distracted

- Early afternoon binge-eating

- Voracious 'eating window' behavior

- Morning hunger signals that seem impossible to ignore

- Headaches, light-headedness, dizziness, nausea, or even dangerously low blood sugar

- Low mental and physical energy during your fasting window

- Low energy for morning workouts

- Constipation

- Quitting before you can experience positive results

That last bullet is pretty key for a lot of people. When you rush into starting or restarting, you run the risk of feeling discouraged and thinking, *This whole fasting thing isn't for me*, or *I can't do this*. You might quit because you hate how you feel when you force yourself to starve for 16 hours (because that's what the internet told you to do).

I'm here to tell you that 12 hours is an ideal target for a beginner, as well as for experienced fasters who've abandoned a fasting habit and wish to return. This gradual approach is especially helpful while you work on that carb-reduction phase explained in Part 2 and eating more nutritious foods, covered in Part 3.

Give your body and brain time to adapt, and you're more likely to enjoy fasting and experience immediate benefits! This also gives you a chance to clean up your diet while your metabolism learns to use stored energy, so fasting feels easy and rewarding.

The easiest way to grasp the importance of a 12-hour starting line is to consider Janet, who's starting a new running habit. Janet doesn't think of herself as a runner because she never really runs or jogs for exercise. Just yesterday, however, she decided to sign up for a marathon because her best friend inspired her by suggesting they run alongside each other.

The marathon is six months away, and Janet needs to start training for it. Does she start running ten miles a day? No way! Even if she was a runner back in high school, she can't just pick up a habit like that without training up to that level again. So, she wisely starts with a one-mile jog for the first week or so. Then she runs one-and-a-half to two miles. Then she runs three miles, she goes to four and five miles, and so on. If she tried running ten miles from the start, she'd likely injure herself and quit before she even got close to the life-changing experience the marathon tempted her with in the first place.

A 12-hour fasting window looks something like this:

- Finish eating dinner (or drinking that glass of wine) by 8 p.m.

- Forego any evening snacks (drink herbal tea if you'd like).

- Fast overnight from 8 p.m. until 8 a.m.

- Don't consume anything in those 12 hours, with the exception of Bulletproof coffee (AKA fatty coffee), black coffee, or unsweetened tea in the morning (read the coffee section ahead in Part 1 to learn more).

  o Herbal tea is also acceptable for the evening. Stevia is an approved sweetener, but use only enough to make it tolerable, not very sweet, and be sure it's not the brands *Pure Via* or *Stevia In The Raw,* which would break your fast as they're made with a glucose-spiking ingredient called dextrose.

Are you ready to get started?

It's time.

Right now, promise yourself a minimum of 12 hours as a daily goal while you train your body and mind to get used to the changes. Everything in your life will influence or be influenced by your new intermittent fasting lifestyle. You'll be glad you took your time to consider and adapt to all the variables involved.

Some variables to consider while adapting:

- When will you eat?
- Where are you in your day when you hit that 12-hour mark?
- Do you have food ready, and do you have time to prepare or eat it?
- How does this affect your morning routine?
- How does this affect your evening routine?
- Is it convenient or inconvenient to eat at that time?
- Did you start fasting too early before bed?
- How were you affected by the eating habits of other people in your surroundings?
- What did you experience in your fasting window that was positive? Negative?
- Does it feel good? Does it feel effortless or difficult?

Even if you don't go any further with intermittent fasting, this 12-hour minimum will enable you to have more energy, heal faster from injury and pain, have less anxiety, get more rejuvenating sleep, lose weight or maintain weight more easily, and live a longer, healthier life!

Stick with a fasting window of around 12 hours until it feels effortless, and then you can gradually increase by 30–60 minutes per week as long as the increment you're at feels nearly effortless before you next increase it. More questions are answered in the action steps located at the end of Part 1. Let's move on to Chapter 4: *Breakfast Myths,* and then we'll learn about your circadian rhythm so you can start to reframe your perspective on the importance of a morning meal, typical breakfast foods, and eating breakfast 'like a king'.

CHAPTER 4

Breakfast Myths

A s you start incorporating fasting into your routine, you can expect some unsolicited comments from others who are puzzled by your choice to skip a traditional meal like breakfast. Members of your household may express concerns like, "Breakfast is the most important meal of the day!" or "Skipping breakfast will slow down your metabolism!"—or "Did you see this?" as they share a clip of this morning's news anchor boasting about another study that reportedly *proves* breakfast eaters are healthier than non-breakfast eaters.

Nutrition research is a messy industry, and the scientific methods used make it difficult to draw real-world conclusions—especially when it comes to our dietary habits. If you're interested in the complex reasons research links breakfast with better health or the absence of breakfast with lesser health, I enjoyed the decent summary in a NYT article titled *Sorry, There's Nothing Magical About Breakfast*. I appreciate the important mentions and terminology used, such as *association, not causation*, and *publication bias*. Although the article serves as an adequate summary, it doesn't even touch on the differences between breakfast-skippers who are fat-adapted versus those who are carbohydrate-dependent. You'll learn to identify and distinguish the two states, fat-adapted versus carb-dependent, in Part 2 of this book.

Lucky for you, my RESET method helps to train your body to become fat-adapted—less carb dependent, less insulin-resistant, and more metabolically flexible—so skipping meals doesn't deserve a second thought except for how much you wish you tapped into this superpower sooner!

Now that I've spent wayyyy too many hours of my time learning about the history of breakfast and trying to sift through the competing facts, studies, and perspectives about whether breakfast is healthy or not, I feel exhausted by this topic. That's when it occurred to me that all you, as the reader, really want to know is:

Is breakfast really that important?

Short answer: It depends on your other eating habits. For some people, breakfast isn't that important. For others, it is.

Medium answer: If you plan to skip one meal every day as part of a new fasting lifestyle, it could be healthier for you to skip dinner, eating only breakfast and lunch rather than skipping breakfast. This is because our bodies are designed to process food more optimally during the daylight hours. The body responds with more healthful outcomes when you stop eating by the time evening sets in.

But—and this is a big but—*it doesn't matter which meal-skipping approach is healthier if you can't stick with it long enough to experience benefits and maintain them.* That's why I gravitate toward breakfast-skipping. It's easier. It feels more natural. In the many years I've been a fasting coach, I've learned the vast majority of people feel the same way. We skip breakfast because it works better with our lifestyles and the timing of our appetites.

A majority of people find it easier to skip breakfast rather than dinner because:

- Hunger-stimulating hormones are lowest in the morning between 4 a.m.–9 a.m. [12] Thus, it's easier to skip breakfast and put off eating until afternoon.

- Skipping breakfast gives you one less thing to do in a hectic morning routine.

- It leaves you with one less thing to figure out during those groggy first hours of the day.

- Morning routines usually include coffee or tea drinking, both of which help curb hunger (and give you something to look forward to besides food).

- Evening time means increased appetite hormones, decreased willpower, and an increased desire for personal autonomy (like eating or snacking freely while at home).

- In most households, dinner is a coveted time for family or social connection, and it's the meal most associated with pleasure.

What to Expect In This Chapter

There's still much to consider on this topic, so let's review what's coming. I'll introduce you to some key periods in human history that culminated in popular breakfast beliefs and the unhealthy breakfast habits of today. Then, I'll take a swing at the destructive American breakfast foods so you can consider whether a high-carb meal is ever advisable for breakfast (or for dinner).

You're likely wondering, *Is breakfast the most important meal of the day? Should it be the largest meal of the day?* To help answer those questions, in the next chapter, I'll teach you about your internal clock called the circadian rhythm. This will give you an understanding of one of the most influential facets of your health and functionality—and it's pretty foundational to any conversation about meal timing.

First, we should get clear on what you literally mean when you use the word *breakfast*.

Breakfast, to you, might mean one or more of the following:

1. **A meal comprised of breakfast foods**—socio-cultural foods from the breakfast 'category' which is primarily made up of typical American breakfast foods (like eggs, bacon, breakfast sausage, pancakes, waffles, hash browns, cereal, bagels, coffee cake, oatmeal, toast, English muffins, pop tarts, blueberry muffins, scones, orange juice, etc.).

2. **The morning meal**—a meal consumed within two hours of waking.

3. **The first meal** of the day.

4. **Ingestion that breaks the fast**—food, drink, or caloric content that technically breaks the foregoing fast.

I'd like to bring your attention to numbers 3 and 4 on that list. Consider how the first meal you eat is often the thing that *breaks your fast* (i.e., #3 can also be #4—as long as you don't break your fast before your first meal—like by adding sugar or milk to your early-morning coffee). In a fasting lifestyle, you might call your first meal breakfast, regardless of the time you eat, because that meal literally breaks your fast. That meal is also the first meal of your day, but it's not necessarily comprised of typical breakfast foods, and it's not necessarily in the morning (list items #1 and #2).

Ahhhh semantics. Gotta love it.

Let's look at the history of a morning meal so you can decide whether a meal with typical breakfast foods (#1) and a morning meal (#2) carry any power in shaping your healthy journey ahead. What you're about to read is going to open your eyes to a whole new point of view.

History: Paleolithic Times

Some people find history boring. I know. At times, though, it sure helps put things in perspective like nothing else can. By learning a bit about the history of American breakfast and how our human ancestors ate throughout our ancient past, you'll have a new opportunity to determine what makes sense for your own way of eating versus just doing things everyone else thinks are best.

How about we first think back to our oldest human ancestors—way, way, way back to our hominin and *Homo sapiens* ancestors who roamed this planet during the Paleolithic era, before we became a civilized species. They were nomadic, always on the move, never settling down in one place, and only eating whatever they could scavenge, forage, and hunt in their tribe's surrounding area (a range of 7–500 square miles).

There was no meal ready to consume in the morning. For a tribe to eat first thing, considering the lack of secure food-storage solutions during these times, ancient humans would need to first forage, gather, or prepare that food for safe consumption. Any easy-to-grab insects, grubs, roots, and leaves were prepared for the children who were no longer breastfed, and the remaining tribe members would split off to start on their daily chores (women and children weaving baskets, repairing or making clothing, prepping animal hides, harvesting berries, drying herbs and leaves, acquiring fresh water, while men went off to scout new land, hunt and catch dinner with a trap, net, bow, spear, or whatever means their culture had advanced to at the time).

The only meal enjoyed together as a family or tribe was one around the fire at the end of the day or following a successful hunt. There was no 'three meals a day'. There was no breakfast. Everything was about survival first. As you read this book, keep in mind that the Paleolithic era spans around two million years. In the latter 65,000–300,000 years of this time period, the human species, *Homo sapiens,* was being encoded with the DNA recipe that determined the genetic blueprint we're all made of today. And that's why, even if you couldn't care less about paying attention in history class (like me), you might want a basic understanding of this stuff.

Your genetic code is nearly identical to that of our ancestors living in the so-called caveman days.

Our DNA simply hasn't had enough time to evolve with the changes of modern life. That means your body's hardware is designed to work with the same inputs people were exposed to during primitive times—and if you want your hardware to function optimally today, you'll need to put some effort into learning what inputs your DNA requires.

That ain't easy, considering *everyyyything* has changed and advanced in modern societies today. The good news is that *what* you eat and *when* you eat are two of the simplest things to tweak and satisfy those inputs your body needs to thrive.

Once humans began to settle into civilized nations, like the start of the Roman Empire around 400 A.D., breakfast was still practically non-existent. Records show that people across Europe and Egypt woke up super early before the sun rose, and before noon, they had nothing but coffee and a pipe to smoke.

Imagine what it was like in that Game-of-Thrones-like era. Leading civilizations were primarily governed by Christian principles above all else. Europeans saw a morning meal as an act of gluttony, a deadly sin. They believed they were more in alignment with God by resisting temptations to sin, which included unnecessary food consumption. Regardless of the outdated moral viewpoints these concepts were founded on, the truth still remains. Breakfast wasn't a thing.

Although breakfast wasn't a thing back then, certain people still ate in the morning. It was socially acceptable for laborers to eat a morning snack to fuel the back-breaking exertion of the day ahead. It was also expected for young children, the elderly, and the physically weak or wretched to consume food in the morning. Still, this wasn't breakfast—or any actual meal. It was something small like a piece of bread or a piece of cheese. Even ale or wine was consumed to supply simple caloric energy.

Remember, there weren't any refrigerators, preservatives, or foods-in-a-box at this time. So, a morning breakfast meal was impractical and unattainable for most.

The Term *Breakfast* Emerges

Looking at historical records, it's apparent the term breakfast began to appear in 15th-century English, where it was defined as a morning meal that literally broke the fast endured through the night. Interestingly, most people tried to avoid it.

According to the Wikipedia article on medieval cuisine, "…men tended to be ashamed of the weak practicality of breakfast."[3]

In his book *Food & Feast in Medieval England*, P.W. Hammond explains, "Eating breakfast meant that one was poor, was a low-status farmer or laborer who truly needed the energy to sustain his morning's labor, or was too weak to make it to the large, midday dinner."

By the time we get to the 18th and 19th centuries, people still only sat down for one formal meal per day, known as *dinner*. After the Industrial Revolution shook things up in the 19th century, dinner shifted to the evening time because factory work made it unfeasible to consume a main meal during the middle of the day. Until then, however, dinner was eaten around noon. Interestingly, according to Abigail Carroll in her book, *Three Squares: The Invention of the American Meal*, it was considered the most important meal of the day because it "…bridged the gap from dinner one day to dinner the next."

Our ancestors fasted most of the day, eating *one meal a day*. In the fasting community, we abbreviate this as OMAD.

Once we were in the early 20th century, times massively changed. The American breakfast at first became quite an indulgence. There was more freedom and possibility in the development of American culture, so if a large morning meal made people happy, then that's what they adopted. Americans faced massive social and cultural shifts as a result of economic threats, modern inventions of this time, and other significant events that ultimately left them desperate for household conveniences. That's where the business-savvy food inventors, like John and Will Kellogg, found an opportunity to position their new *breakfast cereal* of sugar-laden cornflakes as a solution for the modernized consumer.

The Kelloggs and other food innovators claimed breakfast cereals were lighter, healthier, and faster to prepare, and they promoted their products as the answer to pretty much every health and lifestyle pain point of this time. The busy housewife and modern worker were promised less time in the kitchen thanks to that so-called complete meal in a box. From this point forward, the American breakfast was reinvented. Americans ate it up. Literally. They trusted the Kelloggs' marketing slogan, "Breakfast, the most important meal of the day," and passed on this faux wisdom for many more generations to come (and counting).

And so it began. The average American household turned to packaged foods and nutrition claims rooted in deceptive marketing campaigns. Families rose and shined with a meal of mechanically processed carbohydrates—like Carnation's instant breakfast or some sugar-laden breakfast cereal disguised as a health food—in place of traditional foods like eggs, cheese, wild berries, cold meats, and ham or beefsteak, oatmeal, stone-ground cornbread, and johnnycakes.

Which sounds better to you? Those old-time favorites? Or a box of grass seeds that have been milled, extruded, tempered, dried, baked, spoiled, and sweetened to hide the taste of rancid fatty acids. Yup, it's pretty nasty when you consider all that mechanical processing required to turn grass seeds into breakfast cereal—a food I consider unworthy of human consumption, even though it's a nostalgic food that, just like you, I find enjoyable to eat.

Allow me to challenge you to reconsider the significance of a routine morning meal. Particularly, in the next chapter, let's reflect upon the consumption of culturally relevant breakfast foods that are inherently unhealthy and misaligned with your genuine health aspirations.

CHAPTER 5

The Dangers of a High-Carbohydrate Breakfast

Throughout this book, you'll learn about the hormone insulin and the effects it has on your experience of gaining weight, losing weight, and maintaining a healthy weight. One thing to keep in mind for now is that no other nutrient spikes glucose or insulin more than carbohydrates. I'm referring particularly to sugars and starches, not fiber. Therefore, a high-carbohydrate breakfast is less than ideal for almost anyone with access to healthier options.

A high carbohydrate meal, in general, isn't ideal because excess carbohydrates drive insulin production, fat storage, increased appetite, relentless cravings, energy dips, inflammation, anxiety, and more.

Let's say one enjoys a breakfast of two slices of whole-grain toast with butter and one tablespoon of jam. Even with the whole grains, that's a considerable load of quick-burning carbohydrates for breakfast—like over 40 g of carbohydrates in one sitting. In response, your body must ask itself, *Where do I put all this excess sugar so I can get it out of my bloodstream ASAP!?* Since carbs convert to sugar, and too much sugar in your bloodstream is toxic, this job is quite urgent.

Insulin shuttles some of that sugar out of your bloodstream and into storage as quick-burning carbs called glycogen. Then, it helps convert the excess carbs into slow-burning body fat. What happens next is usually a steep drop in your blood sugar levels—which is why you might feel *hangry*, moody, or light-headed, craving a routine pick-me-up snack or drink to help you function for the next few hours.

This vicious cause-and-effect relationship results in a destructive metabolic cycle that's harmful if it happens so regularly. Yet, still, this is a typical experience for a majority of Americans today. What are some of the lesser-known outcomes we suffer from when we're trapped in this vicious cycle? That steep drop in blood sugar stimulates fight-or-flight stress hormones, which heighten anxiety and make it difficult to manage. It's not only anxiety that's triggered by today's American diet; we also see increased impulsiveness and ADHD symptoms, as well as massive cravings that resemble addiction.

Your brain has genetic presets that make it very rewarding to eat carbohydrates and sugar. Over time, it takes more and more of those foods to give you the same dopamine reward you're jonesing for—which explains why you crave carbs or sugar more and more, and you wind up feeling addicted to these foods.

I've been known to say that by serving kids a breakfast of pancakes with syrup and a glass of orange juice, you might as well be giving them a breakfast of frosted birthday cake. The dangers of dessert-like breakfast dishes were even recognized in an 1898 parenting manual, which warned that pancakes are "...part of a 'graveyard diet' and 'one of the worst things that a child can put in its stomach under the pretense of food.'"

Same goes for adults, for whom it can be more damaging to the metabolism. Even now, there's hardly a difference between your bagel or scone and a piece of cake. You could be setting yourself up for disaster. Orange juice? Don't even get me started! It's pure sugar. Cereal? Still sugar. Even whole grains are mostly sugar and quite inflammatory. Oatmeal? It's slightly better, but still sugar.

We're consuming breakfast foods that marketers have cunningly enticed us into eating. We're caught in a collective habit of eating specific foods at designated mealtimes. This behavior is largely driven by society's norms, manipulated science, the addictive influence of carbohydrates, and our limited awareness.

When we look to ancestral health for answers, it would make sense to eat your first meal later in the day because that would give you the morning to gather or hunt for food in the wild. Maybe you'd be picking at some berries or wild fruit you found along the way. Then, you'd have lots of protein in your primary meal, which occurs around midday because it's time to feast on the results of your successful hunt or fishing trip. At other times, you'd be fasting more often than not—especially in the winter when food was scarce.

Without modern factories and farms manufacturing food so cheaply today, it would be impossible to enjoy bagels, pasta, breads, and sweets so routinely. That's why I'd describe most such foods as *treats* (and sometimes even junk!). They don't belong as a staple of your diet, no matter what the breakfast industry tries to tell us with their heart-healthy labels.

We shouldn't even have oatmeal every day when healthier options are available. Think about it. Long ago, you'd only have oats available every morning during harvesting season, and you'd have to spend many of your waking hours harvesting those tiny grains by hand. Then, to reduce the toxic compounds in those seeds (which you'd know about because of the wisdom gained by living in harmony with nature), you'd soak and ferment the oats before cooking. That's what our ancient ancestors did. They knew how to treat such plants so the food became more digestible.

Before I became a health coach, I was a food blogger at *mylongevitykitchen. com*. My most popular blog post is titled *The Truth About Overnight Oats*. I created that post because of how many people I saw praising overnight oats as a healthy breakfast solution. Overnight oats is uncooked oatmeal mixed with a liquid (like water, milk, or plant milk) and soaked overnight in the refrigerator so the oats have softened enough to eat by morning.

You can imagine why that article is popular. It's a shortcut—overnight oats—and many so-called health enthusiasts claim that it's a nutritious breakfast. Don't fall for this new age wishful thinking. Cook your oats, every time, or eat them less frequently. The best oatmeal to try would be sprouted or fermented. Sprouting or fermenting helps reduce toxins and release more of the nutrients that are otherwise trapped inside the seed. Both sprouting and fermenting also increase our ability to digest the oats properly.

What To Eat For Breakfast

If you're a breakfast eater, I recommend your meal be comprised mostly of whole foods. **Here's such a breakfast meal:**

- Eggs
- Meat (uncured, nitrate-free, antibiotic-free)
- Seared cherry tomatoes
- Sliced avocado
- 1 mini tangerine

Breakfast could also be something like a smoothie or soup. Such options are easy to digest and, thus, won't disrupt your daytime concentration and energy as much as a normal meal would. Try to think outside of the breakfast box. The foods you eat for your first meal don't have to be from the breakfast category. Leftovers make some of the best breakfast meals, especially because it doesn't take much to satisfy us in the morning!

When it comes to your weekly rotation, do your best to avoid packaged 'breakfast' foods, pastries, and grain-based breads of any kind. Save those foods for special occasions, and instead, choose leftovers or cook some eggs (and eat the yolks!) and veggies, like the good ol' days. If you can't eat eggs, try some uncured breakfast ham with avocado stacked on top of a sweet potato or with organic cottage cheese if you're eating low-carb.

The most important macronutrient for you to consume in the daytime is protein. When you eat enough protein, it keeps you full for hours after your meal and supports your body with enhanced metabolic health.

When it comes to carb-rich foods, anything made with flour, or food and drinks sweetened with sugar (including 100% fruit juice, concentrates, the syrups in your fancy coffee, and synthetic sweeteners like aspartame), we'd all be wise to save those things for a consciously welcomed treat.

When you break your fast with quick-burning carbs, it sets you up for decreased glucose tolerance the rest of the day, no matter what your meals look like for lunch/dinner.[4] What this means is that your body is more stressed by the high carbohydrate load, which equals more inflammation, more fat storage, more insulin resistance, and less reliable energy to get you through the day. What you break your fast with determines whether you improve or worsen your glucose tolerance for the rest of the day. Keep in mind there's hardly a good time of day to routinely eat a carb-heavy meal. Our body's response only worsens the later we eat it unless it's following a strenuous bout of exercise, a time when your glucose tolerance is significantly improved.

Breakfast Like a King (Intro)

Are you familiar with the saying, breakfast like a king, lunch like a prince, dinner like a pauper? Before we wrap up the conversation about breakfast myths, let's explore this popular advice that breakfast should be the largest meal of the day.

Is it best to eat your largest meals early and your smallest meals later in the afternoon and evening?

Short answer: Yes. That regressive order of meal size is ideal for our metabolic health and for maintaining good balance in our circadian rhythm. So that you can understand why and how this may pertain to you, it's time to learn about your circadian rhythm.

CHAPTER 6
Circadian Rhythm and Meal Timing

What is the Circadian Rhythm?

There's a fascinating relationship between the daily rise and fall of the sun and our body's internal clock. We all have a powerful 24-hour cycle that's regulated by sunlight, and you might be surprised by the significance of this system. These rhythmic 24 hours orchestrate various bodily systems that control the metabolism, the release of stress hormones, hunger hormones, digestive enzymes, energizing hormones, even sex hormones, and neurotransmitters (the messaging hormones that transmit information between neurons and brain cells, dictating your alertness and mood, your ability to think clearly, your motivation, and much more).

The circadian rhythm is vital, complex, and essential to acknowledge if you want better control of your health. In other words, you might be tempted to ignore this because it sounds too *sciencey* or because you want things to be simpler. Maybe your work-life demands have you working swing shifts, so you'd rather hide from the truth than see the real-time negative impacts this has on your health. I get it. It's tough to face the facts sometimes. Ultimately, however, they cannot be ignored without suffering the consequences of an out-of-sync circadian rhythm.

Common Symptoms and Effects of a Disrupted Circadian Rhythm:[5]

Short-term effects

- Insomnia
- Fatigue
- Decreased mental focus
- Exacerbated ADHD symptoms
- Headaches or migraines
- Irritation or moodiness
- Heightened anxiety
- Indigestion
- Constipation
- Muscle fatigue

- Increased joint pain
- Dysregulated hunger/fullness cues
- Dysregulated cortisol stress response
- Decreased insulin sensitivity
- Stomach pains or increased bloat/gas
- Elevated fasting glucose
- Decreased immunity

Long-term effects

- Gastrointestinal disease
- Diseases of immunity (including autoimmune disease)
- Metabolic diseases (including obesity, type 2 diabetes, high triglycerides, high blood pressure)
- Infertility and reproductive disease
- Neuro-degenerative disease (including Alzheimer's, dementia, schizophrenia)
- Chronic inflammation
- Various cancers

I was living this very scary reality. A life with a completely messed up circadian rhythm that stemmed from constant eating and horrific sleep patterns, resulting in chronic fatigue and high oxidative stress markers in my lab results—a flashing sign for chronic inflammation, cellular stress, and advanced aging that must be addressed.

I'll never forget my worst experience. I suffered with debilitating jet lag after a two-week trip visiting my husband's home state of Hawaii. We jumped five time zones in a non-stop, east-bound return flight to get home. When I tried to get back to work during the first few days that followed, I was an emotional wreck, and my brain was entirely useless. I napped, I cried, and I knew there was a lesson to be learned there. Thanks to that experience, I've since solved the problem by using a jet-lag prevention app called Timeshifter, which helps me prepare for the time change by modifying light exposure and sleep habits so my body can adapt more swiftly after travel.

Between the debilitating jet lag and other horrible crap I went through (thanks to my messed up sleep-wake habits and ignoring my circadian rhythm), I've become pretty passionate about these topics. It took for me to be scared for my life on more than one occasion, but now I can say I no longer suffer the consequences of an out-of-sync internal clock.

It's your turn to gain awareness of the looming threats circadian disruption may be triggering in you. Take charge of your health here, where it has one of the greatest impacts of all. The 24-hour circadian clock in your brain sends daily rhythm signals to every other region in your brain and every organ in your body. It controls when you want to sleep or wake, your preferences for timed eating and drinking, your moods and emotions, your core body temperature, your metabolism, and the release of numerous hormones.

Every cell in your body has an internal clock telling it the time of day. Isn't that amazing? When you're living in accordance with your circadian rhythm, your body's systems will be more properly coordinated. But when your circadian rhythm is disrupted—like when you eat right before bed or you wake up at different times throughout the week—immune function is impaired, symptoms start to manifest, and disease may eventually ensue.

Circadian Fasting and Timing Your Largest Meal

Okay. So, you're getting the idea that your circadian rhythm is really important, and it's related to (pretty much) everything to do with your health and body.

*Now, **how does this relate back to intermittent fasting?***

There's a popular term for intermittent fasting called time-restricted eating, or TRE for short. Sometimes, you'll hear it specified as eTRE, early time-restricted eating, to emphasize an early eating window. I've even heard it called circadian fasting and reverse fasting. The commonalities between them are prioritizing an eating window that occurs while the sun is out and a fasting window starting before the sun sets.

Why would the position of the sun dictate when you fast or eat?

Because, *ages before you were even conceived,* your internal clock was programmed to coincide with the position of the sun. It's how we're all built as human beings. Your body isn't designed to digest food after the sun sets or while you sleep. When you eat a massive dinner in the evening or snack until you fall asleep, you can experience almost immediate consequences on your health, like insomnia, elevated heart rate and body temperature, inadequate deep sleep, irritability and a lowered stress tolerance, impaired mental sharpness, inflamed arthritic pain, increased appetite, decreased glucose tolerance, delayed ketone production, and increased insulin resistance.

When you eat more than once per day—as you'll do with intermittent fasts ranging from 12–20 hours a day—your metabolism will respond best when you eat a larger meal first and save the smallest meal for last. The later it gets, the smaller that meal should be. The more metabolically f*cked up your body is, the more this matters. Big time.[6,7]

Time and time again, we see that by adopting any degree of intermittent fasting—even with only 10 hours of daily intermittent fasting,[8] with or without low-carb dieting,[9] and with or without an early eating window[10]—metabolic health markers do improve.

Regardless, obese people who eat a larger breakfast (compared to a larger dinner) may experience a dramatic improvement in insulin sensitivity. Studies show an average improvement of 163 percent in insulin sensitivity in obese women who ate a large breakfast, mid-sized lunch, and small dinner versus an average 56 percent improvement in the group who ate a small breakfast, mid-sized lunch, and large dinner.[11] What a difference!

Particularly when a larger amount of protein is consumed at breakfast, people feel more satisfied and report fewer hunger signals, which is explained by reduced concentrations of ghrelin—an appetite-regulating hormone that makes food more enticing. What's more is the increase in our satiety hormone, leptin, which makes a person feel satisfied.[12,13]

Things to consider for yourself regarding the timing of your eating window and the largest meal of the day

Because you want results *right now*, I'll bet your mind immediately wonders, *What is ideal?* The problem with this eagerness is that you need to walk before you run. You need to standardize before you optimize, meaning you need to think practically about what can work for you as a starting point before you try turning your life upside-down to implement what is ideal. Why? Because that's how you figure out what works, and that's how you create a plan that's ultimately effective and sustainable.

If you take on too many changes too fast, you might not make it long enough to see the improvements you seek because you jumped in with both feet before you—and your mind and body—were ready. Thus, you quit before it pays off.

Instead, with the long-game strategy I'm teaching you, you'll train your body to make these changes. By training your body, you're working with its thermostat, so to speak. You're working with your body's continuous homeostatic reactions by giving it time to adapt and become accustomed to the changes. This way, you'll suffer few-to-no consequences, you'll see and feel some incremental progress, and you'll feel entirely capable and willing to continue and achieve your goals because you enjoy it and it improves your life without disrupting it.

More things to consider:

People naturally eat more calories for dinner (30–50 percent of daily intake) and fewer calories at breakfast and lunch. This could be another reason we see better results in people who skip dinner and do eTRE. They break their fast in the morning, when appetite hormones are still low, which inclines them to eat a smaller meal. Then, they eat a large lunch, and they start fasting (by skipping dinner) before the sun sets.

Alternatively, breakfast skippers tend to wait until lunchtime to break their fast. They might eat a medium or large-sized lunch. Then, they'll eat dinner before closing the fasting window at a time when appetite hormones are at their peak. The increased appetite leads the person to eat more calories than they otherwise would if they shifted their eating window to occur earlier in the day (essentially, skipping dinner instead of breakfast). Even though the dinner skipper wakes up to an empty stomach, they still experience low hunger signals in the morning. We all do because of our circadian rhythm. That explains why they might, naturally, eat a smaller breakfast even though they haven't eaten since lunch the previous day.

Here's the thing. You'll hear me say this throughout the book: your fasting habits should work around your life instead of the other way around. You need to figure out how to reasonably integrate a fasting schedule into your life without disrupting the natural flow and routines essential in your personal relationships and routine lifestyle—especially the things that bring you peace and contentment.

For most of my clients, that means starting out by skipping or postponing breakfast. They simultaneously work on improving their nutrient intake (which you'll learn more about in chapters ahead), and they reduce snacking habits while also improving their sleep. Then, they're ready to tweak and optimize their fasting routine as they experiment and gather more insights, increasing self-efficacy over time.

In the words of fasting trailblazer Dr. Jason Fung, "Skipping breakfast is usually easier, but skipping dinner is usually more effective."

Since around 2014, I've been skipping breakfast most days of the week. I do that because I have *way* more energy, better concentration, and I'm more productive. I even sat through two EEG brain scans to see if my experience could be proven[i]. Turns out my brain is a lot easier to work with while I'm in a fasted state. You know you're doing something right when you feel better all around.

So, if you're not eating breakfast, or you're not eating at all in the morning, can you drink coffee? Sure you can! The next chapter will open your eyes to the many ways your morning coffee habit can make or break your daily fast.

---

i   In February 2020, I underwent two EEG brain mapping sessions with clinical psychologist Dr. Sam Effarah, who specializes in neurofeedback and quantitative EEGs, to confirm or refute my hypothesis that eating exacerbates my ADHD symptoms. The first brain map was conducted in a fasted state, and the second occurred thirty minutes after I consumed a nutritious meal of salad, homemade dressing, and sardines. The hundreds of pages of results confirmed that my ADHD symptoms were substantially exacerbated after eating. I share more details on a dedicated episode (#88: Fasting for ADD/ADHD and Mental Energy) of my former podcast, The Foundation of Wellness. Corresponding images from my brain scans can be viewed on the YouTube video for episode #88.

Coffee Guidelines for Intermittent Fasting: A Brief Overview

It's pretty fantastic that you can still drink coffee during a fast. Like most things in health and nutrition, however, there's plenty of nuance to consider. **The goal for these next two chapters is to provide you with enough details to help ensure that you don't:**

✓ Accidentally break your fast with your *coffee

✓ Become unnecessarily restrictive with something you enjoy as much as morning coffee

Notes: * *When I say 'coffee' in this book, I'm also referring to decaf coffee and plain tea (black, white, green, herbal, whatever plain tea you enjoy that contains zero sugar or sweeteners). Not a coffee drinker? If you don't drink coffee, tea, energy drinks, or anything with an ingredient list in the morning, you can skip this chapter and head to Chapter 9: What Breaks a Fast.*

How about a quick overview of the coffee guidelines I've given my clients for years? In the next chapter, we'll get into the nuance and circumstances that call for a stricter habit.

General Coffee Guidelines

Continue reading the rest of this section for expanded explanations and nuance for each of the following guidelines:

1. Black coffee might be your best choice overall.

2. **Bulletproof-style coffee might be the best way to start or restart with IF.

3. High-quality MCT oil might enhance your fast.

4. Most coffee creamers (dairy or non-dairy) will break your fast.

5. Protein, collagen powder, and amino acid blends technically break your fast.

6. Sugar or carbs ≥ 1 g will most likely break a morning fast.

** Bulletproof is a brand name and a trademarked coffee recipe that consists of low-toxin black coffee blended with unsalted grass-fed butter and MCT oil. For flexibility from the original recipe, I'll be referring to this as fatty coffee some of the time.

Not So Strict

Most fasting advice out there says you can't drink anything besides water, black coffee, and plain tea during your fast. Welp, I've got a handful of reasons you might consider that advice to be unnecessarily strict.

- Many people can achieve most of the same benefits of water fasting even when they consume fatty coffee or coffee with some of the approved ingredients I share in this section.

- Pure fat, in the absence of carbs and protein, doesn't stimulate insulin production. And in the absence of insulin, ingesting pure fat can actually increase the metabolic rate by 15–20 percent because the body starts metabolizing those fat calories, creating ketones for energy.

- If one of the following descriptions fits you, you might increase your chance of success with fasting when you include fatty coffee or other approved creamy coffee in your fasting plan. This applies to beginners just starting out, someone who has taken a long break and is restarting a fasting habit, or when recovering from a recent COVID-19 infection or other debilitating illness, injury, or setback.

5 Reasons Fatty Coffee Can Be Helpful During a Fast:

1. It gives you something delicious to look forward to, helping you feel less deprived during the fasting window. This leads to increased follow-through and commitment.

2. Fatty coffee or coffee with MCT oil can help a beginner have more energy available while training their body and brain to start using ketones for energy. This means they experience fewer cravings and feel more satiated. They experience increased self-efficacy (*I can do this!*) and a greater chance at success because they're more likely to stick with the plan.

3. For individuals advised to take medications or supplements with food (including fat-soluble vitamins like vitamins D, K, E, and A), added fats in the coffee can ease the logistics of fasting. Dietary fats facilitate the absorption of key nutrients and medications and prime the stomach to help prevent feelings of nausea. This might also be helpful for individuals advised against drinking coffee on an empty stomach.

4. Fatty coffee can help you fast more comfortably, thus helping you increase your fasting window sooner, with less effort required.

5. MCT oil can increase fat burning and weight loss compared to fasting without, because, in the absence of insulin, the metabolism will increase to make ketones from the MCT oil. Ketones are energy molecules produced when the body runs on fat, rather than sugar, as the fuel source. Fat burning or weight loss is indirectly boosted for

the following reasons. First, for those who suffer with constipation, MCT oil stimulates bowel movements, which can release several pounds of backed-up crap at a time! Another reason is that MCT's isolated fats are like a safety net for the metabolism, preventing it from slowing down (as it wants to do when you restrict too much too soon or too frequently).

Continue on to Chapter 8 to dive deeper into the six general coffee guidelines introduced in this chapter.

CHAPTER 8

Expanded Coffee Guidelines for Intermittent Fasting

1. Black coffee might be your best choice overall.

If you like black coffee, then great! If not, you probably think it's nasty. I know for me drinking black coffee used to cause this unpleasant sensation that felt like instant heartburn. I don't experience that anymore, thanks to my black coffee hacks (see #1 on my list of *7 Black Coffee Hacks To Make You Hate It Less* at *marisamoon.com/notsofast/resources*).

Don't worry. You don't have to start out drinking black coffee, and you may never need to switch to it. Like every recommendation in this book, it depends on your goals and your changing circumstances. In many cases, with intermittent fasting, black coffee is ideal. It contains 0 g of fat, 0 g of sugar, 0 g of carbs, 0 g of protein, no amino acids, and no sweeteners. This means it's basically like drinking water with beneficial polyphenols (botanicals) and the boost of naturally-packaged *caffeine. Note that decaffeinated coffee is acceptable, too (Swiss water and CO2 extraction methods are the safest sources). I personally drink decaf coffee most days of the week because by cutting back on caffeine, my body's stress response has greatly improved.

I do not recommend consuming products that contain added caffeine, even if it's a natural caffeine source like coffee bean extract or green tea extract. If caffeine is listed in the ingredients of your energy drink, drink powder, pre-workout drink, bottled drink, electrolytes, etc., you should consider switching to caffeinated coffee or tea. Mother Nature provides us with caffeine—in the coffee berries, tea leaves, and cocoa beans—packaged up with beneficial polyphenols that change the way the caffeine affects your system. When it's consumed as an additive or extract, however, it can lead to more of the negative side effects that caffeine is known to have: increased anxiety, emotional instability, panic attacks, lowered stress tolerance, adrenal fatigue, feeling wired-but-tired, increased caffeine addiction, insomnia, and more.

Coffee on an empty stomach?

Certain individuals with adrenal fatigue (physiological burnout), autoimmune flare-ups, thyroid dysfunction, taxing PMS, or morning anxiety may be advised against consuming coffee on an empty stomach. Without food in your system, caffeine can be quite a blunt force to your adrenals (your stress hormones), worsening or prolonging the states I just mentioned. In such cases, black coffee would be too harsh, and fatty coffee would be a more reasonable way to start the day. If you need food with your coffee, then you're better off skipping dinner instead of skipping breakfast.

Caveat aside, many people see increased fat burning when they switch to black coffee.

2. Bulletproof coffee might be the best way to start or restart with IF.

Fatty coffee, AKA Bulletproof coffee, might be the best way to start or restart a fasting lifestyle. Let me break it down for you.

What is Bulletproof coffee?

This trendy-ish coffee recipe combines low-toxin coffee blended with unsalted grass-fed butter and MCT oil. It was created by biohacker and author Dave Asprey from *bulletproof.com* to help boost ketone energy, pleasure, and cognition in a fasted state. Asprey's inspiration came from drinking traditional yak-butter tea in the high-altitude Tibetan mountains. Since then, he's popularized this coffee in the biohacking, fasting, and paleo communities.

Many variations and monikers exist today for Bulletproof-inspired coffee, such as butter coffee, fatty coffee, and keto coffee. Because I'll encourage you to consider variations of the original recipe, I'll most often refer to it as fatty coffee.

Variations I recommend may include one or more of the following ingredients blended with coffee:

- Grass-fed or European unsalted butter

- Grass-fed, low-salt cultured butter

- Ghee (clarified butter) or lactose-free butter

- Unrefined coconut oil

- Brain Octane C8 MCT Oil (by Bulletproof, or a comparable version of C8-dominant MCT oil such as Keto Brain)

- InnerFuel Prebiotic Powder (by Bulletproof)

For my clients on a weight loss journey, I typically recommend starting by keeping added fats below 1.5 tablespoons (total combined servings during the fast) and working their way down to a max of 2–3 teaspoons. Some may eventually cut it out altogether and opt for black coffee if needed to dig out of a plateau or switch things up.

I'll be honest with you. A majority of the fasting community thinks this has no place in a fasting window because they assume it breaks a fast, or they fear saturated fat or think they won't lose weight while consuming fats. Well, hopefully, by the end of this book, you'll understand why these concerns may be overgeneralized and based on misinterpreted facts. My experiences beg to differ from conventional opinions.

I began intermittent fasting somewhere around 2013, drinking Bulletproof coffee every morning during my fast. I found this style of fasting so effortless and enjoyable that it blew my mind, further propelling me into the study of ancestral health. In 2017, I started teaching a four-step introduction to my intermittent fasting method, and since then, hundreds of my clients and followers have succeeded at losing weight and sustaining a fasting lifestyle with Bulletproof or fatty coffee during their fasting window.

> *"Today, I'm officially down 20 lb. I was at a plateau going up and down a few pounds for the last few months, but on your program, I'm down 6 lb and feel great. Bloating gone. Also, some skin lesions on my legs were getting to be a concern and are now almost non-existent. No breakfast, just bulletproof coffee mostly, and the occasional black coffee with cinnamon. Thanks for all you do, Marisa!"*
> - Karen

Plain and simple, starting or restarting with intermittent fasting is easier and more enjoyable when you do it with fatty coffee. It also helps you more effortlessly increase your fasting window, providing your brain and body with quick ketone energy—even when you're not yet fat-adapted.

3. MCT oil might enhance your fast.

MCT stands for medium-chain-triglycerides, which naturally comprise certain saturated fats like coconut oil and palm oil. MCT Oil is a supplement made from mechanically isolated fats that don't require digestive enzymes or bile to digest and break down for absorption. The MCTs you ingest with MCT oil are metabolized only by the liver, and within minutes of ingestion, they can be made into ketones for clean, sustainable cellular energy.

Even though MCT oil is high in calories (130 calories per tablespoon) and comprised almost entirely of saturated fat (13 g per tablespoon), MCTs can actually *increase* body fat burning around the clock and prevent fat storage.

> *"MCTs enhance thermogenesis and fat oxidation, which suppresses*
> *the deposition and accumulation of body fat."*
> - Dr. Dominic D'Agostino

Not so fast with the MCT oil.

Should you take too much before your gut is adapted, you can experience what some people call disaster pants. This is because MCT oil goes through the GI (gastro-intestinal) tract unabsorbed, and until you build up a tolerance in your gut, it can have an osmotic effect, drawing water into your colon like a laxative—which means it can give you urgent diarrhea. Although it's pretty harmless to experience, it's so unpleasant when it does. Even if you don't have that reaction, you might feel nauseated. That's why you'll want to start slow with MCT oil.

Start with a serving size of 1 teaspoon of MCT oil (preferably a *C8-dominant MCT oil). Over the next few weeks, gradually increase the serving size to > 2 teaspoons, depending on your goals. The serving size is important to consider when you're a newbie because your gut needs to adapt to these fatty acids before you jump to a 2–3 teaspoon habit, which is a standard serving size recommendation (the latter equal to 1 tablespoon).

How to incorporate MCT oil:

MCT oil, as well as butter, typically requires a blender to mix into your coffee. Otherwise, the oil will float at the top, and your coffee will taste greasy. It shouldn't taste greasy whatsoever. It should taste rich, smooth, and creamy.

A prominent new product on the market is powdered MCT oil. Since we don't yet have the scientific research on powdered MCT oil, I can't be sure it's harmless or that it produces the same effects as the fluid version.

MCT Oil Benefits include:

- ✓ Fasting longer with ease

- ✓ Instant ketone energy in the brain and body (more mental and physical energy)

- ✓ Reduced cravings

- ✓ Reduced likelihood of plateaus or slowed metabolism

- ✓ A richer-tasting coffee (when blended in, with or without other fats or cream)

- ✓ Increased gut motility and bowel movements

- ✓ Help with stabilizing blood glucose and reducing fasting blood sugar levels

- ✓ Increased fat burning (lipolysis) and thermogenesis (metabolic rate during digestion)

- ✓ Improved gut microbiome and anti-inflammatory pathways.

"MCT oil gives me energy, and I swear it helps me lose more weight. The trick that helped me a ton was MCT oil in my tea around noon to help me keep fasting and get back on track more easily. Without MCT, I have more cravings and wanted to break my fast hours sooner…it helps me readapt and get free ketones."
- Ashley

4. Most coffee creamers (dairy or non-dairy) will break your fast.

If you're opposed to trying the fatty coffee or drinking it black, then the next best thing would be to try Nutpods original creamer. Here in the United States, it's easy to find Nutpods on Amazon or at large grocery store chains. Nutpods stands apart from the majority of plant-based and dairy creamers because it contains 0 g of carbs and 0 g of protein per serving size. This tells me it must be comprised of more water than other brands—but it doesn't taste water-based because it's thickened by natural gums that emulsify the 'milk', making it a richer, creamy consistency.

I co-coach a group program called My6Method, where we've successfully coached over a hundred clients to achieve results with intermittent fasting even when they fast with coffee containing 1–4 servings (1–4 tablespoons) of Nutpods original creamer.

If you're not willing to blend your coffee with fats like butter, ghee, coconut oil, or MCT oil, Nutpods is the easiest way to transition from regular coffee creamer because it doesn't require a blender.

Note: I do not recommend anyone drinks oat milk (not even oat milk products by Nutpods) because oat milk definitely breaks your fast as it contains too many carbs and natural sugars. Look for the Nutpods original line, which is the unsweetened coconut/almond milk recipe. Unsweetened flavored Nutpods is also acceptable.

5. Protein, collagen powder, and amino acid powders/drinks (BCAAs or EAAs) technically break your fast.

Benefits await when it comes to supplementing your diet with collagen protein, protein powders, and amino acid powders. There's a time and a place for these supplements, but they will definitely break your fast and blunt autophagy (a cellular recycling process inhibited by the presence of insulin, thus amplified during a fasted state). That isn't always a big deal because, well, it's a matter of the pros and cons of your situation.

Sometimes, the benefits of fasting with these supplements outweigh the risks of fasting without them. If it aligns with your current health priorities, they can warrant a strategic place in your fasting routine. For now, skip the added proteins unless you're an athlete, if you lift (heavy) weights and are prioritizing muscle building, or if you're recovering from injury, surgery, COVID-19, or other illness.

Note: It's fine to take isolated amino acid supplements—such as capsules with L-tryptophan or L-theanine, for example. Single amino acids are not enough to break your fast because the body needs a certain quantity and combination of various amino acids to blunt autophagy (disrupt ketone production by triggering insulin) and break the fast. If you take one to three individual amino acids in capsule form during intermittent fasts, it's probably nothing to give a second thought.

6. Sugar or carbs ≥ 1 g in your coffee or creamer will break your fast.

This is the most basic concept of fasting you'll want to grasp. You need to avoid sugar and carbs during your fast because it will cause a glucose and insulin response, which turns off the fat-burning systems and knocks you out of a fasted state. It's especially crucial to avoid consuming sugar or carbs in liquid form because your body will hyper-respond to them.

When new clients enter our group program, it's not uncommon for some to say, "I guess I've been fasting all along, and I didn't even know it." They *think* they've been fasting because coffee was all they consumed before 11 a.m. But, as soon as I ask a few questions or look at their food journals, we discover their coffee is made with creamer, plant milks, sugar, or collagen peptides—or they take gummy vitamins in the morning. They weren't in a fasted state, after all.

Making this small change makes all the difference. You want to get this right. Otherwise, you may end up thinking, *No matter what I do, I can't lose the weight!*

Sweeteners

If you want to sweeten your coffee, your best bet is to use pure stevia, pure monk fruit, allulose powder, or erythritol. Whatever product you consider, you *must* read the ingredient list to check for any of the common additives that technically break a fast. Food manufacturers and marketers are tricky, sneaking sugar-like fillers into otherwise sugar-free substances like stevia packets or monk fruit sweetener because it improves the texture and flavor profile and reduces the cost. That's why you must read the ingredient lists and, by using the lists in Chapter 9: *What Breaks a Fast*, confirm whether it will or will not break your fast.

Try weaning yourself entirely off of sweeteners if you're:

- Carrying excess weight primarily in your abdominal region (visceral fat, the most concerning fat accumulation site)

- Insulin-resistant, pre-diabetic, or have type 2 diabetes

- At a weight-loss plateau for three weeks or longer, and want to know if sweeteners have been hindering results

- A self-proclaimed sugar 'addict'. Fasting and weight loss may come easier if you eliminate sweeteners altogether

- Hungry during the fasting window or frequently distracted by a desire to eat. Sweeteners consumed in the fasting window can trigger hunger and cravings in certain individuals

Confused about what breaks a fast? Let's move on to the tips and handy lists I've created to help you decipher which ingredients are worth fussing over and which ones I consider fair game.

CHAPTER 9

What Breaks a Fast

I wish I could be definitive here and tell you *exactly* which foods and substances will break a fast or knock you out of ketosis. Sure, some obvious things like sugar or protein will technically break an intermittent fast. But when we consider the effects caused by seemingly minor things—such as chewing gum, taking supplements, ingesting 1 g of carbs, or drinking a splash of heavy cream in your coffee—the effects vary from person to person and situation to situation.

Dozens of variables exist that are unique to you and your current circumstances. When consuming what I'll call 'gray area' stuff during the fast, **the following variables can dictate whether or not you stay in ketosis and a fasted state:**

- Your age
- How insulin sensitive you are (or how insulin-resistant you are)
- Other metabolic health factors (like the health of your mitochondria, liver function, cardiovascular health, and how fat-adapted you are)
- Your activity level this day or the previous day

- Your body composition, especially how much muscle you have

- How much body fat you have to spare

- What you ate the night before

- What your diet has been like the last few weeks

- How long you're fasting that day

- How early or late in the fasting window you're consuming gray area stuff

- Your current state of gut health

- Your current degree of pro-inflammatory conditions

- The medications you take

- Your history of dieting and yo-yo weight gain and loss

- How much sleep you've gotten the past night or two

- How in sync you are with your circadian rhythm

- Your current state of hormonal health

- How stressed you are (physically or mentally)

I'm sure more variables exist, but as you can see, there are a lot of factors that make this question of "What breaks a fast?" tough to answer. That explains why you'll see not one list of things that break a fast but four:

1. Never Breaks a Fast

2. Rarely Breaks a Fast

3. Likely Breaks a Fast

4. Definitely Breaks a Fast

Even within certain lists, you'll see *asterisks* which can guide you to consider further nuance to determine how strict you might be in your fasting window. I work closely with my clients, helping them consider adding or removing any gray area stuff, depending on their current challenges, immediate priorities, and goals. Certain individuals may need to be more strict and stick with the Never Breaks a Fast list, like people with insulin resistance, pre-diabetes, type 2 diabetes, or metabolic syndrome. This is because the body's insulin response may be exaggerated compared to someone without severe insulin resistance.

I'm writing this book for people who prefer flexibility and want to craft a sustainable fasting lifestyle while improving their relationship with food and dieting for good. I aim to avoid unnecessary restriction whenever possible. That said, if you're reading this and are more desperate for hard-and-fast rules and quick results—and you're self-motivated to persevere in the face of challenges—then you might also prefer to stick with the *Never Breaks a Fast* list.

NEVER Breaks a Fast

- Water
- Lemon/lime/mint/cucumber water
- Black coffee
- Tea leaves or herbal tea (no fruit), unsweetened
- Electrolytes (unsweetened, ≤ 10 calories, 0 g carbs/protein)
- 100% creatine powder/capsules
- Vitamin/multivitamin tablets/capsules (excluding collagen or protein)
- Fish oil supplements
- MCT oil

- Coconut oil (< 1 tablespoon)
- Ghee or butter (< 1 tablespoon)
- THC/CBD oil capsules or tinctures (unsweetened)
- Herbal supplements (≤ 10 calories, 0 g carbs/protein)
- Probiotic/prebiotic supplements
- Medication (pill forms or injections that don't contain insulin, glucose, or stimulate insulin in a fasted state)
- Apple cider vinegar

- Pickle juice (made without sugar/sweeteners)
- 100% pure mushroom extract
- Cinnamon, spices

RARELY Breaks a Fast

Consider removing these items to break through a plateau, increase insulin sensitivity, or accelerate results.

- Stevia (excluding Stevia In The Raw and Pure Via)
- Electrolytes (stevia-sweetened)
- ** Sugar-free gum made with stevia, xylitol, erythritol, isomalt, allulose
- Allulose sweetener
- 100% monk fruit
- Sucralose, although it's not recommended (note that Splenda breaks a fast)
- ** Vitamins made with food powders 0 g protein, ≤ 1 g net carbs (e.g. green powders, beet powder, blueberries, wheat grass, etc.)
- Medicinal mushroom powders (≤ 1 g net carbs, depends on formulation, serving, length of fast)
- ** Natural Vitality CALM magnesium drink powder (flavored)
- ** Heavy cream (≤ 1 tablespoon)
- Veggie broth (≤ 0 g protein, ≤ 1 g carbs)
- ** Sugar-free drinks (0 g carbs, made with stevia or monk fruit only)
- ** Unsweetened Nutpods creamer (max 2–4 tablespoons)
- 100% cocoa powder (serving size ≤ 1 teaspoon)

**Depends on serving size, length of fast, and bio-individual variables; may be beneficial to include at times, depending on current challenges and goals (see Example 9.1 below)

LIKELY Breaks a Fast

- Nut or plant-based milks (sweetened or unsweetened, ≥ 1 g carbs/sugar/protein per serving consumed)

- Dairy or non-dairy creamer (sweetened or unsweetened, ≥ 1 g carbs/sugar/protein per serving consumed)

- Chewing gum (made with sugar, aspartame, or xylitol)

- Electrolyte powders made with fruit/veggie powders, or ≥ 1 g carbs/sugar/protein, > 10 calories)

- Certain green powders (including chlorella/spirulina/algae, ≥ 1 g carbs/sugar/protein, > 20 calories)

- ** Xylitol

- ** Certain vitamin supplements, capsules, or tablets (≥ 1 g protein per serving, e.g. moringa, chlorella, spirulina)

- ** Sugar-free energy drinks or diet soda (made with any sweeteners other than stevia or monk fruit)

**Depends on serving size, fasting length, and bio-individual variables; sometimes beneficial to include, depending on fasting goals and challenges

DEFINITELY Breaks a Fast

Occasionally, I may suggest certain clients include an item on this list even though it will technically break a fast. The reasons for that are based on individual circumstances (mentioned in Example 9.2 and Example 9.3 below)

With intermittent fasting, most items above 200 calories will definitely break a fast. Exceptions could be made for calories derived entirely from fats. For 36-hour fasts, like with alternate day fasting, the daily guideline is 500 calories or less.

- Most items > 1 g sugar, > 1 g net carbs, or ≥ 1 g protein (unless lab-tested to prove they're compatible with fasting) don't result in elevated blood glucose or elevated fasting insulin and don't disrupt ketosis

- Sorbitol or maltitol (found in sugar-free chewing gum and certain packaged foods designed for low-carb and keto diets)

- Dextrin or maltodextrin (found in most packaged foods, Splenda sweetener, Stevia In The Raw, Pure Via stevia, and many zero-calorie products)

- Gummy vitamins

- Milk

- THC/CBD edibles or gummies

- * Protein powder

- * Colostrum

- * Collagen powder

- * Amino acid supplements (containing three or more different amino acids)

- * Broth (such as bone broth or veggie broth > 1 g carbs/protein per serving)

- Sugar-sweetened drinks or electrolytes

*Sometimes beneficial to include, depending on fasting goals and challenges (see Examples 9.2 and 9.3 below)

Example 9.1

Natural Vitality CALM magnesium drink powder is a widely available supplement used to help promote relaxation or sleep. This product is made with magnesium citrate powder and is typically flavored, combining stevia leaf extract and natural flavors. It seems that, besides in the most insulin-resistant people, this product can be consumed at night during a fasting window without breaking a fast. The benefits of taking magnesium—for balancing stress, promoting healthy bowels, and sleeping better—typically outweigh the concern and low probability that it breaks a fast.

Example 9.2

It may be beneficial to consider fasting with bone broth, veggie broth, or collagen, depending on the individual's circumstances, goals, and dietary preferences. Individuals who meet one of the following criteria may consider this modification:

✓ Impaired digestive health

✓ IBS or IBD (irritable bowel syndrome or disease)[14]

✓ Difficulty fasting longer than 16 hours

✓ At or close to maintenance weight

✓ Healing from an injury, surgery, COVID-19, or other debilitating illness

✓ Primary goal is to improve joint health, skin, or gut lining (leaky gut)

It may be beneficial for certain individuals to consider a modified fast or fasting with some food or food-like supplements so more nutrients can be obtained in an otherwise insufficient diet. Bone broth, some protein powders, and some supplements can enhance fasting benefits while only temporarily disrupting certain fasting-induced processes (such as autophagy). More on this in Part 7. Individuals who might try these modifications would typically match one or more of these criteria:

✓ Over seventy years old, when we're most susceptible to sarcopenia (age-related progressive muscle loss)

✓ Eating a nutrient-poor diet

✓ Immunocompromised

✓ Certain cases of neurodegeneration or neurological dysfunction

✓ Healing from an injury, surgery, COVID-19, or other debilitating illness

The longer a fast is, the more these modifications can be beneficial, helping to reduce inflammatory compounds and protect the mucosal lining in the GI tract.[15]

Example 9.3

If a client's goal is to build more lean muscle, and they're exercising in a fasted state, I may introduce them to the benefits of taking amino acid supplements immediately following, during, or up to 30 minutes prior to a workout. This may technically break a fast, but it's temporary, and the benefits far outweigh the concerns for individuals who want to preserve or gain muscle mass and continue their fasted training regime.

Now that you've got my *What Breaks a Fast* lists, coffee guidelines, and a new perspective on the tradition of breakfast, we're ready to wrap up Part 1 and finish with action steps. The following action steps will help you put the most important things into practice—right now—starting with the first phase of my RESET method.

Part 1 Action Steps:
Train Your Fasting Muscles

You're ready to take what you learned in Part 1 and put these concepts into action! First, it's time to start training your fasting muscles. Here are four steps to get you started.

Action Step #1:

Get your coffee situation figured out.

Over these first couple of weeks, if needed, test out new things in your coffee to be sure you can enjoy it while also staying in a fasted state. Refer to the coffee guidelines and *What Breaks a Fast* lists from the previous chapters.

Action Step #2:

Download the Life Fasting Tracker mobile app (or similar fasting tracker).

It's quite effortless and motivating to use a fasting tracker. You tap the screen to start and end your fast, and there's a progress meter to motivate you to continue. Even if you forget to start or stop the meter, you can manually adjust the times. Using a tracker is a smart move. Sure, you could rely on your memory—trying to recall what time it was when you finished your last after-dinner snack—but trust me, as we get further along, you'll wish you'd started using the tracker from the beginning.

Action Step #3:

Starting tonight, establish a comfortable baseline fasting window.

Train your body and mind for daily intermittent fasts, and be patient as you *oh-so-gradually* increase this fasting window following the guidelines below.

Not so fast. Start by using the fasting tracker every day. Try to stick with your initial baseline fasting window for 7 days, or a minimum of 4 days, before increasing the length of your daily fasts by 30 minutes at a time. This allows you time to experience variations in your schedule, mood, and life so you can assess how different circumstances, emotions, and schedules affect your ability to fast comfortably.

Beginners:

At first, it's a good idea to stick with routine start and end times for your fasting window. Be as consistent as you can while working with the time constraints of your day-to-day obligations because this will make it easier to adjust. The older you are, or the more digestive symptoms you have, the more important routine is at this stage.

Example of a beginner routine:

- ✓ Fast 12 hours each night from 8 p.m.–8 a.m. for the next 4–7 days.
- ✓ Do your best to break your fast around 8 a.m. each day.
- ✓ Do your best to finish eating and snacking by 8 p.m. each night.
- ✓ Your body appreciates the predictability as it gets accustomed to these changes.
- ✓ Your circadian rhythm and digestive health are improved with this routine.

Later in your journey, I'll encourage you to mix it up and avoid being so rigid with your fasting times because that's a better long-term strategy once you have more metabolic flexibility.

How do you know what your baseline fasting window is?

Your baseline fasting window feels comfortable and mostly effortless. A key sign you're at the appropriate fasting window for your current state is that you feel really good during the fast and you're not starving when you break it. You shouldn't have the desire or impulse to binge eat when your eating window opens, and you shouldn't be relentlessly distracted by hunger or cravings during your fasting window. Those are signs you're pushing this too fast.

TO ALL EXPERIENCE LEVELS:

Once you're comfortably and effortlessly fasting in your current window for 4–7 days in a row, and you've tested it out on weekends and weekdays, that's a good time to try increasing the fast by 30 minutes at a time. Repeat the same process every 4–14 days, or however long it takes, until that fasting window feels comfortable and practically effortless. Wait to increase your fasting window until the current window feels consistently good. See Jacob's story in Case Study 10.1 to help you appreciate this pace.

Not so fast. Take your time. It'll be worth it.

Case Study 10.1 **Jacob's Experience of Action Step #3**

Jacob started out fasting for 13 hours, Tuesday to Saturday, roughly between 8 p.m. and 9 a.m. He felt great. He followed the coffee guidelines and used the *Life Fasting Tracker* to confirm his consistent efforts. The fasting window worked out fine in most situations, and he felt confident it was time to increase it on Sunday.

So, on Sunday, Jacob increased his baseline window to 13.5 hours. He sometimes went to 14 hours if it felt good in the moment, but reminded himself that 13.5 hours is still an improvement. He recognized weekends can be tricky, so he stuck with 13.5–14 hours for the entire week, Sunday through Sunday, to be sure it would become nearly effortless for him.

By Saturday, the kids had a bunch of activities, Jacob was short on sleep, and his in-laws invited the family to brunch on Sunday. Needless to say, the weekend didn't go as smoothly as he'd planned. He decided to stick with 13.5–14 hours for another week to make sure he could be consistent through the following weekend.

Jacob continued this baseline process, using the fasting tracker, checking in with himself daily, and meeting weekly with me. He learned to be patient along the way as he trained his body and mind for a fasting lifestyle. One month later, he was fasting comfortably for 16 hours per day, shifting the start and end times of his window to adapt to his daily circumstances. Over the next 3.5 months, Jacob was able to see an average loss of 1.5–2 lb a week.

Bonus Action Step #4:

Continue reading to finish *Part 2: Reduce Your Carbs*.

Ideally, while training for daily fasts, you'll start your 21-day carb reduction journey. You'll find it described in the action steps at the end of Part 2.

Part 2 is a powerful piece of the puzzle, so don't hesitate to get started. By training your body to operate on fewer carbs, fasting becomes easier to do.

PART 2

Reduce Your Carbs

RESET

Reduce Carbs

E Eat Nourishing Foods

S Start with 12 Hours

E Extend Your Fasts

T Thoughtfully Adapt

CHAPTER 11

Training For Your Metabolic Muscles

An Intro to Carb-Reduction

It's time to get realistic about how much of your diet is made up of carbs. Simultaneously, while starting with the action steps from Part 1, you'll enhance the training of your fasting muscles by reducing your daily carbohydrate intake. The chapters that follow in Part 2 will set you up for a 21-day carb reduction journey.

Carbs! (Insert: drooling emoji.)

I knowww. You love carbs. You don't want to give them up. And you shouldn't have to.

Instead of diving into a restrictive keto, low-carb lifestyle from the start, I'm going to teach you gradual, strategic carbohydrate reduction so you can test out carb moderation to see if it works for you. You can always progress to that level of restriction once you're fat-adapted and more metabolically flexible. Your body and mind will appreciate your patience in this graduated approach!

Before we move into the meat of this topic, let's get one thing straight: I like to use the words carbs and sugar interchangeably. So, while you're reading, you can think in these terms:

Carbs = Sugar

Sugar = Carbs

Glucose is what we call blood sugar, which is carbohydrates in the bloodstream.

It's true that all sugars are classified as carbohydrates, but technically speaking, not all carbohydrates are sugar, nor are they all converted to glucose in your bloodstream. For a carbohydrate to wind up as sugar in your bloodstream, it must be absorbed through your GI tract after being eaten. *Fiber* and *sugar alcohols* are categorized as carbohydrates, but they typically *aren't* absorbed or converted into glucose in your bloodstream. All other forms of carbohydrates are.

Science Lesson

Certain carbohydrates don't get absorbed through your GI tract. Thus, they don't turn into sugar in your bloodstream or make you fat. The carbs we're talking about here are classified as fiber and *sugar alcohols, which, instead, are eaten up as prebiotics by the microbes in your gut or otherwise eliminated in your urine or stool.

*Not all sugar alcohols behave this way. Erythritol, xylitol, isomalt, and allulose are the best types of sugar alcohol for carbohydrate reduction because 50–90 percent of the carbohydrates present in these forms won't be absorbed or contribute to elevated blood glucose levels. Other commonly used sugar alcohols, like sorbitol and maltitol, are either mostly absorbed and converted to blood glucose, just like sugar, or cause gastrointestinal upset and increased insulin levels.

Although a small percentage of the carbs you ingest might not contribute to blood sugar or weight gain, I use the terms carbs and sugar interchangeably throughout this book because it keeps things simple and emphasizes the long-reaching effects of this lifestyle change.

Sweet tooth, carb-a-holic, bread lover, rice devourer, or snack addict—we're all the same because we're stuck in sugar-burning mode. Are you stuck in sugar-burning mode? Let's find out because, on discovering you're mostly a sugar burner, you'll learn how much power you have over your appetite, your energy, and your waistline by taking this journey along with me. The best news is that simply by reducing how many carbs you consume, fasting will be much easier for you.

CHAPTER 12
Sugar Burner vs. Fat Burner

Are you currently a Sugar Burner or a Fat Burner?

Until you start intermittent fasting with some regularity or commit to a lower-carb diet, you're a sugar burner. We all are at some point in our lives because modern society has molded us into being sugar burners. This is thanks to industrialized, processed foods, biased national nutrition guidelines, and the Big Food industry, which intentionally exploits the basic human instinct to prefer carbolicious foods. As a result, we crave, seek out, and overeat the foods that make big food corporations rich.

A sugar burner is someone who has become metabolically dependent on carbohydrates. In this state, their body is entirely dependent on the quick-burning energy derived from eating carbohydrates. The person must eat every 2–4 hours, or they'll feel irritable, hangry, and taken over by their desire to eat. In those moments, they feel as if they're *starving* even though their body has plenty of energy stored as fat to use in place of the next meal or snack.

A fat burner is someone who's operating with the factory settings we're born with as humans. Native to the human genome is this ability to store body fat for future energy needs and a factory setting that enables us to burn that stored fat for energy whenever food is scarce.

The body is designed to fuel itself from two primary sources: carbohydrates (technical term: glucose) and fats (technical terms: ketones and fatty acids). Your metabolism breaks down these different fuel sources and turns them into cellular energy needed to stay alive and thrive. When you abuse your body long enough on a high-carb diet—like we've done as a culture since the days of industrialized and processed foods—and couple that with eating all the frickin' time, you start to screw up your factory settings.

Genetic Switching

The body has genetic switches—like light switches—that determine which genes are being expressed or which light is switched ON. One of our factory settings is a fat-burning switch that, when turned ON, will metabolize body fat and convert it into usable energy. Efficiently, cleanly, and painlessly. You want your body capable of switching this fat-burning gene ON whenever it's needed.

When the body has been abused for so long by decades of bagels, sandwiches, donuts, pasta, candy, soda, pizza, BBQ sauce, etc., the genetic switch that burns body fat for energy is stuck in the OFF position. And the gene that relies on glucose for energy is stuck in the ON position. This leaves a person entirely dependent on carbs, AKA sugar, for fuel. The result? The person becomes a sugar burner, reliant on frequent snacks and carbs to keep them even-keeled.

For a sugar burner, no degree of willpower or portion control will stop the vicious cycle of cravings, appetite, and stuffing down those carbs/sugars. They quickly burn through that fuel and store the excess as body fat—all the while imprisoning pre-existing body fat in long-term, stubborn storage.

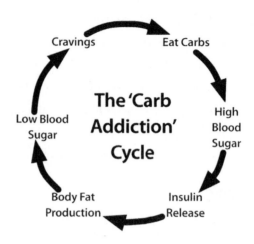

An Intro to Metabolic Flexibility

The term *metabolic* refers to your metabolism—the process by which your body converts food and nutrients into energy. For many people, the term *metabolism* itself has been limited to those functions. In reality, your metabolism is a complex series of systems and processes. Yes, it breaks down the food you eat, but it also breaks down cellular components, hormones, and chemicals that provide energy to your body. It also repairs and protects your cells and tissues while removing waste. Your metabolism allows your body to function and thrive through this intricate network of chemical reactions.

All you need to think about right now is how your metabolism makes the food you eat—or your own body fat—into energy it can use and energy you can feel! Your metabolism is designed to work with two primary fuels at any given time: carbs, in the form of glucose, and fat, in the form of ketones or fatty acids. But, because of the way our Standard American Diet has placed carbohydrates on a pedestal, we've become a nation of eaters who are addicted to carbs and are metabolically *inflexible*.

What do I mean by metabolically *inflexible*?

Think of your metabolism like a car with different gears to drive in. High gear, low gear, etc. Your metabolism is meant to function using different gears at different times, depending on how much fuel you have, what kind of fuel you give it, what kind of load you're carrying, the speed you're driving, etc. It's very likely that right now, your metabolism is stuck in high gear, burning through fuel at an unsustainable rate, not allowing you to cope under different circumstances by switching into lower gears.

For the standard American eater, being metabolically inflexible means your body is a sugar burner—stuck in a metabolic gear that can only burn carbs for energy. It burns 'em fast and creates more 'exhaust' or inflammation and stress in your body. Being stuck in this gear makes your metabolism reliant on more carbs and more frequent meals and snacks, while it can't possibly switch into the lower, fat-burning gear. You'll learn about metabolic flexibility later in Part 5.

The more frequently you eat and the more carbs you eat, the more stuck you are in a metabolic state that depends on the quick energy of carbohydrates and glucose. In turn, that means you're constantly hungry, constantly eating, and constantly storing more body fat—or at least preventing the body fat you already have from being burned.

> *"It's years of repeated daily spikes that slowly increase our fasting glucose level, a pattern we discover only once that level is classified as pre-diabetic (a state of insulin resistance that's type 2 diabetes on the horizon)."*
> - Jessie Inchauspé, *Glucose Revolution*

The wonderful news is that you can get back to your factory settings. You can turn the ideal genetic switches back on so you can burn body fat, stop feeling so damn hungry all the time, and experience real food freedom that gives you more resilient health, enjoyment, and confidence in your relationships with food and mealtimes, as well as more confidence in your body.

15 Signs You're a Sugar Burner

Those who struggle with three or more of the symptoms listed below may be eating a diet that's dangerously high in sugar and carbs. This suggests they're a sugar burner—meaning their body has become entirely dependent on frequent meals, snacks, and carbohydrates for energy. This person is almost certainly insulin-resistant as a result.

Are you a sugar burner? Review the following list, and place a checkmark beside each symptom you currently experience.

- You're hungry or tempted to eat all the time.

- You crave sweets daily and must have dessert/something sweet after every meal.

- You experience daily mood swings and irritability.

- You suffer from depression or tiresome anxiety.

- You experience energy crashes (no matter how much you sleep).

- You experience brain fog and have difficulty concentrating or articulating thoughts.

- You've experienced significant weight gain.

- You have excess weight accumulated in the abdominal region, and your waist circumference is larger than your chest or hip circumference.

- You've been warned about/diagnosed with pre-diabetes or type 2 diabetes.

- You have high triglycerides (fats in the bloodstream measured by standard cholesterol and lipid tests).

- You have high blood pressure.

- You frequently get sick (cold/flu/repeat infections, or sinus problems).

- You have gut issues (including gas or bloating).

- You get *hangry* or anxious when you don't eat soon enough.

- You wake hungry in the middle of the night.

- You urinate frequently (including more than once during the middle of the night).

Notice that some of those symptoms listed above are also factors used to determine a diagnosis for metabolic syndrome—a cluster of three or more criteria of the five metabolic risk factors (all of which are measured at annual doctor visits as part of routine lab work).

The five metabolic risk factors for metabolic syndrome diagnosis include:

1. Low HDL cholesterol

2. High triglycerides

3. Obesity (specifically waist circumference)

4. High blood pressure

5. High blood sugar (elevated fasting glucose, pre-diabetes, type 2 diabetes, or elevated HbA1c levels).

Many of my clients are surprised to learn that all those symptoms are due to metabolic dysfunction. The symptoms are exacerbated or even caused by a high-carb, high-sugar diet that includes eating too often. Such dietary habits result in an inflammatory cascade of consequences for the cardiovascular system, hormonal and metabolic systems, and even the neurological system, which greatly increases one's risk of all chronic diseases—and death. And quite frankly, it's safe to conclude that for most individuals, all of those factors are initiated by a state called insulin resistance—which you'll learn more about in this book.

Looking back to the list of signs you're a sugar burner, how many of the symptoms did you check off? These days, it's not uncommon to experience most or all of these symptoms at once. Good news is, you will find relief once you've adopted a low-sugar, moderate-to-low-carbohydrate diet—especially when you include intermittent fasting and moderate physical activity.

It is possible to turn your health around, and it is liberating! Free yourself from the grips of a relentless appetite and experience the optimal settings you were born with. Simply by following the 21-day carb reduction action steps at the end of Part 2, you can experience the life-changing effects of becoming a fat burner—being more metabolically flexible and more insulin sensitive (the beneficial state that's opposite of insulin resistance). These are the ultimate outcomes needed to give you back more freedom with your diet and resilience with your health.

CHAPTER 13

What Fasting Is Like Without Fixing Your Diet

O ther fasting methods skip the step of carbohydrate reduction. They tell you it's okay to eat whatever you want, like the wildly popular method *Delay, Don't Deny*. Well, in my experience as a food lover, an intermittent fasting coach, and a professional food addiction coach—for most people, this is a recipe for disaster.

Imagine you start right now with fasting 16 hours a day, and you don't change a thing about the foods you eat. Then, next week, you push yourself to fast for 18 hours on most days. You have a goal to fast 22 hours every day by the end of the month because you've heard that's what it takes to lose the excess pounds. This is one meal a day (OMAD) fasting.

Guess what that experience would be like? For most people, especially women, it's gonna suck! It'll feel like every single day is a battle. It would feel like you're at war with your inner cookie monster, and you'd probably binge out every night when your eating window finally opened. You'd be relying solely on willpower and grit to get you through those long daily fasts because every other biological signal would tell you to *EAT! FIND FOOD NOW!*

Ummmm…. That's the last thing you want.

You want to be free from your obsession with eating. You want to feel good in your body and get on with your life without depending on willpower to get you through each day—and without diving face-first into a pint of Talenti Gelato Layers as soon as someone pisses you off (or immediately after the kids are asleep. *Ahem. Parents, I'm talking to you!*).

When you fast without reducing your carb and sugar intake, it's as if you're driving with your right foot on the gas and your left foot on the brake pedal—at the same time! You're sending stress signals to your body while you force it to fast, and your body is sending you signals to eat, find food, cry, quit, and take a nap. It's completely unsustainable, cruel, and contradictory, all in one day. On repeat.

Your body would be too stressed. Your metabolism would eventually slow down. It's also likely you'd experience constipation, keto flu, and more unwanted side effects because you did too much, too fast. Your daily stressors would compound, and soon, you'd be abandoning the diet because it's all too much in the context of your busy life.

If, instead, you work on reducing your carb and sugar intake to something more natural for the human body and you increase your intake of nutrient-dense foods (in Part 3), you'll gradually lead your body back to its factory settings. This means you'll reduce the demand for insulin, allowing your body to burn excess fat whenever food is scarce—just like it was designed to do. Your metabolism will also be in balance, knowing there's plenty of fuel to sustain you—right there on your lovely love handles!

Not so fast.

Even in the books by one of my favorite fasting experts, Dr. Jason Fung, he encourages 36-hour fasts and 72-hour fasts, both in an effort to force your body into ketosis without changing your diet. This works for Dr. Fung and his team because they're in a clinical setting. They specialize in working with sick patients who are running out of time to turn their health around. With the limited time he has to influence an individual's eating habits and make such life-changing adjustments to their diet (like those I suggest in this book), Dr. Fung's way is a shortcut, indeed, and it works for many people who are desperate for rapid change.

That shortcut, however, leaves many others feeling inadequate or discouraged because they have no desire to fast for > 36 hours at a time. Even if they do try, they criticize themselves for not having either the discipline or the willpower to continue this as a habit. They feel like failures because it's simply unrealistic to continue consistently enough to induce lasting change.

I'm assuming you're not interested in doing a 36-hour fast to force yourself into ketosis at this stage you're in. Sure, it may seem alluring because, in some ways, it sounds easier. But, you know yourself. Would such a shortcut work for you?

Let's imagine what it would be like for you, shall we? Tonight, after dinner, you'd start fasting. Tomorrow, you can't eat anything. Afternoon and night, you fight off the endless urges to eat something. You go to sleep tomorrow night and try to sleep through the night just so you can finally break your fast after 36 hours without food. Could you do that? Would you want to at this stage? And then what? You go back to eating whatever you want as long as you suffer through those 36-hour fasts two or more times a week? Meanwhile, you're constipated, exhausted, hungry, irritable, and debating whether you should give up or hire a fasting coach. (Trust me, I know, because nearly half of my private clients come to me after trying and failing at Delay Don't Deny fasting or the extended fasting methods from Dr. Fung's books.)

So, what if you took your time instead, and this whole thing was so much easier on your mind and body? So much more enjoyable. Less disruptive. Requiring less willpower. More flexible and sustainable for your lifestyle. It's a practice that *becomes* an actual lifestyle and gives you lasting results. And you patiently created this lifestyle with habits and characteristics that reflect your newfound dedication to healthier living.

Sounds good to me.

You're taking an active role in your personal health, no longer playing dumb when it comes to your own body. Without taking ownership of your health, you're headed toward disease. I don't care if your great-aunt Carmen ate a bunch of junk food and lived comfortably until the impressive age of ninety-five. Times are changing. Our environment and food system are seriously messed up. Our bodies are burdened by far too many things outside of our control today, which is why it's time we take control of the things we really have the power to change.

Consider this simple concept known as The Illness-Wellness Continuum.

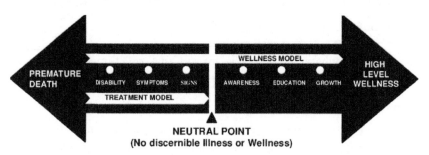

The Illness-Wellness Continuum is a graphical illustration to demonstrate that wellness is not merely the absence of symptoms or disease, but also a dynamic process that leads to premature death or high-level mental and physical wellbeing. Original Source: John W. Travis, M.D. 1972, 1975, 1981, 1985, 2004.

If you were living with virtually no symptoms, you wouldn't be reading this book. So, let's presume you live with nagging symptoms, which places you on the left side of this spectrum. Symptoms are your body's way of sending you messages that something is dangerously wrong. If left unresolved, symptoms will likely lead to disability, diseases, or disorders (which you may already have). This diagram makes that connection, following the arrow toward the left, which eventually leads to premature death. *Screw that!*

What if, instead, you take an active role in your health. You look at those signs, symptoms, or diagnoses as a cry for help from your body. This is a wake-up call for you to become more aware of your current state of health and disease. Look at the center of the spectrum moving toward the right. You'll see *awareness* and then *education*. That's what you're doing right now, for you. You're here, facing your symptoms and educating yourself on what you can do about it.

Notice the direction the right arrow is going toward *growth* and eventual *high-level wellness*. That's where you'd rather be. Wouldn't you? By taking an active role in your health and taking responsibility for certain eating habits that are detrimental to your health, you'd reverse the direction you were headed. You'd start traveling to the right, toward wellness you can feel and exude. You *can* change your health around. And that's why you're here.

~

2 Common Dietary Extremes

People come to intermittent fasting from one of two extremes: aggressive fasting or aggressive (ultra-restrictive) dieting. To put this in perspective, let's consider the following scales:

Dietary Restriction on a scale of 1–10

1 = no dietary restriction whatsoever

10 = the most restrictive diet

Fasting Intensity on a scale of 1–10

1 = the least amount of fasting (fasts of about 10 hours)

10 = the most aggressive amount of fasting (OMAD, or weekly extended fasts ranging from 36–72 hours)

Here's how I'd describe the two extreme approaches people first come to me with:

Person A:

They're at level 1 on the Dietary Restriction scale and level 9 on the Fasting Intensity Scale. They start fasting without changing a single thing about their diet, and they eat like crap. The whole reason they're attracted to fasting is because they think, *Finally, I can eat whatever junk I want as long as I fast every day for 20 hours or start doing 72-hour fasts every week. Yippie!* No wonder they eventually fall off the wagon, right?

Person B:

They're at a level 9 on the Dietary Restriction scale and maybe a 6 on the Fasting Intensity Scale. This person is totally new to fasting. After committing themselves to a full-on keto diet or low-calorie diet, they attempt to do daily 16-hour fasts. They hear about the benefits of both fasting + keto, or fasting + calorie restriction, and they join one of those huge keto fasting Facebook groups or plant-based fasting groups that are flooded with misinformation and extreme dieters. They're under the impression the only way to make progress is to cut out all carbs or slash calories every day while consistently fasting 16–20 hours right off the bat. That's a lot of restriction, no matter which way you slice it.

Talk about completely flipping your life upside down! In the case of keto fasting, not only are you skipping most meals of the day, but when you do eat, you aren't supposed to touch a piece of fruit or a grain of rice for weeks, months, or seasons at a time? K, bye-bye food freedom. Bye-bye family dinners. And hello to headaches, keto flu, frustrated family members, constipation, constant nagging from the devil and angel on your shoulder, and carb-loading binge sessions on the privacy of your couch.

You might be thinking, *It's worth it to push myself through those challenges and do whatever it takes to achieve my weight-loss goal.* What happens after you've achieved the weight loss? Which, by the way, you may still not achieve because the strategy is too aggressive, and your body won't like that. You gradually—or abruptly—go back to eating a non-keto diet, fasting less and less as your life goes back to normal. Before you know it, two years have passed, and you've gained back 40 lb. You think to yourself, *How did I let this happen? I don't feel I've been that bad. Maybe I need to stay keto for the rest of my life if I want to lose it again and keep the weight off!*

Screw that.

Not only is it tiresome to uphold such eating habits and so defeating to experience such oscillating body weight, but it's also detrimental to your metabolism. It influences your body weight set point and your resting metabolic rate. In other words, yo-yo dieting or back-and-forth weight gain and loss results in a slower metabolism and a heavier baseline body weight than you've ever had before. It's like a contingency plan your body reacts with to protect you from future threats—like extreme dieting.

Screw that, big time. My solution is simple and sustainable. It lies in the middle of the spectrum, between those two extremes. It's what I call carbohydrate moderation, and it's something you can make your own.

CHAPTER 14

Carbohydrate Moderation

I usually cringe when I hear the word *moderation* because moderation isn't for everyone, yet it's been forced down our throats by dietitians and weight-loss gurus for decades. But, in this instance, it's the most precise way to describe what I'm talking about. Carb moderation implies that you eat around 50–130 g of *net carbs per day. Where you'll fall in that range depends on your current experience level, how much you're fasting, and how active you are.

Public health officials actually consider that range to be low-carb. In the keto community, however, low carb would imply that you stay under 20 g of net carbs per day, which is way lower than the starting point I recommend. With my approach, you'll learn to gradually moderate your carb intake. For starters, you'll cut out half of the bread, pasta, and other flour-based foods you consume daily, along with fried foods and most treats or sweets—but you won't be on a keto diet. You can have up to five times as many carbs per day as you do on a keto diet and up to two-and-a-half times as many carbs as you can have on a typical keto IF diet.

This moderate version leaves space for so much flexibility and variety in your diet. You'll enjoy the process while still training your metabolism to stop

90

depending on carbs and sugar and rather start using body fat for energy like it was designed to do.

> *We're not designed to thrive on any-and-every*
> *modern Frankenfood we can get our hands on*

To understand why we can't just eat whatever we want, whenever we want— or why and how your metabolism got so far out of whack in the first place— you'll need to know the basics about how energy storage works in the body.

Storing Away Those Excess Carbs

Body fat serves as a survival advantage ancient humans needed to protect them from famine and starvation. Humans can store endless amounts of body fat. Have you ever seen one of those TV shows like *My 800 lb Life*? The body continues storing energy that never gets put to use!

Our fat threshold differs from person to person, however. This explains why some individuals may never become morbidly obese, but by consuming excessive carbs and nutrient-poor foods long enough, that fat starts to accumulate inside their liver (non-alcoholic fatty liver disease) and in the visceral abdominal region surrounding the organs. You've seen those skinny guys with giant 'pregnancy' bellies. Once the abuse persists long enough, type 2 diabetes, metabolic syndrome, cancer, and cardiovascular disease (just to name a few) are forming, regardless of a person's personal fat threshold.

Where does all the excess body fat come from?

Contrary to what we were told in the '90s and 2000s, excess body fat doesn't accumulate because a person consumes too much dietary fat or even necessarily from eating too many calories, which we discovered during that low-calorie, low-fat societal craze when everyone slashed calories but still gained weight and had trouble losing the excess fat.

Excess body fat comes from abusing the metabolism. For most Americans and members of other Westernized societies, it's primarily from consuming too many carbohydrates or too much sugar—particularly in the context of a high-fat or nutrient-poor diet—and from eating too frequently and/or abandoning a formerly active lifestyle.

When you consume more carbohydrates or sugar than your body needs, where does it go?

Since carbohydrates (glucose) are prioritized as quick energy, and they're toxic when they linger in the bloodstream, the body tries to get them out of there right away. If you don't need the energy and use those carbs right now, your body checks if there's room to store them as glycogen in your liver and muscles. Then what?

If there's no space left to store them in your liver and muscles, those excess carbs are converted into *fat*. Yup. Triglycerides. And triglycerides can increase inflammation in your bloodstream, increase plaque and dangerous cholesterol, and contribute to a fatty liver. Carbs are turned into fat and stored in the liver since there's not enough muscle to store them in, and there are too many carbs. Oh, and those triglycerides are stored as body fat inside your fat cells. Keep snacking all night long and keep eating those excess carbs, and your fat cells will grow in size and number. Every single day.

Now, back to the conversation about endless body fat storage. We know the body can store a seemingly limitless amount of fat, but it has limited storage space for carbs. That's why **leftover carbs are converted to body fat for long-term storage**.

Before I became a health coach, my eyes used to glaze over whenever someone tossed around words like glucose, glycogen, triglycerides, etc. I felt as if it was too much information for me to concern myself with, and I needed a clearer picture to help the concepts make sense and stick in my mind. Finally, when I saw the numbers, I was able to grasp it.

The average adult's body can only store around 100 g of carbs in the liver and 400 g of carbs in the muscles at a time, depending on how active they are, their age, and how much muscle mass they have.

If you think of your carb storage space as *luggage* with a limited capacity—like 500 g of carbs—you can begin to understand why your body needs somewhere else to put the excess carbs you consume. When your luggage is full because you rarely unpack it by fasting or burning stored carbs through exercise, and you don't have enough muscle tissue to increase the capacity of your luggage, *and* you keep adding more crap to your luggage, your body ends up looking for other *suitcases*, like fat cells and fat in your liver where it doesn't belong, in which to store the overflow.

The 500-gram capacity in your carb luggage equates to somewhere around 1,600–2,800 carbohydrate calories. The higher the number, the better. The more muscle you have - the more carbs your muscles can store - the more luggage space you have for excess carbs you eat. This also means your body is less likely to store them in your fat suitcases, which is yet another reason you want to prioritize protein intake and strength-training exercises.

This tells us we're designed to have a decent amount of muscle mass. Furthermore, because excess carbs are converted into body fat, and we can store an endless amount of body fat, it becomes obvious that the human body was designed to utilize fat as our most dependable energy source.

An Evolutionary Mismatch

Humans are extraordinarily predestined to coordinate with nature in a seasonal, cyclical way. Back in the day, when summer weather culminated in an abundance of carb-rich plants to engorge ourselves with, for example, the body stored fat in preparation for the upcoming cold season and imminent food scarcity. In today's modern societies, however, this feature of human design isn't doing us many favors.

Have you faced circumstantial starvation or significant food scarcity in your adult life? Thankfully, most of us can answer "No". Odds are, everywhere you turn, there are cheap carbs and tempting foods within arm's reach, available all hours of the day or night and any season of the year. This presents a modern-day problem, and you're living it. On the daily. For decades on end.

Understanding this *evolutionary mismatch* is one of the keys you need to achieve greater health management and food freedom in today's world. Let's dig deeper, shall we?

CHAPTER 15

The Carbohydrate Curve

Our ancient human ancestors lived throughout what's known as the Paleolithic era, a pre-civilized period that predates both the agricultural revolution and the advent of industrially processed foods. In pre-civilized times, there were no refrigerators or chemical preservatives to make food last in storage. There were no corner shops or drive-thrus. No delivery services to get food whenever someone was hungry. Ancient humans had to find food in the wild. They needed to hunt and fish, gather and find things in their surroundings. And they shared or rationed their food among their families or tribes.

Historically, humans have always cycled between unpredictable feasts and food deprivation. When a person found a lot of food—like when nature rewarded them with a big bounty of fruit on an orange tree or a big bison kill on the hunt that day—there'd be lots of food or a *feast*. These same humans would go through periods of food deprivation or starvation where they couldn't find any food at all. That's the kind of rhythm the human body has evolved to cope with over hundreds of thousands of years. This rhythm gives us health even in times of deprivation because we're built to deal with that duality. The feasting *and* the fasting.

It may come as a surprise to you, but our genes are nearly identical to those of our Paleolithic ancestors. Our genes simply haven't had enough time to evolve much since then, which is why an evolutionary mismatch matters. That's why our modern-day diets and habits can be so destructive when forced up against our ancient ancestral genes.

For most of us, the evolutionary mismatch is why we get into trouble consuming so many simple carbohydrates, starchy foods, and high-sugar foods, and it's also why we're so friggin' attracted to those foods in the first place. It's why we can't healthily consume so many grains, seeds, or even nuts that are un-sprouted or unfermented (the old-fashioned food-processing methods needed to increase digestibility and nutrient availability in such foods). Our guts aren't yet evolved for these dietary staples.

The evolutionary mismatch also explains why we can't eat all the friggin' time. Our genes don't have the programming to deal with constant eating and constant carbs without resulting in a fat or sick human. You see, ancient humans would've been *really* lucky to have food every single day or even to have one meal every day. Summers and early fall could be pretty bountiful in nature, indeed. Yet there were wars, droughts, and freezing prolonged winters—even an ice age!—famine, and, you know, just unlucky surroundings in different climates making it impossible for people to have bountiful food every day, all year round. It'd be impossible to sit on their asses all day, too.

Picture those ancient humans struggling to find food In the morning, the afternoon, all day long, or for days at a time. During times of starvation or manageable food scarcity, you'd think their energy would have suffered. But it didn't. They needed energy and brainpower to continue the search for food while they starved. That's why we've evolved with another survival advantage that equips us with some amazing mechanisms to ensure we can find food and have enough energy to thrive under such circumstances (such as going for days without food).

So, you see, our bodies are designed to fatten up for the winter. When our ancestors encountered abundant seasonal fruits, starchy tubers, and vegetables in their surroundings, they'd gorge on them, storing away excess energy for the coming starvation of winter.

If you've ever grown your own fruits or vegetables before, you know most plants give you all the goods at once. In abundance. You're gonna get all your bananas at one time, all your avocados at one time, all your walnuts at one time. Nature just bombards you so you can gorge yourself on certain nutrients before the season ends. It's when we fattened up for the winter. That's why we have a never-ending capacity for body fat because the body is reliant on it when food is scarce.

Here's the mismatch. In our modern lifestyles, we never experience a winter, *per se.*

Well, then, how can we eat in a way that's more aligned with the way our bodies were designed? How do we include the foods of modern society without sabotaging our efforts to be healthier?

A great starting point is to go back to how many carbohydrates the human body can realistically and safely process each day. You'll then compare these guidelines to the way you typically eat. A cornerstone resource for this is a simple chart known as the Primal Blueprint Carbohydrate Curve (Figure 15.1 below).

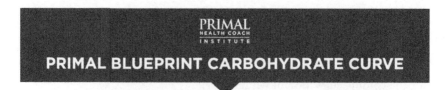

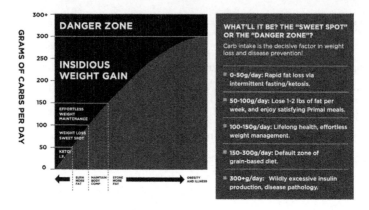

Figure 15.1. This chart, by primal nutrition pioneer Mark Sisson, was designed to illustrate the cumulative impact daily carbohydrate intake can have on a person's weight and their propensity toward disease. Today, it's not uncommon for the average American to consume over 250 g of carbohydrates per day on a regular basis. If you consider the tiers on this carbohydrate curve, 250 g of carbs is likely to lead to insidious weight gain, inching you toward wildly excessive insulin production and disease pathology.
Source: *The Primal Blueprint by Mark Sisson*

How easy is it to fall into insidious weight gain territory even while trying to eat what public health authorities and mainstream nutrition guidelines advise as a healthy diet? It's easier than you'd think. Check this out:

A day of healthy-ish eating that easily leads to weight gain:

Breakfast:

- Bowl of quick-cooking plain oatmeal, sweetened with stevia and 1/2 sliced banana

- 1 cup of coffee with 4 oz of Califia Farms unsweetened oat milk creamer.

Lunch:

- Turkey bacon sandwich with low-fat mayonnaise, tomato, lettuce, and 2 slices of whole wheat sandwich bread.
- 1 serving of sweet potato chips
- 1 serving of strawberry Chobani yogurt

Mid-day Snack:

- Starbucks chai tea latte made with coconut milk

Dinner:

- 1 serving of whole wheat couscous
- 4 oz roasted chicken breast
- Sauteed spinach and peppers

After-Dinner Snack:

- 1 serving of Justin's dark chocolate peanut butter cups

Would you believe this example will take you over 255 g of carbohydrates in a day? Here you are, trying to eat healthier, following mainstream dietary advice, and still, the weight piles on, and it won't come off. Even by controlling the portions of these foods, you're gaining weight, you're hungry all the time, and you're fighting an uphill battle. In the final chapter of Part 2, I'll share with you some action steps to reduce your daily carb intake without restricting your diet too much. This way, you can still enjoy many of your favorite foods throughout the change process and adapt to the changes in a reasonable time.

Carbs Per Day

Figure 15.1, the Primal Blueprint Carbohydrate Curve, is a good guideline to reduce your daily carbohydrate intake to something more moderate, such as under 130 g of carbs per day when you're fasting ≤ 14 hours and fat loss is your goal.

When you start fasting around 16 hours or more—and fat loss is still your goal—you might consider keeping daily carbs under 100 g per day to accelerate results. You'll see more guidelines for such modifications in the action steps at the end of Part 2. If you have high fasting blood glucose, your goal might be to reduce your carbohydrate intake to a level that keeps your glucose under 120 mg/dL after a meal.

If you're here for health and weight maintenance, you'll still want to embark on the 21-day carbohydrate reduction journey described in the upcoming action steps. Then you'll become more fat-adapted and ready to create a sustainable lifestyle plan that, ideally, keeps your daily carb intake below 150 g per day. This leaves plenty of room for nutrient-rich veggies, fruits, nuts, and a few of your favorite safe starches and carbohydrate-comfort foods in the regular rotation. This moderate carb intake is a sustainable solution for weight management, disease prevention, and an enjoyable lifestyle.

Carbs Per Meal

One thing to keep in mind as a helpful guideline for mealtime is to aim for meals under 40 g of total carbs. This makes sense when you're on a fat-loss journey, you're fasting less than 18 hours a day, and you're *not* exercising in a fasted state for longer than 60 minutes of exertion. This recommendation also helps keep insulin levels lower as part of a reasonable maintenance and longevity plan.

≤ 40 g of carbs is an important threshold because we can only expect to metabolize 40 g of carbs within the safe two-hour insulin window that follows a meal. This general guideline is helpful for those eating three meals a day, especially for packaged foods, restaurant foods, and anything that contains starchy carbs or sugar. More on that in a bit, but starchy carbs are primarily foods made from flour, grains, potatoes, and starchy tubers like cassava, yuca, plantains, and taro. The amount of added sugar or total sugar (including syrups, fruit juices, dried fruit, or concentrates) is factored into the carb count, too.

Look at the packaged foods you include in a meal—the bag of sliced bread, the box of oatmeal, the frozen pizza box—how many carbs are in the serving size you actually eat? Don't rely on nutrition claims from the front of the package or the amount per serving without considering the nutrition facts along with the serving size you eat.

Front labels and packaging can be VERY misleading:

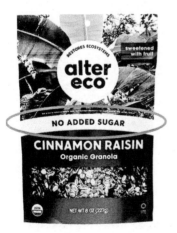

Let's say a product you like states the total sugar = 6 g per serving, *but* there are 8 servings in the package...

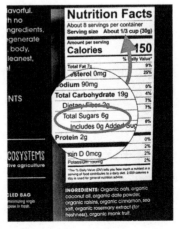

...which means if you ate *half* of the package, you just had 24 g of sugar and 68 g of net carbs in one sitting!

When you go to a restaurant or fast food joint, look on the website for the nutrition facts (or use a free tool like *myfitnesspal.com* or *fatsecret.com* to search for the item you're ordering) so you can take charge of your health and only order foods that won't hinder your goals.

Popular meals and snacks that can easily go into weight-gain territory

Food Item(s)	Brand or Restaurant	Total Carbs
6" Tuna Sub on 9-Grain Bread + Baked Lay's Chips	Subway	65g
Pumpkin Spice Latte (grande)	Starbucks	52g
Grill Chicken Club Sandwich + Fruit Cup side	Chick-fil-A	59g
Tonkotsu Ramen Noodle Soup	Santouka	111g
Sourdough Breakfast Sandwich	Dunkin	58g
Plain Bagel + Cream Cheese	Dunkin	67g
Cauliflower Crust Pizza (6 pc or personal pan)	Blaze Pizza	96g
Falafel Pita Wrap	Roti Mediterranean Grill	109
Impossible Burger with Fries	Wahlburger	95g
Bacon Turkey Bravo Sandwich	Panera	104g
Citrus Asian Crunch Salad (with dressing)	Panera	50g
Vegan Pepperoni Pizza (frozen, serving 1/2 of whole pizza)	Daiya	91g
Fried Chicken (2 piece white) + Cole Slaw + Corn	KFC	59g
Spinach Artichoke Dip + Flatbread Crisps	Olive Garden	75g
Vegan Lifestyle (Burrito) Bowl	Chipotle	88g
Hummus (1 cup) + Pita Chips (1 serving)	Sabra + Trader Joe's	51g
2 Grilled Fish Tacos dinner with Rice and Beans		86g

Meals That Are Supportive For Fat-Loss and Improved Insulin Sensitivity

Most of these examples are made without any starchy carbs, which means they're naturally low-carb. You don't need to waste time or energy counting the carbohydrates or including them in your daily carb count since they're inherently low in starchy carbs. *The ones with an *asterisk*, however, do contain starchy carbs and should be included in your daily carb count.*

- 🍲 **3 egg omelet with baby spinach and feta** (no hashbrowns)

- 🍲 **Avocado toast made with Base Culture keto bread**

- 🍲 **Subway No Bready Bowl** or **Protein Bowl** (no teriyaki or BBQ sauce)

- 🍲 **Chipotle Lifestyle Bowl:** keto, paleo, or Whole30 versions

- 🍲 ***Panera Mediterranean Bowl with Chicken**

- 🍲 **Mexican fajitas** (ask for no rice, beans, or tortillas – substitute with avocado and pico de gallo on the side, or eat at home with Trader Joe's Spicy Mexican Cauliflower Rice)

- 🍲 **Spaghetti Squash Pizza Bake** from *paleomg.com* (use a zero-sugar tomato sauce)

- 🍲 **Homemade miso salmon** (* no sugar) **and steamed baby bok choy** with garlic and sesame oil

- 🍲 **Homemade 'ramen' soup with kelp noodles or shirataki,** AKA Miracle Noodles

- 🍲 ***Shredded rotisserie chicken and pesto smothered cauliflower gnocchi** from Trader Joe's or Whole Foods Market (1 serving gnocchi)

- 🍲 **Slow-cooked beef chuck roast with roasted turnips and carrots** (beef that's humanely raised with no added hormones or antibiotics)

- 🍲 **Shrimp stir fry** (no sugar or added starch) **with broccoli, snow peas, and red bell pepper**

By now, I hope you're getting pumped and ready to get carbs out of your way. There's something pretty major we haven't covered yet, though. It's time to learn about the one thing you can take to help your body adjust to carb moderation and intermittent fasting without the crappy side effects like low-energy keto flu or persistent sugar-withdrawal headaches. After coaching hundreds of clients through this stage, I have no doubt electrolytes are a game changer worth trying.

CHAPTER 16

Electrolytes

When I started coaching groups through my intermittent fasting method combined with an elimination diet, I noticed a pattern where some individuals would experience headaches, muscle cramps, and even nausea in the first few weeks after cutting out sugar and excess carbs. That's when it became obvious to me that their bodies needed electrolytes to help smooth the adaptation phase for this new way of eating.

Up until then, electrolytes seemed to me like this elusive concept people promoted willy-nilly without a real need for it. Unless you're nursing a hangover or recovering from the stomach flu, I thought the body would regulate electrolytes without you needing to interfere. Welp, I was wrong to assume that's the case for everyone. Many of my clients do need to supplement with electrolytes. And once we recommended that in our group program, the benefits were undeniable!

"I tried the electrolytes you told us about. What a difference! I sweat a lot, and I mean a lot. I've been having major salt cravings at night and alcohol cravings. The electrolytes seem to have helped with both of those issues. I'm telling you, I felt immediately energized. There's definitely something to these electrolytes.

105

I wish I discovered this earlier."
- Melissa

If you've been eating bread, sugar, and other carb-o-licious foods on the daily, then you're about to take your body through some major changes. That's our clue that an electrolyte supplement may be necessary to help your body adjust and avoid the unwanted side effects listed here:

- Headaches
- Irritability
- Low energy, lethargy, fatigue (more than usual)
- Muscle cramps (typically a sign magnesium is needed)
- Achey, sore legs
- Frequent urination
- Excessive hunger
- Nausea
- Constipation (worsened or new)
- Specific cravings
- Fog brain (reduced mental energy and sharpness)
- Dry lips

What are electrolytes?

Electrolytes are key minerals inside your cells that also circulate in your bloodstream. Electrolytes get their name from being—literally—electrically charged. These key minerals are responsible for sending electrical signals to all different parts of your body, from head to toe.

Electrolyte minerals include sodium, chloride, potassium, magnesium, and calcium. Your levels of these minerals will fluctuate regularly, although, thanks to homeostasis, your body works hard to maintain balanced levels. Sodium is the most important electrolyte because it seems to be the only one that's inadequately balanced by your body in response to dietary changes.

Electrolyte levels, especially those of sodium, can become significantly imbalanced in response to any of the following:

- Sudden low-carb dieting and drastic sugar reduction
- Intermittent or any other fasting as a sudden change
- Over-restricting of dietary sodium
- Sweating
- Increased water intake
- Vigorous exercise
- Endurance exercise
- Fasted exercise
- Moving to a higher elevation
- Blazing heat or humidity
- A drastically cold environment or after cold therapy
- Breast-feeding

Why do those circumstances lead to an imbalance in your electrolytes? To help explain it, let's consider the behavior of drinking water. You've probably thought to yourself at some point, *I need to drink more water if I want to get healthier.* You're proud of yourself for increasing your water intake, but you're not necessarily feeling better. In fact, you wonder, *Why am I feeling so lazy lately? Isn't all this water supposed to energize me?* Well, water and sodium have an important reciprocal relationship inside your body because their balance helps maintain the right consistency in your blood and the overall hydration of your organs and cells.

When you increase your water intake, your electrolyte levels are diluted, and increased sodium intake may be necessary to return your body to balance—especially when you simultaneously reduce your carb intake, increase exercise, or incorporate longer fasts. Try some sea salt on your tongue and wash it down with a glass of water. *Ahhhh…. Now that's better.*

Additionally, when you reduce carbs enough and/or integrate intermittent fasting, some interesting changes are underway. By switching your diet in this manner, changes occur where your cells no longer require so much water to assist in energy metabolism. As your cells release that excess water, you might suddenly lose 5–10 lb and feel quite encouraged by these new changes. The reason this initial weight loss occurs so swiftly compared to successive losses is that it's caused by your body releasing sodium and water weight.

You've probably heard that phrase before. Water weight. That water was packaged up in your cells with stored carbohydrates called glycogen. After cutting enough carbs in your diet or fasting long enough, your body depletes stored glycogen, and your cells no longer need the water it's packaged up with. Thus, you pee it out. This also explains why a cheat day of excess carb intake can result in an acute, drastic gain of ≥ 4 lb; it's the water weight going right back into storage with that glycogen. Interestingly, this can also result in even greater losses on the scale once you swiftly return to a low-carb diet.

When you lose water weight, you also lose sodium, as both are released from your cells and kidneys as you incorporate new dietary changes. Thanks to the reduced carbs in your diet and/or the reduced food intake (fasting), your pancreas makes less insulin and makes it less frequently. Less insulin means less water and sodium being stored in your kidneys. Thus, you pee out that excess water and sodium.

The thing you want to remember is that the more you fast and cut carbs, the more sodium and water are depleted in your body. Your body works hard to accomplish a balance between sodium and water, and negative symptoms will manifest when your assistance is needed to reach optimal balance.

How to increase your sodium or electrolytes

You might only need a 1/8–1/4 teaspoon of sea salt washed down with some water, and boom, you're all good. Some fasting enthusiasts enjoy taking a shot of pickle juice (sugar-free) to meet their sodium needs without breaking the fast. Others who exercise more, sweat more, fast for longer periods of time, or implement lots of changes at once may consider a higher-sodium electrolyte supplement like LMNT by Elemental Labs. Even the flavored

LMNT packets (which are sweetened with stevia) have helped dozens of my clients get great results.*

Experiencing muscle cramps? It's likely you're low on the electrolyte magnesium. Try soaking your feet in water with Epsom salts or magnesium salts. Thanks to magnesium's relaxing effects, this is especially great at night to help decompress and get ready for bed. You might also try a topical magnesium oil or lotion like the products made by Ancient Minerals. Any magnesium remedy can provide instant relief and restore balance.

> *"Wow! Electrolytes were a huge difference for me. I had an extremely long day at work, and typically, I get very sore, and my body feels worn down (I work in a chemistry lab on my feet testing and running around the lab). The electrolytes came at 3 p.m. today, and as soon as I added them, within zero minutes, that feeling went away! Thanks, Marisa!!!"*
> - Ashley

No Pain, No Gain?

If you feel like crap before or during a workout—nauseated, have zero energy, muscle spasms, or inflamed injuries—it may not only be electrolytes you need to worry about. I urge you to strongly consider how your sleep and stress are affecting your body's ability to perform at the level you're forcing it to. The no pain, no gain mentality is BS because the more pain you're in, the more likely your body will do whatever it takes to stop you from hurting it further—which means fewer gains, less progress, and more fatigue, hunger, and injury. If you're not sure why you feel like crap and you want to push through, start with electrolytes. For a lot of people, that will do the trick.

CHAPTER 17
Part 2 Action Steps:
How to Reduce Sugar & Carbs in 21 Days

Y ou've got body fat there to burn as an energy source, but your metabolic switch could be stuck in the OFF position, leaving you dependent on carbohydrate energy—even though all that body fat is ready and waiting! That's why it's time for your 21-day carbohydrate reduction. It takes a minimum of 21 days to reset your genes and flip your metabolic switch ON for fat-burning efficiency.

Starting now, you'll simultaneously train your fasting muscles while gradually reducing your carbs. Those two phases work together to help you achieve metabolic flexibility more effortlessly and with fewer side effects.

Not so fast….

The side effects people may experience when they rush into a super low-carb diet (< 50 g total carbs per day) or try to consistently fast 16 hours before their body is ready:

- Intense cravings

- Binge-eating when breaking a fast

- Keto flu

- Constipation

- Frustration and feelings of deprivation

- Irritability and mood swings

- Dizziness

- Headaches

- Nausea

- Increased anxiety

- Fatigue and exhaustion

- Self-doubt or perceived failure that may result in a desire to quit

- Hormonal dysregulation, such as low thyroid hormone or disrupted menstrual cycle

Those symptoms are no joke. Yet they're commonly experienced in this field because most people take on the changes much too fast. You'll be particularly susceptible to the negative side effects if you're coming from a standard carbohydrate intake of ≥ 250 g per day, like most Americans—or if you have a daily dependence on diet soda or diet energy drinks or a daily habit of consuming excessive sugar—and you go against the general advice in this book and rush through the process.

It's more realistic and enjoyable to take your time. It's ultimately more effective, too, because it increases the likelihood you'll stick with it and your body will adapt appropriately. Taking your time now and listening to your body will reward you during weeks two to six and beyond.

Simple Guidelines for a 21-Day Carb Reduction Journey

These are general guidelines for new fasters and dieters who aren't in ketosis.

Overview of Part 2 Action Steps:

Action Step #1: Choose a starting date for your 21-day carb reduction.

Action Step #2: Get real about your current carb intake.

Action Step #3: Start your 21-day carb reduction.

Action Step #1

Choose a starting date.

Looking at your calendar now, choose a nearby date to start your 21-day carb reduction and implement the next steps.

Fill in the blanks: *Starting _____(date) I will begin my 21-day carb reduction. I put it on my calendar because this is important to me. It's important to me because I care more about feeling/achieving/overcoming _____ than I care about eating excess carbs and staying stuck in my ways.*

Action Step #2

Get clear on your current carb intake starting today.

It's important to wake up to the reality of your situation and be clear on the average number of carbs you habitually consume before you start the 21-day reduction plan. It's beneficial to know this because you need to know where you're starting from. If and when you experience setbacks or side effects, it will be useful to assess how drastically you've changed your diet and lifestyle. The more drastically you change things, the more likely setbacks and side effects become, and the more patience is required from you during these few weeks ahead.

How to get clear on your current carb intake?

For the next 3–5 days, consider tracking the carbs you eat and drink. You won't need to change anything about your diet just yet, but you do want to decide if and how you'll track your carbs.

Choose one of the following three variations (A, B, or C):

Variation A: Tracking net carbs

To track, consider using an online food tracker and database, such as Carb Manager or MyFitnessPal, both of which are available as free apps and desktop browsers. They can help you track your net carbs (total carbs minus fiber and sugar alcohols), which is great if you enter everything you eat or drink daily. If this variation sounds good to you, start logging everything you consume for the next 3–5 days. I don't recommend tracking longer than 5 days unless it's a habit you already have in place or have enjoyed doing in the past.

Note there's no need to track *non-starchy* vegetables like leafy greens, cabbages, broccoli, cauliflower, celery, or green beans (because those carbs don't raise insulin)

Variation B: Tracking total carbs

Do you prefer the simplicity of note-taking on your phone's notes app? Or maybe you like the ol' pen-and-paper method. Either way, designate a specific note or notepad for this. Be sure it's somewhere you'll see it throughout the day, so you remember to write down whatever you eat. With manual tracking like this, it's easier to track total carbs rather than net carbs (since you won't be using an app or tool to track and calculate it for you). You won't need to calculate much or write down *every single thing* you consume. **Take note of the total carbs (in the serving size you consume) from any of these food categories:**

- **All packaged or processed foods** (boxed/canned/jarred/bagged foods, ranging from salad dressing and frozen dinners to chips, bread, and protein bars; also including fast food, items from restaurants, coffee shops, etc.)

- **Grains** (corn, masa, rice, wheat, etc.)

- **Beans and lentils** (including hummus, chickpeas, falafel)

- **Sugary fruits** (basically all fruit besides fresh whole berries < ½-cup portion)

- **Sweetened drinks of any kind**

- **Starchy vegetables** (potatoes, sweet potato, plantain, green peas, beets, winter squash, cassava, taro)

Read the nutrition labels of all packaged foods. US nutrition labels disclose the total carbohydrates and the serving size that correlates. How many servings did you eat? Keep that in mind as you note the total carbs in each meal or snack. Whether you eat restaurant food or something homemade, do a quick Google search, like, *total carbs in Dunkin' multigrain bagel* or *total carbs in one medium baked potato.*

A day of total carb tracking in iOS notes app:

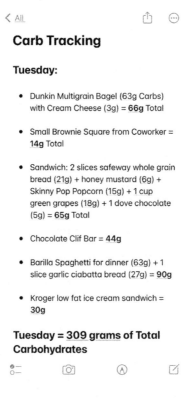

> ‹ All   ⬆   ⋯
>
> ### Carb Tracking
>
> **Tuesday:**
>
> - Dunkin Multigrain Bagel (63g Carbs) with Cream Cheese (3g) = **66g** Total
>
> - Small Brownie Square from Coworker = **14g** Total
>
> - Sandwich: 2 slices safeway whole grain bread (21g) + honey mustard (6g) + Skinny Pop Popcorn (15g) + 1 cup green grapes (18g) + 1 dove chocolate (5g) = **65g** Total
>
> - Chocolate Clif Bar = **44g**
>
> - Barilla Spaghetti for dinner (63g) + 1 slice garlic ciabatta bread (27g) = **90g**
>
> - Kroger low fat ice cream sandwich = **30g**
>
> **Tuesday = 309 grams of Total Carbohydrates**

Variation C: No tracking, just read labels

Tracking can be tedious or triggering, and it's not for everyone. Maybe you know there's no way you'll track everything you're eating or remember to track it, even if it's only for a few days. Maybe food tracking is triggering for you because of a history of compulsive overeating or an eating disorder. Daily carb counting isn't required or recommended if it doesn't feel supportive to you.

If you prefer not to track at all, you can skip tracking and commit yourself to tips #1 and #2 listed below under Action Step #3. Furthermore, when eating packaged foods like frozen meals or rice, corn, pasta, soup, crackers, bread, etc., look at the nutrition facts label and aim to keep your serving of total carbs < 40 g per meal. That guideline, combined with tips #1 and #2, will get you on the right path to reset your metabolism—without the need to track and tally your daily carb intake.

Action Step #3

Start your 21-day carb reduction journey.

Follow these tips to effectively reduce carbs and train your metabolism for more fat burning:

- **Tip #1: Commit to < 10 g of total sugar for all packaged foods and < 5 g of sugar for all drinks.** Ideally, you eliminate all sugar-containing drinks and greatly reduce diet drinks, too, because, in the long run, both will only hinder progress and promote more cravings and insulin resistance.

- **Tip #2: Swap flour-based foods, rice, and potatoes (or similar starches) out of at least one meal a day.**

- **Tip #3: Consider purchasing electrolytes.** Taking electrolytes or salt in your fasting window helps you to ease more comfortably into the carb/sugar-reduction phase and avoid unpleasant side effects.

- **Tip #4: Reduce your daily net carbs to < 130 g per day or total carbs < 150 g per day.** Stick with that number for the first 7 days if it feels good, or up to 14 days if you need more time to adapt.

- **Tip #5: Once you feel good at the current carb range, around days 7–14, try reducing net carbs to < 100 g per day or total carbs < 130 g per day**. You're reducing carbs over these few weeks while simultaneously getting accustomed to intermittent fasting and patiently increasing your fasting window.

- **Tip #6: Don't count calories.** It's usually detrimental to your progress if you concern yourself with calorie counting while reducing carbs and eating more nutritious foods. This often leads to under-eating, which, as a result, leads to increased hunger, a desire to quit, plateaus, and even a slowed metabolism that can cause permanent damage.

Cutting carbs can be a big lifestyle change. Free yourself from the expectation that this will be a straight and narrow journey, and think of it as an experimental process. There's no doubt you'll have lots of questions along the way. Rest assured, you'll learn much more about how to eat a nutritious diet later in Part 3.

Meanwhile, **keep the following nutritional adjustments in mind as you embark on this carb-cutting road ahead:**

- Increase your intake of colorful vegetables and berries

- Include veggies at every meal, with variety being a top priority.

- Aim for a minimum of 25 g of animal protein at every meal.

- If, until now, your diet has been fairly low in fat or you've been watching calories, increase your intake of quality fats like extra virgin olive oil, cultured organic butter, avocados, MCT oil, coconut oil, and a variety of roasted nuts eaten in single servings. Note that peanuts should be reduced or avoided entirely due to their inflammatory, addictive nature and natural sugar content.

- If carbs and sugar have been a major part of your diet until now, it's wise to consider adding electrolytes to ease this transition into a lower-carb lifestyle.

Maybe you read that checklist, and your eyes glazed over. Give yourself a reassuring hand-hold, knowing change takes time. You can still make massive progress if you only do the action steps from the first two parts of this book. Things will be different now. No doubt about that. Your meals will look so different because there'll be less white stuff on your plate and more colorful foods. You'll probably use more bowls than plates and a fork and knife instead of two slices of bread to handle your food.

From here on out, you'll be shopping for more fresh groceries and putting a little more time into planning your meals and cooking them. Not in the habit of cooking regularly yet? Start small by cooking two or three times a week. No time for cooking much at all? Then it's quite likely your solution is to source healthy pre-made meals to have ready and waiting for you. Either way, be patient with yourself as you experiment with what works and get accustomed to this new way of living, eating, and prioritizing your health.

To ease this transition, I've put together some helpful tools and food lists like my favorite carb swaps, photos of my favorite meals, and more at *marisamoon.com/notsofast/resources*.

Scan this QR Code to visit the resources page for this book:

One of those resources I highly recommend during this stage is what I call *Are you an Abstainer or Moderator?* That worksheet helps you identify and tackle your tripwires, so to speak. Which foods can you realistically eat in moderation, and which foods are you better off cutting out of the picture altogether? There will be challenges. There will be a little devil on your shoulder saying, *Screw it. Eat all the carbs!* This is part of the process, and I'm here to guide you through it.

PART 3

Eat Nourishing Foods

RESET

Reduce Carbs

Eat Nourishing Foods

Start with 12 Hours

Extend Your Fasts

Thoughtfully Adapt

CHAPTER 18

Nutrition:

The Transformative Key to Sustainable Fat Loss, Food Freedom, and Lasting Health

Nutrition. You wish it didn't matter.

For decades of your life, you've either reassured yourself or been influenced by others that:

- You don't have time and energy to care about nutrition.

- You'll find an easier way to lose weight rather than fuss about nutrition.

- Maybe nutrition doesn't even matter that much (*after all, your grandfather lived a pretty good life, lasting until he was ninety-one on a diet primarily made up of frosted coffee cake, Kentucky Fried Chicken, fettuccine alfredo with unlimited garlic bread, and the annual trash-can-sized Christmas tin filled with caramel popcorn*).

If you care about nutrition already, I'm impressed. If you don't care about nutrition, that doesn't surprise me, even though I don't know you, because, odds are, you have a similar line of thinking as most of the folks who ask me to help them lose weight.

Which line of thinking do you relate to the most?

- **Person A:** A nutritious diet, in your mind, means boring food, deprivation, and diet foods that take the fun out of life.

- **Person B:** You view nutrition as a privilege you simply cannot have. From your perspective, a nutritious diet is something others can have when they're privileged with more time or money, better access, or know-how.

- **Person C:** In general, you respect the critically important role nutrition plays in optimizing your health, whether or not you currently eat a nutritious diet.

Whether you're like person A, B, or C, I'm sure you find it pretty challenging to care about healthy eating or to prioritize it because it seems like a complete overhaul of your diet and lifestyle is needed. This feels too daunting even to consider, let alone put into action. And that's why you continue to avoid it, falling for any alternative scheme you encounter.

For decades, it's this wishful thinking that's got you desperately seeking weight-loss shortcuts, falling for dietary falsehoods and empty promises that claim to help you reach your health goals some other, *easier* way. You're allured by such promises because you *realllly* hope you don't have to overhaul your diet and lifestyle. Prioritizing nutrition is a formidable task to undertake, so you try to avoid it, even though, ironically, it could address the root of the very problem you've been battling all along.

Let's celebrate the fact that you're here. You're ready to take ownership of your health. You're open to reading about nutrition with me, and I encourage you to read with curiosity. Pause whenever you feel your attention repeatedly drift toward mindless tasks like checking social media or online shopping. That's a sign your brain needs a break, and you'd be better off closing the book for ten minutes, or even a full day, and coming back to this content with fresh eyes. Do come back!

Think of this section, this book, as a resource that's always at your fingertips should you wish to revisit the concepts or dive deeper as your journey deepens. Even though I've been passionate about nutrition since my late twenties, it was an absolute necessity to have repeat exposure to basic concepts and terminology about nutrition, especially from an ancestral health perspective, which is a key vantage point of this book.

Patience and self-compassion are also imperative in the learning process. Our brains need time and space to process, interpret, absorb, and apply the things that we learn long before we can expect ourselves to remember the concepts off the top of our heads. I don't expect you to grasp or remember at first all the things you read in this section, and you shouldn't expect that of yourself either. Take your time and think of how the intake of new information plays into your big picture. Months from now, you'll be pleased if you've successfully grasped, implemented, and remembered just a few major concepts from this section on Nutrition.

Over time, as you conceptualize things you learn here and begin to incorporate or experiment with them, you'll be more and more capable of building on that knowledge, diving deeper than ever before. It's a journey that will bring you compounding knowledge, confidence, and rewards over time. How great is that?

~

Around the years 2014–2018, as I journeyed into food blogging and health coaching, my passion was fueled by a scarcity mindset. Even though I felt so empowered by my new understanding of nutrition and ancestral health, I didn't recognize the person at the wheel. *X foods will give me cancer*! *Y foods will make me insulin-resistant*! *Z foods will cause an autoimmune disease*!

Who is this person I've become? I contemplated. I learned the hard way that the persona I started showing up with was so vastly different and more fearful compared to the person I always had been. I no longer enjoyed being with myself. Others no longer enjoyed eating around me as much. I was a pain in the ass. *Little Debbie Downer.*

It was a hard lesson I needed to learn so that I could reinvent myself. I needed to rediscover the role food played in my self-identity. Food, for me, is a hobby in every way. It's a hobby through my love of eating, my love of fasting, my love of cooking, travel, nutrition, and more.

I'll never make that mistake again. I won't allow my consideration for nutrition to take away from the overarching recognition that food is an invaluable pleasure in the experience of life. In the big picture, what matters just as much as the nutrition in your diet is that you have a feel-good relationship with food. As Dr. Bill Schindler explains in his book *Eat Like a Human*, "It's important to remember that food is more than nutrition. It's also a cultural experience that's invaluable to our health and happiness."

CHAPTER 19

An Evolutionary Perspective on Nutrition and the Human Diet

We modern humans are so confused about what to eat. No other species faces such a dilemma. *What should I be eating? Is this going to make me fat? I just need to control my portions. Maybe I should drink celery juice every morning.*

Consider yourself lucky if you're not burdened with overthinking every meal and every snack. Food and mealtimes have become their own chronic stressor for so many adults today. In fact, people discover the reason they love intermittent fasting so much is because it removes some of the decision-making required when they eat more frequently throughout the day.

Here's the thing, though. Even if that voice in your head has other priorities, your human body has some requirements that need to be met. Evolutionarily, humans have lived through some key, formative conditions that shaped *your* biology *today*. Your biology requires certain inputs. Certain nutrients, behaviors, and conditions are required to promote your health span or the length of time during which you're generally healthy. If you want to increase your health span—the number of years during which you feel pretty darn good in your body—you'll need to acknowledge some basic human needs, inputs that keep you and your DNA functioning adequately.

Okay, okay, Marisa. Tell me what to eat, and I'll do it.

Okay, okay, Reader. Every day, eat a wide variety of vegetables, seasonal fruit, plenty of herbs and spices, some nuts and seeds, a variety of clean animal protein, and enough minimally-processed healthy fats to keep you satiated.

Simultaneously, there's a debate happening with the voice in my head: *Should I also mention staying away from tap water? You might want to avoid GMOs, or genetically modified crops, because of the gut-destroying chemicals that come along with those, too. I should mention it's possible that nuts and seeds are too inflammatory for you. You might want to avoid all grains, or at least avoid gluten—or at least be sure your grains are fermented or sprouted and organic. You might want to avoid factory-farmed fatty meats and nitrate-cured meats and start to prioritize humanely pasture-raised meat and wild seafood that's low in mercury. Oh, and avoid that deliciously crusty surface you love on a seared steak or blackened salmon. Always avoid the temptation of deep-fried foods. Did I mention you should avoid the endless array of convenient, packaged, and processed foods that tempt you everywhere you turn? Even if they're keto or the label states they're healthy? I know. Those packaged foods are cheap, they make your life easier, and they explode your taste buds, sending a reward to your dopamine-loving neurons. But cut those out.*

Blehhhh (insert frustrated emoji). It's too much, right?

Eating can be complicated in today's modern society for two main reasons.

1. Our food system has changed dramatically, which means our actual food has changed dramatically, too.

2. We each have individual wants, needs, and limitations to consider—which only increases the internal conflicts we face about food.

Regarding reason number one, food in America is a major issue that contributes to all of your frustrations as a dieter. Not only is the conventional farming industry a hot mess in this country—including everything from corn and wheat to strawberries and concentrated animal feeding operations (CAFO) beef. Even the so-called healthy foods, like vegetables grown on conventional farms, are low in nutrients because most farming methods are so destructive to the soil. Remember, the soil provides the plant with nutrients that we depend on for our nutrition once we eat that food. What's worse is farming methods are massively dependent on the use of chemicals, like synthetic fertilizers, that mess with our hormones.

Even if farming wasn't a major issue for us, it's very likely that on a daily basis, you consume processed foods or fast food. Many of the processed foods you crave and have easy access to are categorized as *ultra-processed foods*. Let's talk about these Frankenfoods for a minute.

Ultra-processed foods are "a broad class of food products that are not merely processed (in the conventional sense to lengthen shelf life), but are modified to maximize flavor, visual appeal, texture, odor, and the speed with which they're digested. These foods are made by deconstructing natural food into its chemical constituents and modifying these into new forms that bear little resemblance to anything found in nature. So radically are they altered that nutrition scientists have given them a new name: ultra-processed..." - Newsweek article[16]

And guess what.

Dr. Ashley Gearhardt, Associate Professor of Psychology (food and addiction) at the University of Michigan, says most ultra-processed foods are irresistible and addicting because they've been meticulously engineered to "directly target the vulnerabilities of the human brain—in particular, to exploit the way the brain processes pleasurable sensations. They often deliver a signal to the brain's reward centers so quick and potent, some neuroscientists believe, that many people find it as addictive as opioids or nicotine. (These processed foods are) so much more rewarding than anything our brains ever evolved to handle. That's why so many of us can't stop eating them."

Food addiction is an emerging term in the fields of psychology and substance abuse today. As I learned in my training to become a certified professional food addiction coach, food addicts suffer from intense cravings, a loss of control while eating under various circumstances, and signs of withdrawal.[17] Understandably, most of the addictive behavior occurs in response to hyperpalatable foods. Hyperpalatable foods are designed by food scientists to contain combinations of fat, sugar, carbohydrates, and/or sodium that are likely to make people eat more in one sitting and crave more in response. What's not so obvious is that everyday foods which have become a normal part of the diet—like bread, pizza, popcorn, and ice cream—are indeed categorized as hyperpalatable foods.[18]

As explained in a 2023 research report[19] by Tera Fazzino, professor of psychology and a leader in addiction research, "These foods have combinations of ingredients that don't exist in nature. They can excessively trigger our brain's reward system and disrupt our fullness signals, which is why they're difficult to resist."

The truth is, hyperpalatable foods are the ones we see everywhere. They're easy to grab, and they're convenient. The foods that are not hyperpalatable, like fresh fruits, vegetables, and wild protein, are not just harder to find, but they may require more effort, and they cost more money. I'll help you begin to find solutions and experiment in ways that feel rewarding to you. Odds are you've wasted a lot of time and energy in your past by counting calories, trying shake diets, doing *Insanity* workouts, or forcing yourself through longer and longer fasts rather than deny yourself addicting convenience foods. How about I help you stop wasting your time and energy on those inhumane solutions?

Good news is, once you minimize your intake of highly processed foods in favor of whole foods, you'll start to crave more whole foods. Highly processed foods will appeal to you less and less. Your taste buds will change. Your microbiome—the microbes that populate your digestive tract, or *second brain*—will change, too. As a result, your appetite and energy will change. Your health and mood will improve, and so will your relationship with food.

It just takes a bit of effort from you in the forms of:

1. Intention

2. Persistence

3. Time

Notice, we're talking about being *persistent* here, not *consistent*. Most people I coach have told me they need to be more consistent. Sure, that would be nice, but it's unrealistic for most of us. What is realistic and necessary is persistence. You need a willingness to ride the roller coaster toward food freedom. You'll make progress, you'll experience a lapse in behavior or fall into old patterns, and once you accept and reflect on that, you'll restart or RESET, making progress again. Lapsing again. Reflecting and restarting again. Persistently, patiently resetting, and all the while, things get easier each time.

Can you count on yourself to be persistent?

I won't lie to you and say this can take a back seat to all the other serious demands on your time and energy. Nutritious eating must, eventually, take a front seat in your life. It takes time to incorporate it, though. It takes time to figure out how this can fit into your life, your relationships, your budget, and your persona(s). Like any passion or hobby that makes you feel fulfilled in your life, you must fit it in with your other priorities. Like I had to, you may need to revise your self-image, so to speak, to feel naturally driven to reach your goals despite the inevitable obstacles you'll face.

Good news is that healthy living is sort of addicting, too. When you successfully adopt one healthy habit, you intrinsically want to engage in more healthy behaviors. Healthy habits breed more healthy habits. Progress, despite the expected setbacks, breeds more resilience and more progress. Soon, you see what is truly possible for you, and there's no turning back.

I want that for you, so let's dive in.

In this section, I'll do my best to give you nothing superfluous. We'll start with the concept of metabolic flexibility and why you want a flexible metabolism. I'll introduce you to these critical energy producers inside you, known as mitochondria. Your mitochondria determine how much energy you can feel and rely on for a longer health span.

We'll then get into the basics of a nutrient-dense diet. What benefits come from eating more ancestral foods, increasing your veggies (even frozen and canned veggies are adequately nutritious and protective). How will you benefit from optimizing your protein intake and prioritizing nutritional diversity by expanding on the variety of foods in your diet? And just when you're tempted to turn away and fall for another shortcut rather than incorporate the nutrition concepts I propose, I'll share with you what intermittent fasting is like without nutritious eating. The unpleasant symptoms and repercussions you'll be destined for if you let your fear of change stand in the way of nutritious eating.

I'll wrap up Part 3 with the top trap people fall into as they try to prioritize nutritious foods. And, finally, I'll give it to you straight in Chapter 31: *Time or Money: Something's Gotta Give*. I'll leave you with specific action steps, of course, and plenty of resources to dive deeper if you're ready to continue learning.

Let's hold hands. I've got you. Here we go.

CHAPTER 20
Metabolic Flexibility

What is metabolic flexibility?

A flexible metabolism is your birthright. It describes your body's innate ability to effectively and instantly switch between burning carbohydrates and glucose for energy to burning fat and ketones for energy. It involves a set of favorable genetic switches we're born with; however, most of us jam those switches because of our chronic, carb-dependent eating habits.

We're designed to work with various energy sources. To understand the positive impact this can have, let's first consider the concept of cross-training in sports. When an athlete wants to improve their performance while also minimizing the risk of injuries, they engage in cross-training, which means they practice one or more additional sports or exercises that enhance their versatility and all-around performance. A football player, for instance, might take up yoga or ballet to help improve their balance, range of motion, focus, and recovery.

Like cross-training in sports, being metabolically flexible implies that you regularly engage different energy pathways, which, ultimately, help to optimize your metabolism's function all around.

When you're metabolically inflexible, however, you're stuck using just one energy pathway. This eventually turns out to be a massive disadvantage. It's inconvenient to be metabolically inflexible: "I can't wait another hour for dinner, I'm starving!" or "I can't have a piece of cake; that will make my blood sugar skyrocket, and I'll feel like shit!" Your eating habits are ruled by your dependence on that energy source, not allowing you to enjoy the benefits of alternate sources as needed.

When your metabolism has been stuck in that limiting state for long enough, cellular dysfunction ensues. **Some consequences of an inflexible metabolism include:**

- Screwed-up appetite and fullness cues

- Increased insulin resistance (decreased glucose tolerance)

- Accelerated mitochondrial dysfunction (think exhaustion, brain fog, weakened immunity, and Long COVID)

- Cognitive decline

- Increased oxidative stress and inflammation (advanced aging and disease processes)

A sugar burner's body (with a metabolism stuck in carb-dependent mode) is so burdened by chronic food intake and excessive carbs that their cells no longer use insulin effectively, blood sugar is chronically elevated, and the fat-burning genetic switch is stuck in the OFF position.

Good news is that changing your eating habits to become fat-adapted means you're more metabolically flexible, insulin sensitivity will be restored, and all those negative effects become old news for you!

"Once you achieve this state of metabolic flexibility, you're in an entirely new, empowered position in your life. You can go long periods of time without having to eat, and you get a handle on hunger, appetite, and cravings; it's an amazing skill that we're all born with. It's in all of our DNA to be able to extract this energy from different substrates. But, most people, for various reasons, spend their lives in a sugar-burning mode where they're constantly trying to stoke the fire and feed their cells energy by eating a high-carbohydrate diet, and they deny themselves the ability, energy, and life force, good mood and healthy metabolism, and a robust immune system and all the things that sort of make for an optimized life."

- Mark Sisson

Ironically, it's not just carb-dependent people who are metabolically inflexible. People who've been on a strict keto diet for a long period of time can become metabolically inflexible, too. They can suffer from something called *leptin resistance*, where the body and brain become ineffective at communicating whether or not the person is full and nutritionally satisfied. Leptin not only signals the brain to help regulate your appetite, but it also plays an important role in your ability to burn fat for energy.

In addition to the possibility of leptin resistance, people on a long-term, strict keto diet can suffer from reduced insulin sensitivity. It seems like a paradox because the keto diet initially improves insulin sensitivity. But, over time, when the body is forced to remain in a continuous state of ketosis for long enough, some individuals may find their glucose tolerance has decreased as a result of this reversed insulin sensitivity.

If and when such a keto dieter finally eats more carbs, their blood glucose spikes higher than normal, and it remains higher for longer because their cells aren't using insulin efficiently anymore. The glucose stays in the bloodstream, and the person feels like crap. There's more inflammation and unpleasant feelings like a rapid heart rate and even shaking.

And you can probably guess what happens to this person who is, to their own surprise, metabolically *in*flexible. They become fearful of carbohydrates. They adopt a disordered relationship with food and carbs because they misinterpret those signs as carbs being toxic and something to fear, whereas, in reality, they simply need to retrain their metabolism to become flexible again.

> *"Metabolic health is kind of a catch-all phrase that encompasses the ability of every cell in the body to function optimally with the amount of energy that it needs (or has access to).... Our ability to supply energy to the cells is critical to our lives—critical to the enjoyment of our lives, mobility, thought; all of these things come back to a central theme, which is access to the energy."*
> - Mark Sisson

How do you know when you're metabolically flexible?

Traits and objective measures of metabolic flexibility:

- Ability to go without food for ≥ 14 hours comfortably, without hunger, and with good energy.

- Ability to unexpectedly skip meals while maintaining energy and physical comfort.

- Feeling physically well after eating a reasonably-sized, higher-carb meal (e.g. > 60 g net carbs).

- Healthy (low normal) fasting glucose numbers (e.g. < 95 mg/dL).

- Healthy (low normal) fasting insulin numbers (e.g. < 8 uIU/mL).

- Healthy Hemoglobin A1c (HbA1c for short), a key metabolic health marker of inflammation that averages blood glucose scores across 2–3 months (e.g. < 5.5 percent).

- Triglycerides < 100 (triglycerides > 100 can be a sign the body is frequently storing glucose by converting it into triglycerides).

- Healthy normal oxidative stress markers, such as high-sensitivity c-reactive protein (hs-CRP) or total serum glutathione (tGSH), among many other lab markers that may be considered in an oxidative stress assessment. (Normal reference ranges are provided by the lab used for testing.)

How to improve metabolic flexibility

So far, I've introduced several concepts and action steps that help you gain metabolic flexibility. Intermittent fasting, carbohydrate reduction, and cyclical keto dieting aren't the only things that help you with fat adaptation and a flexible metabolism. All hormesis-promoting behaviors can increase metabolic flexibility and address energy utilization at your cellular core.

Hormesis. Now, there's a word you may not be familiar with. Hormesis describes a reactive state in the body triggered by a certain type of stressor that results in a beneficial adaptation. The type of stressors that induce hormesis (termed hormetic stressors) confront the body with just the right amount of stress to make it adapt in your favor.

Exercise is one of the most well-known, well-studied examples of hormetic stressor. You'll learn more about hormesis in upcoming chapters, but first, you'll want to learn about the most important players in the body's energy metabolism: your *mitochondria*.

Mitochondria make all the energy inside your cells. When these little buggers aren't functioning properly, your metabolism fights a losing battle. Some experts now theorize that all disease starts by first impairing the mitochondria. The function or dysfunction of your mitochondria may be at the root of metabolic inflexibility. You can support the health of your mitochondria in a big way by becoming more metabolically flexible and teaching your body to switch between fuels. This means that sometimes you run on body fat in the form of ketones, and sometimes you run on carbs or glucose.

"When your mitochondria are sick, they become less efficient at using glucose, often leaving you tired after a meal. Periodic switching into different fasted states creates ketones that will repair your mitochondria and make them more capable of using glucose to your benefit."
  - Dr. Mindy Pelz, *Fast Like a Girl*

Are you ready to start learning more about these fascinating little energy execs known as your mitochondria?

CHAPTER 21

Mitochondria: Energy You Can Feel

Inside most cells of your body live hundreds of these little organelles known as mitochondria. Your brain cells contain thousands of mitochondria per cell because the brain needs lots of energy! We have a quadrillion mitochondria in our bodies. That's 1,000,000,000,000,000 mitochondria energy factories that are responsible for 90 percent of the energy you need to survive!

Ready for this? Gram for gram, your mitochondria make over 10,000 times more energy than the sun—every second![20] Whoa, right?! Without some mitochondria functioning for even a few seconds, the cells (tissues, organs, or the human host) will die because all cellular functions depend on the mitochondria's ability to create energy.

The energy created in your mitochondria is known as ATP (adenosine triphosphate), which is the ultimate gas all of our cells use for fuel. Throughout this book, I've described carbohydrates or glucose as fuel and fat or ketones as fuel, and now I'm telling you ATP is the fuel? Here's why: your mitochondria use oxygen combined with the food you eat—nutrients, enzymes, and the building blocks from carbohydrates, proteins, and fats—to *make* ATP fuel, the only energy source that's ultimately used to fuel your body.

It's sort of mind-boggling to consider energy at its core, so let's spare ourselves the finer details of mitochondrial energy, ATP, and only discuss what we really need to understand.

Your mitochondria are responsible for metabolizing and utilizing the food you consume for energy that your cells can use for EVERYTHING inside your body. Mitochondria are energy factories or the powerhouses of the cells. But that's not all they are.

There's a major function besides energy production that's not (yet) as widely known. Your mitochondria are also threat detectors. Defenders. They detect threats to the health of your cells—sensing and fighting danger, inflammation, toxins, and disease. The mitochondria determine whether to use your energy to feed the immune system in defense of such threats or to make new ATP energy you can feel and thrive on.

Each time your mitochondria are busy cleaning up toxins and excessive inflammation or defending against immune system threats, they provide you with less of the metabolic energy you can actually feel. The mitochondria are vulnerable, and as a result, so are you. When your mitochondria are suffering, over time you become more and more exhausted. You get sick more often because your cells are facing continued, relentless threats. At this point, every effort you make to lose weight or have more energy feels like a losing battle.

Fatigue—whether physical or mental—is a hallmark sign of mitochondrial dysfunction, which, in turn, is a hallmark sign of metabolic inflexibility.

Mitochondrial Threats:

- Chronic stress

- Toxin exposure

- Poor sleep, including insufficient melatonin levels and circadian rhythm disruption

- Poor diet and inadequate nutrition

- Gut dysfunction or dysbiosis (an imbalanced state in the gut microbiome)

- Infections

So what happens when you're stuck in a metabolic rut, being carb-dependent, eating junk, or fighting chronic offenders often enough? Your mitochondria are taxed. They've been spending far too much time cleaning up your messes and defending against relentless threats that they're not only burned out, but many of them are dying off completely.

That right there is the reason you want to prioritize nutrition and nutrient-dense foods (as well as optimizing your sleep). There's no way around it. Everything depends on the health of your mitochondria. When you eat a diet that's carb-centric and highly processed, you wind up bombarding the mitochondria with too many free radicals and not enough protectors. The mitochondria begin to malfunction, die off, and struggle to create energy inside your cells to help you thrive. Disease eventually prevails.

"The food choices we make are of utmost importance. Mitochondria get overloaded and damaged by processed, refined foods, especially those with high carbohydrate (sugar) contents. That means foods like white bread, soda, sugars, and sweeteners are real mitochondria killers."
- Susanne Bennett, *Mighty Mito*

Guess what. Even if you've been a healthy eater for a long time, dozens of other factors may be compromising your mitochondrial health. Simply as a factor of aging, we all experience a decline in mitochondria function. By the age of forty, nearly everyone has what's described as early-onset mitochondrial dysfunction. Most people tend to lose 50 percent of their mitochondrial energy capacity between the ages of fifty and seventy. Yikes.

*"If you want to be healthy, strong, and sharp, then your cells have to
be healthy, and your cells won't be healthy unless your
mitochondria are healthy. That's how you start at the very root,
the very beginning of the dysfunction in your body.
That's how you turn your health around."*
- Dr. Terry Wahls, *The Wahls Protocol*

Dr. Wahls is a medical phenomenon who reversed her Multiple Sclerosis condition from a crippling state to one where her body is fully functioning by focusing on a nutrient-dense diet that feeds the mitochondria.

In her book *The Wahls Protocol*, Dr. Wahls lists the resources and nutrients your mitochondria need to produce the most energy and thrive:

- Glucose and ketones
- Oxygen
- B vitamins: thiamine (B1), riboflavin (B2), niacinamide (B3), pantothenic acid (B5), B12
- Minerals, especially: sulfur, zinc, magnesium, iron, manganese, and selenium
- Antioxidants like vitamin C, glutathione, and antioxidant compounds found in colorful fruits and vegetables
- L-carnitine
- Alpha-lipoic acid
- Creatine
- Ubiquinone or coenzyme Q10

And, of course, your mitochondria need to be protected from toxins, especially lead, mercury, and arsenic exposure.

This is a great segue into the theme of the following topic, nutrient density.

*"More than 250 different nutrients have been identified, and likely
there are thousands more that scientists have not yet identified that
are important to enjoying optimal health."*
- Dr. Terry Wahls, *The Wahls Protocol*

If you want an effective, enjoyable, long-term solution to turn your health around and improve your eating habits, then you *absolutely* want to prioritize the health of your mitochondria. And eat a nutrient-dense diet.

CHAPTER 22

What is Nutrient Density, and Why Should You Care?

The term *nutrient density* refers to how many vitamins, minerals, and other nutrients are present and how concentrated they are in a food per serving or per calorie. Nutrient-dense foods give you lots of vitamins, minerals, amino acids, and antioxidant protectors in relation to how many calories the food contains. Nutrient-poor foods, on the other hand, supply very few vitamins, minerals, and nutrients in relation to the caloric energy they contain.

We're not just talking about macronutrients here, or macros, for short. Macros are what everyone talks about regarding a diet or workout plan—like how many grams of carbs, protein, and fat to include in your diet. But macronutrients only consider those factors: the carbohydrates, proteins, and fats in your food. *Micro*-nutrients, on the other hand, include vitamins, minerals, antioxidants, and even the building blocks of proteins called amino acids, all of which are required for healthy cells, mitochondria, and metabolic health.

Now you're getting it.

When it comes to the science of food, nutrition is kind of mind-blowing. We hardly have a grasp on the many thousands of factors present in foods and how they all interplay in our diet. Which explains why supplements and fortified foods aren't likely to provide the same benefits as whole foods. To give you an idea of how mind-boggling nutrition can be, "more than 70,000 compounds in foods are bound together in a food matrix, which synergistically impacts metabolism and nutrient absorption, and may have beneficial effects on satiety and the immune system, offering protection from disease, among other potentially important health implications."[21]

Nutrient-dense foods not only offer you more nutrition per serving, but they also provide nutrition your body can actually absorb and utilize. That's a critical distinction described as nutrient availability. Let's say you eat 20 g of protein. Just because the food presents with 20 g of protein doesn't mean you'll actually absorb 20 g of protein your metabolism can work with. It depends on the protein's bioavailability and your bio-individual capacity. That's why I favor animal proteins, for instance, because not only are they packed with more nutrients per serving, but animal proteins offer superior *bioavailability* compared to plant proteins.

Bioavailability is also the reason I emphasize the importance of a healthy gut and digestive system because your gut health determines your ability to absorb nutrients. When adequately digested and absorbed, nutritional components from the food you eat will pass through the walls of your small intestine and into your bloodstream for your metabolism to work with.

In 2022, researchers from the Global Alliance for Improved Nutrition set out to determine which foods make up a nutrient-dense diet—with careful consideration regarding the top micronutrient deficiencies in the world and in the United States. The deficiencies they targeted were vitamin A, folate, vitamin B12, calcium, iron, and zinc. This study[22] was exceptional because they also considered how many of each nutrient was bioavailable in the foods they tested.

Let's compare what the researchers analyzed in a nutrient-rich food versus a nutrient-poor food.

Examples of nutrient-dense foods:

- **Bivalves** (oysters, scallops, clams, mussels, cockles)
- **Serving Size:** 3.5 oz
- **Overall Nutrient-Density Score (Per Gram):** very high with a score of 103 (The serving size in grams needed to provide 1/3 of the recommended nutrient intakes of vitamin A, folate, vitamin B12, calcium, iron, and zinc)
- **Iron:** very high
- **Zinc:** very high
- **Vitamin A:** very high
- **B12:** very high
- **Calcium:** very high
- **Folate:** moderate

If we use **mussels** as an example for this nutrient-dense food category, a 3.5-oz serving of cooked mussels provides the following macronutrients:

- **Total fat:** 2.2 g
- **Total carbs:** 3.6 g
- **Protein:** 11.8 g

Examples of nutrient-poor foods:

- **Whole Grains** (oats, barley, brown rice, farro, 100% whole wheat, rye, corn, etc.)
- **Serving size:** 950 g (approx. 5.2 cups of cooked farro)
- **Overall nutrient density score (per gram):** low with a score of 950 (the serving size in grams needed to provide 1/3 of the recom-

mended nutrient intakes of vitamin A, folate, vitamin B12, calcium, iron, and zinc)

- **Iron:** low

- **Zinc:** moderate

- **Vitamin A:** low

- **B12:** low

- **Calcium:** low

- **Folate:** low

Whole grains ranked low in overall nutrient density, which is the lowest category of ranking for this study. Whole grains contain 9.22 times fewer nutrients per gram consumed when compared to bivalves (one of the most nutrient-dense foods). Besides, eating a 5.2-cup serving as they measured would not only pale in comparison for essential nutrients but a serving that size yields over 220 g of net carbs!

Tips to include more nutrient-dense foods in your diet

Prioritizing nutrient-dense foods is much easier when you download my free PDF, *The Nutrient Dense Foods List*. To get your copy, scan the following QR code or visit *marisamoon.com/notsofast/resources*.

On the first page of this resource you'll see a master list of the most nutrient-dense superfoods. The next page offers some guidance regarding which foods are worth the splurge and how to eat more of those superfoods on a budget.

For starters, you'd be right to assume that foods in their whole food form, from a plant or an animal, are likely to be more nutrient-dense compared to most processed or packaged foods. Still, you'll be buying packaged foods, so it's important that you learn to recognize nutrient-poor foods. They sabotage your efforts to get healthy, so it's time to start reading those labels.

What are the ingredients in this food you want to buy? When you're at the grocery store, I challenge you to pick up a box of your favorite cereal or a can of soup your family enjoys. Look at the ingredient list; if needed, bring your reading glasses or look the ingredients up online—no excuses. *What is this food actually made of?*

Red flags in packaged foods:

What clues to look for on ingredient lists that suggest it's not a nutritious food:

- You don't recognize one or more of the first five ingredients? Put it back (exceptions include exotic ingredients that are unfamiliar to you).

- You can't buy those first five ingredients if you want to make it yourself? Consider putting it back.

- In liquids, sauces, and dressings: is one of those first five ingredients a vegetable seed oil? Put it back (check out Primal Kitchen sauces and dressings instead).

- With solid foods, is one of those first five ingredients safflower oil, cottonseed oil, unspecified vegetable oil, or a blend of two to three oils separated by a hyphen (such as canola-safflower-sunflower oil)? Consider putting it back.

- Is the first ingredient any type of flour, starch, or wheat? It's probably *not* a nutritious food (or it's likely to stimulate overeating).

- Does it contain artificial flavors, artificial colors, or FD&C food dyes such as Red #40, Blue #1, etc.? Put it back.

- This red flag is especially critical to avoid for children, adolescents, and people with ADHD or those showing signs of or with a condition of neuro-degeneration

- Does it contain chemical preservatives such as sodium and potassium nitrates or sodium and potassium nitrites, propylparaben, BHA, or BHT? Such artificial preservatives are best avoided whenever possible because they may be cancerous, and the chemicals kill off healthy bacteria in your mouth and in your gut (worsening digestive health, dental health, immunity, and mental health)

- If it's made with > 20 ingredients, it's probably not a nutritious food.

Be curious. Google those ingredients to see what the heck you're thinking of feeding your body or your family. No one is looking out for us, so it's time we look out for ourselves and become more informed consumers.

You're busy. I know. You like shortcuts. You need shortcuts. And the food manufacturers know that. They've trained you to expect shortcuts and to seek them out. While grocery shopping, how much time do you spend inside those aisles with packaged foods instead of buying food from the produce section and the meat or seafood counters? How much of your food is actually fresh, still bursting with nutrients?

It's been reported that nearly 80 percent of the food found in grocery stores today didn't exist a hundred years ago. Our food supply has changed drastically, no doubt. No one can argue that we've messed with Mother Nature, and she's not happy about it. We now genetically modify plants, literally changing the genetic makeup of the living organism. We've demolished the precious ecosystem in our soil because of synthetic chemicals and aggressive farming methods relied upon in industrial agriculture. We raise animal livestock in crowded living conditions, pumping them with pharmaceuticals, oftentimes depriving them of sunlight, and feeding them unnatural processed diets full of toxins.

Plants will grow without chemicals when we follow nature's time-tested strategies. Cows were meant to graze on and eat grass—not bioengineered corn and soy pellets. Chickens thrive in the outdoors, pecking at bugs and seedlings and following herds of cattle as they migrate. Fish were caught wild in the sea, eating a natural diet that's integral to the cycle of all life on Earth.

It was only a century ago when virtually all fruits and vegetables were organic. All beef was grass-fed. All chickens were raised outdoors and free of antibiotics. All fish were wild-caught and less contaminated by man's pollution and chemicals. Now, these nutritious, natural versions of food are the exception. Depending on where you live and the resources you have, it can be difficult to access foods raised in these traditional, healthy ways—and that's another massive societal issue in itself.

Good news is that some of the most nutrient-dense foods we still have access to are those that can save you money. Our ancient ancestors ate the most nutrient-dense parts of animals, like the liver, heart, and bone marrow, as well as everything else, nose to tail. Today? We're wussies. We only eat bone-less skinless chicken breast and perfectly fileted skinless fish, both of which Americans eat in deep-fried form, more often than not. This is yet another reason animal protein gets a bad rap in observational human studies.

Get more nutrient bang for your buck when you seek out organ meats, bones, feet, necks, and whole bone-in chicken so you can save money, and learn to make homemade slow-cooked soups and bone broths that will deeply nourish your family.

Food is *not* anything that's technically edible and referred to as safe (the stuff food marketers encourage us to consume every day). Just because something is edible doesn't mean it should be eaten. Real food is food that nature provides, and humans can make or acquire it with their hands and a few tools—no factory equipment required. Real food is something that's been around for more than a hundred years—and, ideally, for thousands of years!

"If the United States were to receive a report card rating the quality of the Standard American Diet (SAD), it would get a solid 'F' for nutrient density. Despite being high in calories, the Standard American Diet is nutrient-poor. Vegetable oils and sugar, which together comprise 36 percent of the SAD diet, are virtually devoid of nutrients."

- Chris Kresser, M.S., Co-Founder and Co-Director of the California Center for Functional Medicine

Our obsession with flour-based foods must be turned around. Most Americans eat sandwiches, corn masa, fried foods, pizza, or pasta at every meal. These foods are alarmingly low in nutrients combined with too many useless calories. They provide little satisfaction for the metabolism, which leads to overeating, obesity, diabetes, and chronic disease. It's imperative we start eating a diet that's more like a primal human diet, one that's long-preceded the mass production of foodstuff like we see today.

Maybe you're hip to the idea that your diet needs to be nutritious, but you still don't feel motivated enough to make a consistent change. You want more compelling reasons that are meaningful to you. This is a good time to discuss the massive improvement you'll experience with your appetite and hunger when you eat more nutrient-dense foods. These foods satisfy our instinctual urges to eat more, more, more, and they help pave the way to food freedom.

CHAPTER 23

Regulating Hunger With Nutrient-Dense Foods

I know in my heart and in my nutrition-obsessed brain that health starts with real food. I found my way here in 2012 because my digestion was all screwed up. I had embarrassing gas and unpredictable bowel movements that slashed my self-confidence and, at the ripe young age of twenty-nine, concerned me about my long-term health. Deal with that long enough, and you start searching for answers. That's when I found my way to the Paleo Diet. Little did I know it would be fairly simple to resolve my gastrointestinal issues and my lifelong issue of eating-and-eating until I was so full I could hardly breathe.

For as long as I can remember, I ate until I physically couldn't jam any more food inside my belly. My family and friends thought it was cute. Here's this little girl who will eat anything and everything you put in front of her—besides peas (for whatever reason, as a kid, I hated peas). This little girl would eat off of your plate, too! "Are you done with that?" I'd ask. And down it would go. Like a human garbage disposal.

We even used to say my Dad and I were like human garbage disposals. "No food goes to waste over here!" Well, as you can imagine, that was not a healthy relationship to have with food—eating everything within my reach. Lucky for me, it didn't turn into an eating disorder like binge eating, in which a large volume of food is consumed in an unusually short period of time. I didn't even realize it was a problem until I found The Paleo Diet, which, for the first time in my life, helped put my voracious appetite to rest.

Good Lord! I thought to myself. *This is what it feels like to have control around food? This is what it's like to be satisfied after a meal? To be full and to actually choose to stop eating? It's possible for me to go 2 hours without thinking about food or reaching into my purse for a snack?* Finally, I could stop eating before I reached that sickening level of fullness. The more I focused my diet on whole foods, healthy fats, animal protein, lots of veggies, and low-sugar foods, the more I was in control of my appetite. I felt more satisfied by food. I was convinced. There was no turning back. I knew this dietary shift would give me life, and I decided to live this way forever.

There's an almost immediate reward for eating more nutrient-dense foods and increasing the micronutrients in your diet. A nourishing, real-food diet is the key to minimizing cravings and controlling your appetite. When combined with carbohydrate reduction and intermittent fasting, you can eliminate excessive hunger and live in better harmony with food.

That was the ultimate reward for me. Those positive effects helped me stay determined to stick with a low-sugar and lower-carb diet—even though, just like everyone else, I was obsessed with bread, pasta, pizza, McNuggets, french fries, energy drinks, breakfast cereal, Sour Patch Kids, and fancy caramel coffee creations from Starbucks. I wanted to be free from the grips of my never-ending appetite, and finally, I was.

By prioritizing nutrition, you can finally get ahold of your cravings and appetite and stop depending so much on willpower. The brain's appetite system makes you hungry when it senses your body needs more nutrients.

Appetite ends when the deficiencies have been relieved and your brain and body are satisfied.

Eat a bunch of empty calories like simple carbs or sugary treats, and you inevitably eat too much while simultaneously missing out on nutrition. Experts describe a population like ours as a nation of people who are 'overfed and undernourished'. We eat and eat and eat (or at the very least, we think about eating all day long), yet still, we're deficient in nutrients—which perpetuates the cycle in which the brain tells us to find more food!

> *"If the food you're eating is ultra-processed, low in protein, but high in calories and carbohydrates, the brain will tell you to continue eating that food until you reach your protein minimum."*
> - Diana Rodgers and Robb Wolf, *Sacred Cow*

Here's a fascinating finding from a 2010 study[23] that evaluated the effects nutrient-dense foods have on perceived hunger. With a nutrient-dense diet compared to their typical diet, 80 percent of participants (768 in total) reported major differences in their physical and emotional health and hunger. 51 percent of participants reported a *dramatic or complete change in their experience of hunger* when eating the nutrient-dense diet.

Take a look at the graph in Figure 23.1. The lines represent the percentage of participants who experienced hunger pains at different frequencies (*very rarely, occasionally, often, very often, and constantly*). Notice the two tallest bars colored in light gray on the left end of the graph. Those bars indicate a high percentage of people who, on the nutrient-dense diet, experienced *very rare* hunger (50 percent) or *occasional* hunger (approximately 40 percent). Then, notice the last 3 darkly colored bars on the right side, which indicate a high percentage of people who, on their standard diet, experienced hunger *often* (30 percent), *very often* (approximately 40 percent), or even *constantly* (10 percent).

Figure 23.1 Changing Perceptions of Hunger on a High Nutrient Density Diet

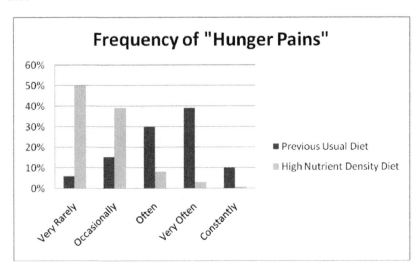

Fuhrman, J., Sarter, B., Glaser, D. et al. Changing perceptions of hunger on a high nutrient density diet. Nutr J 9, 51 (2010)[24]

Researchers concluded that on a nutrient-dense diet, hunger was well tolerated, was *not* an unpleasant experience, and occurred less frequently even when meals were skipped. How friggin' great does that sound? A diet that's high in micronutrients reduces hunger and makes it *significantly less frequent.* And, when you do feel hungry, you easily tolerate it?

The researchers also noted an adjustment period when participants first switched to a nutrient-dense diet since some individuals experienced withdrawal (literally!) from their former, pro-inflammatory diet. But once they'd adjusted to eating them, they were more likely to experience a sustainable eating pattern, prioritizing nutrient-dense foods that lead to weight loss and provide benefits for long-term health.

How Highly-Processed Foods Impair Health and Satiety

Sometimes, the damage from a junk-food diet is irreparable. Consider the case of a thirteen-year-old boy who permanently lost his eyesight after years of eating a junk-food-only diet. The cause of his sudden blindness was determined to be numerous nutrient deficiencies, and tragically, even when they restored his nutrient status, his eyesight never returned (a case reported in the Annals of Internal Medicine).[25]

So, next time you're tempted to fill up on some ultra-processed food because you have a taste for it, I suggest you reconsider. The more crave-worthy you find a food, the less likely it will satisfy your body. Furthermore, after eating highly palatable foods (an industry term for processed foods that send unnaturally high reward signals to the brain), you're prone to overeating when the next opportunity comes along.

Depending on the person, a crave-worthy food could be highly processed, like those irresistible Ritz crackers, or it could be high in fat, carbs, and chemicals, like a crispy chicken sandwich from Chick-fil-A. It can even be something seemingly healthy, like nut butter. Although nut butters can be a nutritious food, the smooth, unnatural richness of the pureed nuts makes it so rewarding to the brain that it often leads to overeating, overconsumption, and reduced food satisfaction for the remainder of the day.

Since we're talking about satiety—satisfaction regarding appetite and fullness—we should chat real quick about the oils used in cooking and food manufacturing. One of the things I'll urge you to avoid is a class of cooking oils known as vegetable oils, or more appropriately described as industrial seed oils. We'll get into details in the upcoming chapter about healthy fats vs. harmful fats. It's important to mention this here because it turns out these highly processed oils and fats have a direct effect on your hunger and appetite.

When you consume healthy fats like extra virgin olive oil or avocado oil (monounsaturated fats) and clean saturated fats like coconut oil or butter, your brain receives a signal that it's satisfied. You're less likely to be hungry or allured by more food. This satiating effect isn't achieved when you consume industrial seed oils (polyunsaturated fats). When you consume inflammatory vegetable oils, like canola oil and soybean oil, your brain doesn't get the signal that you're satisfied. This leads to overeating and a false sense of hunger that derails efforts to obtain or maintain a healthy weight. Cook with quality extra virgin olive oil and avocado oil, natural saturated fats like butter, ghee, and coconut oil, and clean animal fats like organic lard and tallow. Like I said, more on this later.

Let's get back to what I said earlier. The brain's appetite system makes us hungry when it senses the body needs more nutrients. If nutrient deficiencies are the primary driver behind our appetite, then a good strategy would be to optimize nutrition in our diet and lifestyle.

When we look at the US population, we see that about 80 percent doesn't consume enough vegetables. And contrary to public health claims, the average American eats only 5–8 oz of animal protein per day. Most American adults are alarmingly low in vitamin D, especially people who live far from the equator or have naturally dark skin. Americans are also too low in omega-3s, magnesium, calcium, dietary fiber (particularly insoluble fiber naturally found in whole plant foods), vitamins A, C, E, and K, and zinc, copper, selenium, and choline. It's quite common for Americans also to be deficient in iron, B12 (especially plant-based and vegan dieters), and rare amino acids like tryptophan, methionine, choline, and glycine, all of which are best acquired from consuming animal proteins.

One thing that can greatly improve the nutrient density of one's diet is to increase the intake of animal proteins.

"According to the protein-leverage hypothesis, people will continue to eat food in order to satisfy their protein needs…protein is the most

satiating of the macronutrients (carbohydrates, fat, and protein),
and intake of 15–30 percent of total calories can be quite helpful in
regulating appetite by increasing leptin sensitivity (signaling to your
brain that you're satisfied), and inducing weight loss
and blood sugar control."
- Diana Rodgers and Robb Wolf, *Sacred Cow*

If you're eating two meals a day and aim to get around 20 percent of your calories from protein as recommended, then you're eating about 6–9 oz of leaner meats (including red meat), poultry, or seafood per meal. In upcoming chapters, you'll see sample portions of protein intake and how to put them all together for a meal.

Circling back to our conversation about appetite, what I find fascinating is that we see positive hormonal responses when we eat real food. Hormones, remember, aren't just sex hormones or stress hormones. We also have appetite hormones and so much more.

Let's review the various hormonal responses that influence your appetite and energy after eating. When blood sugar levels go up in response to a meal, the hormone insulin is released. It remains elevated for as long as your blood sugar is elevated. Following a sharp spike in blood sugar, which occurs when you consume processed carbs or sugar, there's a dramatic drop in blood sugar to follow. Those glucose swings create false feelings of hunger and wildly fluctuating energy levels and moods. Over time, this creates more ghrelin signals, a food-attraction hormone that makes you sense the need for *more, more, more.* Not only do ghrelin levels go up, but leptin, your satiety hormone, starts working less and less efficiently, leaving your hunger-fullness cues all messed up.

As you can imagine now with this information, hormones can actually trump your willpower, leaving you a victim to endless snacking and cravings while never really feeling satisfied. Have you ever finished a whole bag of pretzels or chips and found yourself searching for something else thirty minutes later?

Many people try to eat less—smaller portions or fewer calories—but eating too much less than what you need long-term can alter those two key metabolic hormones, ghrelin and leptin. Studies have shown that chronic caloric restriction leads to higher levels of ghrelin (the hormone that stimulates hunger) and lower levels of leptin (the hormone that suppresses hunger and boosts fat burning). So, eating fewer calories means feeling hungrier and burning less fat? That doesn't sound too great, does it?

The best diet is the one where you take frequent breaks from eating and aim to optimize protein intake when you do eat, mostly choosing *real foods*—and a variety of them! It's incredible how much the nutrient content in your diet impacts your appetite, your body weight, and your long-term health.

CHAPTER 24

Bioavailability and Food Stressors

By now, you've gotten the idea that our modern food system is messed up. Food companies are packaging together ingredients into things they call food, but it's really just a science experiment on the human population. I know nutrition talk can sometimes be nerdy, especially when we're talking about vitamins and minerals and science and all that. In this chapter and a few to follow, I'm arming you with the real goods. The actual food lists you want to see. I'm giving you actionable advice and helping you sift through the nonsense out there.

One of the core values in my business as a health coach is to *help put an end to the confusion about what's healthy*. Basically, healthy foods are ancestral foods. Healthy foods are whole foods and foods that can be found in the wild, accessible in quantities or frequency at which we consume them. Whenever I get confused about conflicting nutrition claims floating around out there, I remind myself about ancestral health. It's like home base for me.

Ancestral health provides the answer to nearly every modern-day food question.

Is this new plant-based protein healthy?

Is whole-grain brown rice healthy?

Is almond flour healthy?

Are these keto cookies healthy?

Turning to ancestral health principles, I find answers to such curiosities by asking myself these two questions:

Q1. *Would it be recognized as food two hundred years ago?*

Q2. *Could I reasonably grow, harvest, and make it myself to consume the amount I want to consume now?*

If the answers to Q1 and/or Q2 are "No," then I would not describe this food as healthy to consume on a regular basis.

If the answers to *both* Q1 and Q2 are "Yes," then ask this final question:

Q3. *Does my body agree with it?*

Let's try it out together on the first two items:

Is this new plant-based protein powder healthy?

Q1: *Would it be recognized as food two hundred years ago?* **Nope.**

Q2: *Could I reasonably grow, harvest, and make this plant protein powder myself to consume the amount I want to consume now?* **Nope.**

Q3: Not applicable.

Is whole-grain brown rice healthy?

Q1: *Would it be recognized as food two hundred years ago?* **Yup.**

Q2: *Could I reasonably grow, harvest, and make this brown rice myself to consume the amount I want to consume now?* **Maybe, but probably**

not. We'd need enough farmland that's fit to grow rice, and the whole family would need to help fertilize, protect, harvest, dry, and hull the rice. Even then, it would only be available a couple times a year if our climate would allow, and even then, we wouldn't have enough for each family member to eat some every day. It would be near impossible to grow enough for your family to eat regularly. That's why slaves, low-income laborers, massive industrial farms, and now machines are used to grow and supply rice around the world).

Q3: *Does my body agree with brown rice?* **That depends.** How's your digestive health? Do you have an autoimmune disease that's worsened when you eat certain foods? How are your fasting blood glucose and insulin levels? Whole grains can be quite aggressive to the digestive system; they can trigger a leaky gut and alarm the immune system, and they can elevate blood glucose and insulin for too long—depending on the individual, of course. Furthermore, are you able to moderate your consumption of rice, portion-controlling a serving so that you don't mindlessly eat the 100+ grams of carbs served with your Chinese takeout? A serving that exceeds 50 g of carbohydrates in one sitting will surely hinder weight loss and other metabolic health goals.

Now you're getting it! Try it for yourself, asking questions 1–3 to determine if almond flour or certain keto cookies are healthy to consume on a regular basis, and see what you come up with.

Bioavailable Nutrients

The last question, "Does my body agree with this food?" leads us to consider bioavailability, a term I introduced a few chapters back. There's a saying in the nutrition world to help us grasp the relevance we must consider: "It's not about how many nutrients are in a food; it's about how many nutrients you can absorb."

A majority of the time, the quantity of nutrients we absorb is lower than the nutrients in the food, and it varies greatly depending on an individual's state of digestive health, their DNA and gene expression, the way the food is prepared, the presence of other nutrients, and more!

A good example of how bioavailability affects our nutrient intake is that there are 115 mg of calcium in a serving of spinach, but we only absorb around 6 mg of calcium when we eat it. This means you'd have to consume 16 cups of spinach to get the same amount of calcium you get from drinking a glass of milk. I'm not telling you to go drink milk, but I am telling you that this is a massive discrepancy that shows up often in the claims made by vegan, plant-based communities and other popular nutrition resources.

One more example of bioavailability and flawed nutrition advice is that whole grains are high in vitamins and minerals. While whole grains do contain a variety of nutrients, a majority of those nutrients aren't accessible through human digestion. Whole grains and legumes, for example, contain a compound known as phytates, or phytic acid, which binds to calcium, iron, and zinc, making those nutrients less available through digestion. That means that even though the vitamins are present in the food, we cannot access most of those nutrients. That's why I always say, if you're going to consume grains and legumes, they should be soaked the old-fashioned way, sprouted, or, better yet, fermented, like authentic sourdough bread. Those preparations help to reduce phytic acid, ease the digestive process, and unlock more nutrients in the food.

Even without considering bioavailability, all categories of meat and fish, vegetables, fruit, nuts, and dairy are proven to be more nutrient-dense than whole grains. Meat and fish, veggies, and fruit are even more nutrient-dense than beans and lentils when bioavailability is factored in.

Now you can be aware of standard nutrient-density scales that don't factor in bioavailability. Foods like grains, legumes, and even nuts and seeds would rank much lower in nutrition compared to foods with highly absorbable nutrients, like animal proteins and full-fat cultured dairy. The difference is even more drastic when we consider how many nutrients are present in a typical serving size rather than how many nutrients are present per calorie, which is the standard method for measuring nutrient density.

Back in Chapter 22: *What is Nutrient Density?* I shared with you a list of the most nutrient-dense foods. If you pull out that list, you'll notice that plant and animal foods are on there because, together, they make for the most nutrient-dense diet! Animals and plants each contain different nutrients that we require for robust health. I love the way it's explained here:

> *"It's not a competition between these two kingdoms, where one is 'better' or 'worse' than the other; both plants and animals play a distinct but equally valuable role! The fact is there are nutrients we can only get from plants and nutrients we can only get from animal foods. We need both to get the full complement of nutrients that our bodies need to be healthy. Instead of fighting about whether bacon rules and vegetables suck (or vice versa), we should be celebrating the fact that the plant and animal kingdoms are both totally awesome and necessary for health!"*
> - Dr. Sarah Ballantyne

I want you to be eating a wide variety of superfoods packed with available nutrition.

What are *superfoods* really? I'll tell you!

They're the best possible plants and the best possible animal foods available to us. I call them superfoods because they contain a high number of available nutrients per serving. Nutrient-dense superfoods are typically whole foods. They're either unprocessed or they're minimally processed to maximize bioavailability (like the process of fermenting milk to make yogurt or soaking lentils to reduce phytates and enhance digestibility). Typically, nutrient-dense foods are sourced fresh or frozen, locally, in season, and grown sustainably or in the wild to help minimize toxins and maximize nutrients. Ideally, seeds are ancient or heirloom varieties, and milk or animal products are from a heritage breed, wild, or rotationally-grazed animal. Note that the criteria I've shared describe what is *ideal*, not what is necessary. By using my *Nutrient-Dense Foods List* in Chapter 22, you'll have plenty of ideas for eating more nutritious foods on a budget.

But wait. There's more. Another reason to start incorporating nutrient-dense foods into your life is because nutrient-poor foods tend to be stressful on the body. **Three of the biggest food stressors include:**

1. Foods that your body doesn't agree with.

2. Refined sugar (especially high-fructose corn syrup, candy, and any drink made with added sugar ≥ 10 g per serving consumed)

3. Toxic seed oils and trans fats (especially the partially-hydrogenated fats found in processed foods, Crisco/shortening, and margarine, as well as safflower, sunflower, rapeseed, and cottonseed oils, and other polyunsaturated oils like canola, soybean, grape seed, peanut, and corn)

When it comes to food toxins that stress your body, affecting your appetite, gut health, and susceptibility to disease, those aren't the only culprits. **Here's a more expansive list of dietary toxins that stress out your system:**

- Fast-food meals

- Fried foods

- Hard-seared, blackened, charred, or fried animal proteins (including seafood)

- Alcohol

- Fluoridated water

- Trans fats, margarine, and partially hydrogenated oils

- Dried milk powder and powdered creamers

- Heated vegetable oils (AKA industrial seed oils, seed oils, or poly-unsaturated fatty acids—PUFAs), including canola oil, rapeseed oil, soybean oil, safflower oil, cottonseed oil, peanut oil, corn oil, grape seed oil, and sunflower oil

- Artificial sweeteners, esp. aspartame, diet coke, sucralose, and sugar-free energy drinks

- Refined sugars, sugary drinks, and desserts

- Monosodium glutamate (MSG) and cured meats with added nitrates

- FD&C food dyes, especially Red no. 40 or Red 40 Lake (which is currently banned in Denmark, Belgium, France, Germany, Switzerland, Sweden, Austria, and Norway, and for which the European Union requires a warning label on all relevant products that it *may have an adverse effect on activity and attention in children*)

- Modern-day wheat and gluten

- Refined carbohydrates (like every white bread and pasta you eat)

- Excessive carbohydrate intake (exceeding 150 g of net carbs per day)

- Corn, soy, wheat, and grains, especially when consumed in excess without fermentation, and when plants are farmed with glyphosate weed-killer, or when seeds are genetically modified to contain Bt-toxins (toxic byproducts from *Bacillus thuringiensis* bacteria which has insecticidal action that, in some forms, may enter the human bloodstream and cause harm)

This list hints as to why, no matter which whole foods diet you try—like the Mediterranean Diet, low carb, paleo, primal, Whole30, and plant-based—you feel dramatically better *at first*. When you finally cut out all the crap from our food system and start eating more nutrient-dense foods, you've reduced your toxin load dramatically. Unless you fall for a lazy version of those diets—like dirty keto, highly-processed vegan or lazy plant-based diet, or low-protein high-starch Mediterranean Diet—your body will initially thrive. Before the switch, your body was starving for nutrients, and all the dietary toxins were running you down!

In the next chapter, I'll get specific about how to build your plate to eat a more nutrient-dense diet. If the topic of ancestral nutrition intrigues you, and you want to dive into greater depths, I recommend *The Primal Blueprint*, the ground-breaking book that inspired my education as a Primal Health Coach. Despite being a massive 576 pages long, that book has helped millions of people to live and eat more aligned with the requirements of our human DNA and increase their health span as a result. The author, Mark Sisson, has also published thousands of free articles on his wildly popular blog at *marksdailyapple.com*.

Take home message:

Consume real, whole, unprocessed, anti-inflammatory, NUTRIENT DENSE superfoods with plenty of variety. You'll gain control over cravings, rev up your metabolism, ward off disease, improve your energy, and allow your body to be the fat-burning machine it was designed to be.

Meals = Protein + Veggies + Healthy Fats

This chapter is all about simplifying the guidelines for a nutrient-dense diet. I'm answering that burning question, "When I eat this way, what does a typical meal look like?"

Ideal Meals = Complete **Protein** + **Veggies** + Healthy **Fats**

Compare that equation to the way you've probably been eating for most of your life, like:

Meal = Whatever requires the least effort

OR

Meal = Whatever I'm craving

OR

Meal = Whatever my family is eating

OR

Meal = Rice or pasta comprising 50–100 percent of the meal

OR

Meal = A sandwich made with the most highly processed forms of bread + deli meat + cheese + mayo with a side of chips or fries that are laced with toxic seed oils

When you eat the nutrient-dense way, your meals are inspired by *ancestral health*. You eat a more traditional human diet—the way humans ate before industrialized foods. A nutrient-dense plate looks something like the following diagram in Figure 25.1:

The Traditional Human Diet Plate

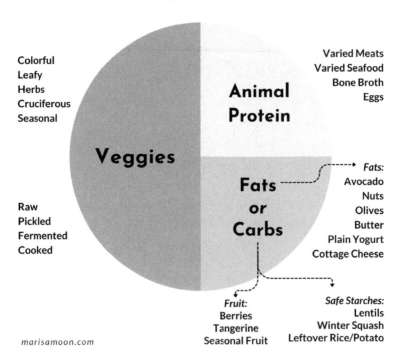

This suggests you aim for 50 percent of your plate's surface to be filled with vegetables. Vegetables (including herbs) can be any combination of cooked, raw, pickled, and/or fermented. More on veggies in a minute.

Animal proteins should comprise 25 percent or more of the surface area on your plate. This can range anywhere from 4 oz of a high-protein cut of meat, like chicken breast or pork tenderloin, or 4 boiled eggs, or a larger 8-oz serving of fattier meats like a grass-fed burger or shredded pork shoulder (skipping the sugar-laden BBQ sauce).

Depending on your goals and personal needs, the rest of your plate may or may not contain starchy carbohydrates, fresh fruit, or satiating high-fat foods to enhance the meal and your eating experience.

At first, this might be way more veggies and animal protein than you're used to eating. Although veggies can require the most effort to prep or include at every meal, protein can be the most confusing and the most important piece to get right. This is why two upcoming chapters are dedicated entirely to protein.

Let's talk veggies.

Most Americans don't eat nearly enough veggies or powerful plant foods like fresh herbs, spices, and seaweed or algae. Furthermore, Americans tend to rotate between the same ten veggies for most of their adult life. According to our nation's 2021 statistics, those oh-so-common veggies are:

1. Potatoes
2. Tomatoes (actually a fruit, but let's call it a veggie)
3. Onions
4. Carrots
5. Bell Peppers
6. Broccoli
7. Cucumbers
8. Salad mix & lettuce
9. Celery
10. Mushrooms

The funny thing is that if I listed beyond the top ten 'vegetables' in the U.S., number eleven would be corn. But corn isn't a vegetable! It's a grain! It's the seed of a grass—which is the definition of a grain. It doesn't count as a veggie. Sorry. Corn is challenging for the human body to digest, like other grains, which is why you might see whole corn kernels in your poop. And that's why traditional societies have strategically soaked, nixtamalized, or fermented cornmeal (to make masa, for example) so the corn can be adequately digested, also making some nutrients more accessible.

If you want to improve your health on every level, you'll need to eat more vegetables (including herbs and seaweed/algae), and eat a wider *variety*. The exception is the Carnivore Diet, a restrictive therapeutic diet that excludes all or most plant foods as an alternative approach to heal an inflamed gut, improve immunity, muscle mass, and more.

Back to that top ten list of the most consumed veggies in America. Let's consider removing potatoes from the list. Unlike most other vegetables, potatoes are comprised of mostly starch, which, unfortunately, makes them less nutritious and more likely to result in weight gain. Potatoes can lead to overeating and insulin resistance. It's best to limit them, especially mashed or fried, while you strive to improve your health.

One significant exception is to consume leftover boiled or roasted potatoes (not mashed) that have been cooled before eating or reheating. This process of cooling cooked potatoes changes the starches into something like fiber that's more resistant to digestion. This means less of it winds up as glucose in your bloodstream. That's why leftover potatoes and leftover rice are recognized as resistant starch. I realize this may be confusing to you, but just know that eating those starchy foods as leftovers—cooled in the fridge or freezer and then reheated or eaten cold, like potato salad—greatly reduces the carbohydrate load and glycemic impact on your body. The food becomes less inflammatory and perhaps more satisfying—but that doesn't necessarily make it nutrient-dense.

So, let's get back to the veggies that are quite nutritious.

40 Lower-carb vegetables to include in your meal rotation:

1. Asparagus (green, purple)

2. Avocado (technically a fruit, but let's say veggie)

3. Artichokes (including artichoke hearts)

4. Arugula

5. Bamboo shoots

6. Bell peppers (red, orange, yellow, green; and baby bell peppers)

7. Beets (yellow or red) (no sugar added)

8. Bok choy or baby bok choy (an Asian cabbage)

9. Broccoli (and broccoli rabe/rapini, broccolini, etc.)

10. Brussels sprouts

11. Butternut squash (no sugar added)

12. Cabbage (red, green, savoy, napa; includes kimchi, kraut, and *living* sauerkraut)

13. Carrots (purple, red, orange, yellow, and parsnips) (no sugar added)

14. Cauliflower (white, yellow, purple, and romanesco)

15. Celery and celery root (celeriac)

16. Cilantro, fresh (AKA fresh coriander)

17. Collard greens

18. Chard - Swiss chard or rainbow chard

19. Cucumber (includes pickles with no sugar added)

20. Chives (fresh), green onions (scallions), shallots, onions (any, not dried)

21. Eggplant

22. Endive (includes curly endive/frisee, Belgian endive, escarole)

23. Fennel bulb (raw or cooked)

24. Garlic (fresh or frozen, not dried or jarred in liquid)

25. Green beans (any variety, not including peas)

26. Hearts of palm

27. Jicama

28. Kale (red/purple, green, curly, dino/lacinato, and baby kale)

29. Kelp, kombu, seaweed, and algae

30. Lettuces (leaf lettuce, romaine, mesclun, baby greens, etc.)

31. (Other) leafy greens like dandelion greens, beet greens, turnip greens, mustard greens

32. Mushrooms (any! button, crimini, shiitake, portabello, enoki, trumpet, maitake, medicinal mushrooms, etc., fresh or dried)

33. Peppers (jalapeno, serrano, banana, Anaheim, poblano, Thai chilies, etc.)

34. Radishes (red, watermelon, daikon, etc.)

35. Spaghetti squash and other winter squashes

36. Spinach or baby spinach (cooked or raw)

37. Sprouts (any green sprouts or microgreens like pea shoots, radish sprouts, arugula sprouts, broccoli sprouts, watercress, etc.)

38. Tomatoes (includes salsa and tomato sauce)

39. Turnips

40. Zucchini/summer squash (yellow, green, Mexican)

Clients who succeed at making their meals = animal protein + veggies + healthy fats tend to eat a veggie and protein-rich salad for lunch and a protein-packed dinner like a stir-fry or salmon with roasted veggies. Some nights, they'll include a small portion of starchy carbs to add variety and make it easier for family dinners. The key is to learn which exceptions work for you in moderation and which indulgences are *worth it*.

Salads for lunch are a great way to consume a wide variety of raw, pickled, or cooked vegetables and save time by using leftover protein (or canned/cured seafood). Then, for dinner, cooked vegetables allow for even more variety and easier digestion before bedtime approaches. For convenience during the work week, consider visiting a salad bar somewhere—like Sweet Greens or a grocery store like Whole Foods Market—where you can craft a nutrient-dense meal in a flash and pour on some olive oil and vinegar to make your own healthy dressing. Additionally, the organic meal kit service, Green Chef, offers 10-minute lunch kits and pre-prepped salad kits for quick and healthy options made at home.

Worried about bloating from eating more veggies? Experiment, little by little, and be curious. Your gut may need time to adapt to changes in your diet. Start slow with raw veggies. Take note of which foods seem to bloat you more (onions are a common culprit!), and remove them for a couple weeks. Soon, you'll be ready to increase raw veggies and reintroduce the ones you've removed. Start with small servings. *It's the dose that makes the poison*, after all. The tricks to adapting your body to this healthier lifestyle include having patience, a curious mindset, and making gradual changes. *Not so fast*, remember?

A sample day of eating:

- Meal 1) Lunch Salad
  - Mixed greens, tomato wedges, diced avocado, scallions, and thinly sliced green cabbage. Top with warm, shredded rotisserie chicken and optional goat cheese crumbles.
  - Finish salad with easy, homemade Italian vinaigrette (fresh garlic, red wine vinegar, extra virgin olive oil, salt, pepper, and dried oregano).
- Afternoon Snack (optional)
  - Yogurt bowl made with organic plain Greek yogurt, sweeten to taste with stevia, and top with 1 serving of Paleo granola and a handful of berries.
- Meal 2) Dinner Stir Fry
  - Saute broccoli florets, shiitake mushrooms, and fresh garlic and ginger. Add thinly sliced sirloin steak strips, season everything with salt and pepper, then mix in homemade stir fry sauce:

organic tamari (soy sauce), rice vinegar, optional Asian hot sauce, and sesame oil. Finish with green onions and fresh basil or cilantro .

- Enjoy with your choice of leftover rice, cauliflower rice, or thinly shredded green cabbage. Bonus points: add a scoop of fermented food, like kimchi.

- Nutrient-Dense Treat:

  - 1 Cutie clementine (mini tangerine) or 1 serving of seasonal fruit.

CHAPTER 26

Healthy Fats vs. Harmful Fats

O ne important element of a nutritious diet is healthy fat. To declare a fat healthy, we should first rule out unhealthy fats. Which fats would I consider harmful, and what makes them unhealthy?

Harmful fats are heavily processed, industrialized seed and grain oils that are unusually high in polyunsaturated fats. These fats or oils promote inflammation, aging, and cancer. They're also shown to directly promote over-eating and insulin resistance.

Harmful fats include:

- **Trans fats and partially hydrogenated oils:**

These scientifically manipulated fats are used in processed/packaged foods, frozen foods, fried foods, fast food, margarine, Crisco/shortening, and powdered creamers. These trans fats cause oxidation, inflammation, free radicals, damage to cell membranes, and DNA mutations—potentially leading to the most harmful effects like heart disease and cancer.

Trans- and partially-hydrogenated oils cause destruction at the cellular and DNA levels. Elimination of these foods is critical for preventing disease and promoting health.

- **Vegetable oils high in PUFAs/omega-6 fats:**

These highly industrialized, liquid cooking oils are ubiquitous in our American food system. They're found in nearly every modern household, commercial kitchens, bottled salad dressing, and packaged, processed foods. They are falsely promoted as healthy, although, in actuality, most of them are easily oxidized during manufacturing and cooking, which causes them to become dangerous to our health.

These pro-inflammatory oils contribute to dangerous cholesterol molecules, the build-up of plaque on arterial walls, advanced aging, and oxidative stress in the body. They screw with energy metabolism in our bodies and threaten the survival of beneficial bacteria in our guts. Ultimately, the inflammatory reactions can lead to all types of chronic disease, especially heart disease, brain-degenerating conditions, and cancer.

It's important to note that although there's danger in overconsumption of high omega-6 fats, a simple remedy may be to increase one's simultaneous intake of omega-3 fatty acids. The goal is to bring our ratio of omega-6 to omega-3 fats down to around 2:1. The typical Western diet achieves a ratio of 10:1 or up to 30:1. That's where the danger truly lies because omega-6 is a pro-inflammatory fatty acid, and omega-3 is the anti-inflammatory fatty acid. They're designed to coexist in our food and in our bodies. We just need to get those ratios right.

Although the inflammatory nature of these oils is most concerning, you might be intrigued to learn that polyunsaturated fats do not have the same appetite-suppressing effects we experience in response to eating monounsaturated or saturated fats. In a 2010 study[26] published in the Journal of Clinical Endocrinology and Metabolism, researchers tested safflower oil, olive oil, and lard to determine certain metabolic responses in human subjects. Both olive oil and lard stimulated two to three times more satiation than safflower oil. Specifically, the hormone GLP-1 was doubled or tripled after consuming the healthy fats. GLP-1 is naturally released by our intestines in response to food and also stimulated by the wildly popular class of weight-loss drugs like semaglutide and other GLP-1 agonist drugs. GLP-1 reduces appetite and hunger through various changes in gastrointestinal function and subsequent metabolic reactions.

Wouldn't you like to be eating foods that naturally stimulate more of that?

Alternative names for *vegetable oil*:

- Toxic seed oils
- Industrial seed oils
- Inflammatory seed oils
- Refined vegetable oils

- PUFAs (poly-unsaturated fatty acids)
- High omega-6 fats

Harmful Fats & Oils To Avoid or Strictly Limit:

- Partially-hydrogenated oils
- Margarine
- Vegetable shortening and Crisco
- Deep-fried foods (including fried frozen foods)
- Most buttery sprays/spreads (typically plant-based)
- Vegetable/seed oils:
  - Canola oil (expeller-pressed canola oil may be the safest PUFA oil regarding the degree of oxidation from cooking)
  - Corn oil
  - Cottonseed oil
  - Grape seed oil
  - Peanut oil
  - Rapeseed oil

o   Rice Bran oil   o   Safflower oil

o   Soybean oil   o   Sunflower oil

I know.

This is one of the most irritating changes to make in your diet simply because these oils are in *everything*—like 99 percent of restaurant food and 99 percent of packaged foods. However, next to reducing the carbs and sugar in your diet, this could be the most important thing you do for your health because of how dangerous oxidized fatty acids really are.

That's why cooking your own food can be critical on this journey. It takes a little more time or a little more money to make these changes, but they're among the most impactful changes you can make for yourself and your loved ones.

It's worth trying, little by little, to make these changes. Starting with the oils in your home, like cooking oils and all packaged foods. Pay close attention to what your household consumes most frequently—especially bottled salad dressings, frozen foods, and sauces and mayonnaise, in which the oil content is quite high.

Why are these toxic oils promoted as heart-healthy on food labels or by organizations like the American Heart Association?

It's complicated. The industry is corrupt, and this comes with quite a history of biased nutrition science and industry corruption. Also, these oils are made from industry byproducts—waste products that are highly profitable for the US economy and agricultural systems. Nutrition science is manipulated, information is misinterpreted, and legislation isn't concerned with our health as much as with industry ties to lobbyists from Big Ag producers and agricultural profit margins.

Vegetable Oils' Deceptive Past

As nutrition expert Nina Teicholz explains in her deeply-researched book, The Big Fat Surprise, the ubiquity of vegetable oils in our food supply stems from a complex history of flawed and industry-funded research, regulatory lobbying, and marketing campaigns by major food corporations. For instance, food companies like Best Foods, Unilever, and other oil giants have long paid "reputable scientists at prestigious institutions to conduct studies intended to find positive results on behalf of their products." From the researchers' perspectives, receiving these industry funds was "considered a necessary evil" given the limited nutrition research funding available. Furthermore, she points out that the troubled history of regular vegetable oils continues to raise health concerns yet remains unresolved even as organizations still advise increasing their consumption. This enduring yet questionable dietary guidance reveals how industry tactics to fund biased research and sustain positive health claims for their products have shaped nutritional policy and science around vegetable oils. The catalog of disastrous consequences continues to plague our population today.

One of the biggest clues that these oils aren't made for human consumption is that it requires a LOT of mechanical processing, chemical intervention, and manipulation to make oil from seeds.

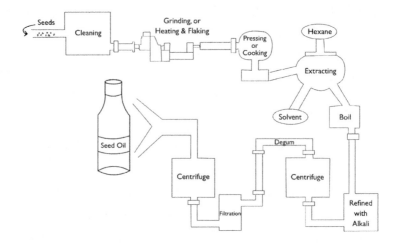

What about Expeller-Pressed Seed Oils?

If it's vegetable oil (AKA industrial seed oil) and has been heated or cooked with, chances are the fatty acids are damaged, oxidized, and dangerous—even when it's expeller-pressed, which is a more gentle extraction method.

It's best to stay away as much as possible, especially cooked foods and processed foods with oil listed in the first few ingredients. The higher the oil is listed on an ingredients list, the greater the quantity per serving.

What about high-oleic oils?

High-oleic oils—like high-oleic sunflower oil—are new solutions in the food manufacturing industry. Although they're not the best options, they're a welcome solution to packaged foods.

Why the new name for those oils?

It's easier to understand if we first talk about seed oils like canola or soybean oil. Our main concern with vegetable oils is that they're high in polyunsaturated fatty acids (PUFAs). One PUFA of particular concern is linoleic acid.

Linoleic acid is exceptionally fragile to heat, oxygen, radiation, and light. This means seed oils contains damaged linoleic fatty acids that wind up incorporated into our cell membranes, causing inflammation, DNA mutations, arterial plaque, and cancer-promoting compounds. It's the linoleic acid that causes a fat to go rancid.

High-oleic oils are the food industry's new solution. They're less inflammatory but still super cheap to make and buy, and they still make use of agricultural byproducts and superfluous supply.

Food producers now make and use high-oleic oils, which are lower in that dangerous PUFA known as linoleic acid. These high-oleic oils are comprised of more beneficial monounsaturated fats (MUFAs) and far fewer PUFAs compared to standard vegetable oils. This means the molecules are more chemically stable and less prone to rancidity and inflammation in the body.

Some high-oleic oils have fatty acid profiles that can rival heart-healthy olive oil and avocado oils. The catch, however, is that they're still highly processed and don't contain the protective plant compounds found in better, unrefined oils. This means they'll never be ideal, although they are indeed acceptable.

Healthy Fats

Once you know why certain fats are bad, you can better appreciate why healthy fats are so good. Good fats are necessary for you to feel satisfied during your meals, to support healthy cell membranes and hormone production, and to provide energy you can feel (especially when you eat a low-carb diet or introduce fasting to your daily routine).

Good fats are bundled up in whole foods (thank you, Mother Nature!):

✓ The omega-3 fats in a filet of salmon

✓ The brain-boosting fats in an egg yolk

✓ The stable saturated fats in a coconut or pastured ribeye steak

✓   The heart-healthy monounsaturated fats in an olive

✓   The complex, heart-protective combination of fats in nuts like macadamias

Toss the toxic seed oils you have at home. That bottle of vegetable oil, corn oil, peanut oil, and even canola oil. They're cheap and likely to cause inflammation, so just throw them away and start anew.

Instead, start cooking with avocado oil from reputable brands such as Marianne's, Chosen Foods, and Primal Kitchen. Note: it's been found that most of the avocado oil on the market isn't, in fact, avocado oil. Instead of being 100 percent avocado, it includes soybean oil or safflower oil and a combination of seed oils (and the company/brand itself may not even know it!). The recommended brands I shared above have been validated to be 100% avocado oil.

Avocado oil and extra virgin olive oil (EVOO) are healthy oils to consume. Even though I'm a huge fan of EVOO, it isn't neutral-tasting or able to complement a variety of cuisines, whereas avocado oil is. Also, EVOO isn't as tolerant of high heat compared to avocado oil. EVOO should only be heated up to a temperature of 375 degrees Fahrenheit, or the fatty acid molecules will degrade and become inflammatory. That's why I recommend every household has a bottle of quality Avocado Oil on hand to cook with. It's great to roast in the oven or grill and cook foods at higher heat.

My newest healthy fat obsession is Cultured Oil by Zero Acre Farms. Cultured oil is very high in monounsaturated fats, is high-heat tolerant, and has a neutral taste. It doesn't solidify in the fridge, like olive oil and avocado oil do. It's made by fermenting sugarcane with a live starter culture like sourdough bread or kombucha fermented tea! This old-fashioned method of generating heart-healthy oil is something to marvel at! If you can afford to try some, I highly recommend it.

Where to start with packaged foods:

Start with the foods you consume most frequently and the foods higher in fat/oil content, such as mayo, salad dressing, and frozen foods. This change takes time. Perfection isn't the goal because it's too unrealistic and stressful. The goal is to be mindful and read ingredient lists, read food labels, and use trusted brands. Be willing to pay a bit extra for non-toxic oils and fats. Keep this a priority on your healthy eating journey, not just for yourself but for your entire family.

2 Key Lessons About Increasing Fat In Your Diet

Key #1: Satiation

When it comes to satiation or the feeling of satisfaction you get from eating, dietary fats have a unique edge. When you eat healthy fats, your brain receives a signal that your meal is providing nourishment. Your level of satiation is a good determiner for how much fat you'd need in a typical meal. If a meal leaves you unsatisfied but physically full, consider topping the dish off with more healthy fats, like a drizzle of extra virgin olive oil or crushed macadamia nuts.

Protein, on the other hand, keeps you full for hours after a meal. Fat satisfies you while you eat, and protein keeps you satisfied between meals.

If, on a daily basis, you find yourself relying on foods like nuts, nut butter, or cheese to satisfy your hunger or cravings, however, that indicates your satiety signals are out of whack due to the habitual consumption of such foods. As I've observed in my clients who have a self-proclaimed addiction to nuts, nut butter, or cheese, when they cut out the food entirely for a couple of weeks, near the end of week one and beyond, they feel free from the addiction. I've had several clients who've experienced this firsthand.

Jody had a relentless appetite for Barney Butter almond butter and would consume just one tablespoon every day. Over time, this habit created a shift in her microbiome—the little microbes that love almond butter started to overpopulate her gut thanks to her habit. I suggested she consider removing nut butter for a couple of weeks to help free herself from the daily craving. Sure enough, one week later, Jody celebrated with me that her cravings for nut butter had vanished!

Key #2: High Fat and Keto Gray Zone

One of the biggest mistakes people make in pursuit of weight loss on a low-carb diet is to intentionally jack up the amount of dietary fats in every meal and snack. The secret to success with keto isn't a super-high fat intake. It's the significant reduction in carbohydrates and the absence of insulin that stimulate ketone production in your body.

While the keto community promotes high-fat foods, remember the goal is to burn your body fat, not the dietary fats you consume. On a low-carb diet, excessive amounts of dietary fat will only encourage a plateau and slow down your weight loss.

One of the biggest traps I see people caught in starts with snacking on high-fat foods like nut butter, cheese, and copious amounts of nuts or coconut products. Cheese and packaged keto bars are a big trap. They're convenient and ready to grab at any urge, and they slow down the rate at which you burn your fat.

Another big trap people fall into is called the *keto gray zone* when high-fat foods and high-carb foods are consumed simultaneously. The trouble is your body produces more inflammation when we combine the two. It forces your body to metabolize both energy sources at once, which increases triglycerides, stalls weight loss, and increases oxidative stress, which ages the body, making you more susceptible to disease. You could approach this meal by meal or day by day, reducing dietary fat in meals that are higher in carbs and vice versa. Ultimately, however, the more exceptions you make by eating a high-carb meal, the longer it will take your body to get back into ketosis and burn the fat you want to lose.

In terms of satiation between meals and weight loss, many people need to increase the protein in their diet. Let's delve into the most essential macro-nutrient, protein, so you can experience greater success with more ease and satisfaction.

CHAPTER 27

Protein Principles

Protein intake is a contentious topic, with no consensus among experts or health organizations. When we throw fasting into the mix, we add to the complexity of this matter. Despite the lack of clear guidelines, there are ways to assess if your protein intake is sufficient, and we'll explore these by the end of this chapter.

Why protein is essential for health:

Of all the macronutrients—protein, carbs, and fat—protein is the most essential for life. To be a fully functional human with biological integrity, we need adequate protein with its building block amino acids. Proteins and amino acids are catalysts for hormones and neurotransmitters, and they're the building blocks of new tissues and old/injured tissues in need of repair. Proteins are critical for immune function and absolutely essential for growth, particularly in children and teens and during pregnancy. Undoubtedly, protein is essential for preserving muscle tissue. By preserving muscle tissue or building more muscle, you can increase longevity, metabolic health, brain function, and so much more.

Cool fact: protein is such an essential macronutrient that the body can use it to make glucose and fatty acids. The same cannot be said for glucose and carbs or fats. This was useful throughout human history because, at times, the only food available would be meat, seafood, or bugs and grubs, while vegetation was scarce. We've evolved with the ability to meet all our nutrient requirements from protein alone if needed. Fascinating!

Signs of *insufficient protein intake:

Insufficient due to a low protein diet, eating the wrong protein sources for one's bio-individual needs, insufficient amino acid intake, or inadequate digestion/absorption of amino acids.

- Hunger between meals or within 2 hours of eating

- Constant cravings or the need for snacks

- Overeating at mealtimes

- Stubborn weight loss

- A decrease in lean muscle mass (or no muscle increase in response to increased resistance training)

- Inability to sustain the energy or strength needed for non-cardio workouts

- Failure of consistent workouts to result in beneficial body composition changes after 4 weeks of a new training regime (you work out more but see fewer/no results)

- Insomnia or trouble getting adequate sleep

- A sudden drop in physical energy during the late afternoon or early evening

- Fasting with only one meal a day, resulting in < 50 g of protein (on most days of the week)

- Thinning hair, peeling nails

- Frequent injuries like strained/torn tendons and ligaments

- Slower than expected recovery from injuries or post-surgery

- Eating less than 25 g of protein in most of your meals

- Craving red meat and rarely consuming it

- Women missing periods or having irregular periods

- Impaired immunity, getting sick frequently, and/or poor recovery

- Long COVID symptoms or daily fatigue since COVID-19 (or other debilitating infection)

- Mental Health:

  o Increased anxiety, depression, or irritability (from unknown causes)

  o Increased brain fog, mental fatigue, trouble learning new things

  o Exacerbated ADHD symptoms (in the absence of major life changes or sleep deprivation)

Digesting Protein

A few key things to know about protein digestion:

1. Proteins are made up of building blocks called amino acids

You can think of amino acids like Lego blocks and proteins like the structures you build with those blocks. Depending on which Lego blocks you have and the combinations you stack them in, you have the potential to build an endless array of structures. Proteins and amino acids offer endless possibilities just like that, and humans need a variety of amino acids in various combinations to function optimally. When certain amino acids are too low or overall protein intake is inadequate, a person can become malnourished and suffer concerning health consequences as a result.

2. How the stomach uses hydrochloric acid (HCl) and pepsin to digest protein

During the first major stage of protein digestion, your stomach and pancreas release stomach acid (HCl, hydrochloric acid) and an enzyme named pepsin to break down the protein structures into building blocks called amino acids. Without adequate digestive resources from your stomach and pancreas, dozens of gut conditions and immune-system vulnerabilities can surely follow. More on that in the sub-section: *Stomach Acid and Digesting Meat.*

3. Plant proteins and animal proteins are different structures made up of different building blocks

You may have heard before that animal proteins provide all essential amino acids, meaning they provide us with the combination of amino acids that our body requires but cannot manufacture internally. That's why they're called essential, and that's why animal proteins are described as complete proteins.

Plant foods, on the other hand, don't contain all the essential amino acids—which explains why they're called incomplete proteins. Technically, however, some plants, like hemp seeds, do contain all essential amino acids, but they fall short in certain amino acid quantities (like not enough lysine and leucine), which means the body won't have enough of the building blocks to prevent malnutrition unless additional sources of the missing amino acids are consumed.

To solve this dilemma as a plant-based eater, one needs to combine different plants to get all the essential amino acids in adequate quantities. This becomes more and more critical the longer someone is committed to a plant-based diet.

The most traditional plant foods to combine are rice and beans because, together, they comprise a complete protein that provides all essential amino acids in fairly adequate quantities. But guess what. For someone to get the same amount of protein available in a (rather small) 4-oz sirloin steak (which contains 30 g of complete protein), they'd have to eat 12 oz of beans (about 1.5 cups) and 8 oz of rice (about 1 cup).

But wait.

What I'm about to share with you is what really shocked me. 12 oz of beans and 8 oz of rice contain 122 g of carbohydrates. One hundred and twenty-two grams of carbs! And those servings aren't very big! Furthermore, the 4-oz steak contains 181 calories, while the rice and beans contain 638 calories![27] *Whaaa???*

Animal protein is superior. Plain and simple. Besides, humans are innately omnivorous creatures. That's how we're designed to coexist with nature, nourish ourselves, and thrive. We'll dive further into the subject of plant proteins in Chapter 28: *Protein Myths, Hacks, and Putting it All Together.*

Proteins and Amino Acid Sources:

This list starts with the most digestible protein sources followed by progressively reduced digestibility as the list continues.

(Note: the order will vary according to quantity consumed, other foods consumed at the same time, and the bio-individual response to each source on this list.)

- **Amino acids** - supplement/powder/drink (EAAs, BCAAs, individual amino acids)

- **Collagen or gelatin protein**

- **Whey protein powder** (isolate or concentrate; cold-processed isolate may be safer for individuals with some dairy sensitivity)

- **Beef protein powder**

- **Egg white protein powder** (only with no suspicion of egg intolerance)

- **Milk protein concentrate** or **casein protein** (*NOT recommended* due to the high probability of immune system dysregulation in the presence of a leaky gut and for large populations unknowingly sensitive to milk proteins)

- **Sprouted plant-protein powder** (digestibility is enhanced in a person with adequate gut health and certain genetics that more adequately convert plant proteins into essential nutrients)

- **Plant-based protein powder (un-sprouted)** (digestibility is enhanced in mixed plant proteins versus single ingredient plant-proteins, and when a person has adequate gut health and certain genetic capabilities to convert plant proteins into essential nutrients)

- **Slow-cooked/pressure-cooked animal protein**

- **Raw/cured seafood, shellfish, and animal protein** (assuming adequate HCl stomach acid to protect from food-borne pathogens)

- **Cooked/canned seafood and shellfish**

- **Cured animal protein** (like deli meat)

- **Lean animal protein** (quick-cooked or dried like jerky) (requires more adequate HCl stomach acid, digestive enzymes, and pancreatic function)

- **Fatty/tough animal protein** (quick-cooked or dried like jerky) (requires more adequate HCl stomach acid, digestive enzymes, pancreatic function and bile salts, and gallbladder function)

Stomach Acid and Digesting Meat

It's not uncommon for me to hear from a client that they love protein or red meat, but they don't eat it much because it weighs them down after eating. They feel too full, and their body doesn't break it down well enough. If this describes you, I can relate. I salivate at the sight of a juicy steak, but I rarely eat steak besides filet (tenderloin) because it can be so tough, chewy, or hard to digest. Even with slow-cooked meats, for years, I felt weighed down after a meal, and it seemed as if the food was in my stomach for a good 4 hours after dinner.

Everything changed once I realized that those are signs of low stomach acid, so I began supplementing accordingly. Since then, I've been a big advocate of these simple, effective solutions to enhance your digestive resources with two key supplements:

1. Digestive enzymes

2. Betaine HCL (HCl, hydrochloric acid)

Contrary to popular belief, it's very likely an adult is low in stomach acid if they:

- Are over the age of thirty-five (especially women)

- Have a history of repeat food poisoning or H.pylori infections

- Have a history of repeat antacid use

- Have autoimmune disease

- Have vitamin B12 deficiency or anemia

- Suffer from chronic stress over a long period of time

- Suffer from gas and bothersome GI symptoms

- Experience feeling heavy in the stomach—like the food just sits there—after eating meat.

What's really wild is that even if someone experiences acid reflux or heart-burn, the root cause is typically *not having enough stomach acid.* That's right. They have heartburn because they're too low in stomach acid.

When you eat a big meal and hard-to-digest proteins, you need adequate stomach acid to speed up the transition from the stomach to the small intes-tine, but without enough acid, pressure builds in the stomach, and gasses rise up into the esophagus, where it causes heartburn and doesn't belong. *Whoa, right?*

Individuals I meet who experience acid reflux are usually taking prescription or over-the-counter antacids because it's supposed to *help* with the acid reflux. It does provide temporary relief, but it actually prolongs the condition since it doesn't address the underlying cause—*it worsens it!*

> *"If heartburn were caused by too much stomach acid, we'd have a bunch of teenagers popping Rolaids instead of elderly folks. But of course, that's the opposite of what we see."*
> - Chris Kresser, M.S., Co-Founder and Co-Director of the California Center for Functional Medicine

So, except for individuals with a history of stomach ulcers or gastritis and persons who regularly take anti-inflammatory medication like prednisone and over-the-counter NSAIDS (like Advil, Motrin, etc., which can all damage the gut lining, increasing the risk of ulcer and gastric bleeding), most adults will benefit from supplementing with Betaine HCl (hydrochloric acid combined with betaine, a natural substance found in plants, and typically formulated with pepsin, an enzyme the body also needs in this stage of digestion). Betaine supports the breakdown of fat accumulating in the liver, and promotes improved hydration and protein balance in the cells.[28]Note that HCl supplements should never be combined with acid-blocking drugs whether over-the-counter or prescription proton-pump inhibitors.

Most of my clients will experience a noticeable difference with 2 or 3 capsules of Betaine HCl taken with a meal, starting with one per meal and gradually increasing until a personally adequate dose is reached, and it can be life-changing! I personally carry around a pill holder with my digestive enzymes and HCl capsules (as well as chlorella to help eliminate ingested carcinogens from charred/blackened meats, fried food, and alcohol).

I take a serving of digestive enzymes at the start of every meal (goodbye gas and bloating! Hello nutrient absorption!) and 1–3 capsules of HCl with every meal and any alcohol (also helpful to prevent gas and bloat caused by undigested food fermenting in the gut). I feel so much lighter after my meals, my energy is more consistent, and my food is done being digested in a reasonable amount of time so I can sleep soundly after dinner, which is where I've experienced the biggest payoff!

Sick of taking pills? This is an area where traditional remedies may suffice. Stimulate more stomach acid production in your body by consuming digestive bitters and vinegar-rich foods at the start of every meal. This may not produce the same amount of relief and resolution you can achieve with capsules, but it will suffice for milder cases.

Stomach acid also plays a critical role in immunity because our immune system relies on it to kill off potentially harmful bacteria before they wind up in our GI tract, where they will multiply and make us very sick (food poisoning or H. pylori infection, anyone?). Not only does it help protect us from pathogenic infections, but stomach acid also helps prevent nutrient deficiencies, leaky gut, and gut dysbiosis, as well as these all-too-common conditions that can result from undigested foods entering the GI tract: IBS or SIBO conditions (got bloat? got gas? got diarrhea?), skin problems, autoimmune conditions, and more.

Proteins Require More Bodily Energy to Metabolize

Another benefit of eating protein is that, out of the three macronutrients (protein, carbs, and fat), protein requires the most energy to digest, metabolize, and store. This is known as the thermic effect of food, or TEF. It's beneficial to have higher TEF foods (like more protein) in your meals because this helps raise the thermic effect of the entire meal.

Let's think about it in numbers. If fats have an average TEF of 2 percent, carbs have a TEF of around 7 percent, and proteins have a TEF of around 25 percent, then a meal higher in protein will help bring the average TEF somewhere around 10–15 percent—which would help explain why people who eat a lot of protein rarely gain weight as a result. The body uses more calories to digest the food.

This is one of the reasons, too, that explains why you can't just count calories to try and lose weight. All calories are not created equal. 200 calories from protein might leave you with only 150 calories of protein stored (thanks to the high TEF and caloric energy needed to digest and metabolize it), whereas 200 calories of carbs could leave you with 185 calories stored.

Protein is an exciting topic, and we're about halfway through the discussion now. Ready for more?

CHAPTER 28

Protein Myths, Hacks, and Putting it All Together

Plant proteins evolved to serve as one of a plant's top defenses. The proteins in a plant seed are evolutionarily designed, by nature, to inhibit digestion in the human body (and in animals and insects) so the seed can pass through the digestive system relatively unscathed and wind up in the soil where it can grow into a plant—its ultimate biological destiny.

Plant proteins include a pesky class known as *lectins*. The most infamous group of lectins is *gluten*. Humans simply cannot digest lectin plant proteins. It's only a matter of digestive integrity, stress load, and immunity that will determine how offensive lectins and plant proteins will be for an individual at any given point in their lifetime. Let's not forget I suddenly became gluten-intolerant in my late twenties. Gluten is a lectin and a plant protein!

Many health experts theorize it's the indigestible proteins in plants that are to blame for the alarming number of life-threatening plant food allergies today—corn, peanuts, soy, wheat/gluten, and tree nuts.

Animal-sourced top food allergens are shellfish and eggs, especially egg whites, which may also have been triggered by our consumption of isolated egg white proteins during the past few decades of the low-fat, low-cholesterol diet craze. The whole egg is meant to be eaten at once!

Animal Protein Myths and Misconceptions

Prior to 2020, no one had thoroughly and convincingly debunked the numerous misconceptions about meat as a nutritious and sustainable dietary staple. This changed with the release of the extensively researched book and its accompanying film, *Sacred Cow*, which presented an unprecedentedly clear and comprehensive summary of the topic.

Authors Diana Rodgers and Robb Wolf tirelessly combed through the research and statistics, interviewing experts around the globe, to ultimately provide an unbiased summary or rebuttal of the following myths and misconceptions—and more:

Myth 1: We eat too much meat

Myth 2: We eat too much protein

Myth 3: Red meat causes chronic disease

Myth 4: Meat eating isn't environmentally sustainable

Myth 1: We eat too much meat

According to *Sacred Cow*, the national statistics that claim Americans eat an average of 265 lb of meat a year are false because that number doesn't take into account the many losses that should be factored in—like the large percentage of meat used for pet food, the organs, skin, and fat discarded or repurposed from a meat processing plant, the meat that spoils in the grocery stores or is never sold, the pounds of moisture lost during cooking, etc. In reality, the average American is consuming about 130 lb of meat per year, not 265. *Sheesh.*

Myth 2: We eat too much protein

Numerous large-scale and rigorous human studies have demonstrated the health and weight-loss benefits of a higher protein intake, yet false claims still exist to spread the nonsense that we eat too much protein. In a 2005–2014 National Health and Nutrition Examination Survey[29], data from 11,680 adults over fifty years old were investigated regarding meeting or not meeting the national protein recommendation. Some age groups only consumed up to 46 percent of the RDA minimum protein intake recommendation, which is around 70 g of protein per day for an average American man weighing 195 lb and 60 g of protein per day for an average American woman weighing 166 lb.

But what you may not know about the U.S. Dietary Guidelines for RDA (recommended daily allowance) is that those numbers are a minimum requirement. *Minimum.* In other words, what's the *lowest* amount you could consume daily to prevent disease caused by malnutrition. I don't know about you, but I don't want to know the minimum needed to prevent me from dying a slow death; I want to know the amount that gives me increased health and vitality.

Nearly half of American adults over age fifty don't meet the RDA minimum requirement for protein intake, and we have large-scale human studies to show there are measurable health consequences, including insufficient nutrient levels of fiber, thiamin, niacin, vitamin B6, folate, choline, vitamin C, vitamin B12, vitamin A, vitamin D, vitamin E, vitamin K, zinc, calcium, phosphorus, magnesium, iron, copper, and selenium. [30]

> *"Overall, adults not meeting protein needs have much higher likelihood of lower micronutrient intakes (on the day of intake), and nutrient deficiencies, combined with a lower protein intake, in older adults may increase risks of common issues, such as falls, pressure sores, osteomalacia, osteoporosis, hip fractures, muscle weakness, and mortality."*
>
> - J. L. Krok-Schoen et al.[31]

Needless to say, most adults don't eat enough protein and/or enough bio-available protein. Most adults probably need around 100 g of protein per day in the context of a 2,000-calorie diet or 30 percent of total daily calories coming from protein. I hate talking about calories because it can contribute to the mindset that calories should be counted (which is a losing game in most cases), but using calories to do some math here makes sense to help determine how much protein we're talking.

For someone practicing intermittent fasting as a lifestyle who eats two meals a day and around 1,600 total daily calories, 480 of those calories would be coming from lean animal protein. This turns out to be a 7–8-oz serving of lean animal protein per meal, which gets you around 45–50 g of protein per meal and 90–100 g of protein per day.

> *"A lot of people (especially women) push back and feel like this is too much. However, once people actually get this level of protein in their diet, they generally feel a lot better and eat fewer calories because they feel so full. (Because protein is highly satiating, when we increase our protein intake, our overall caloric intake generally reduces.)"*
> - Diana Rodgers and Robb Wolf, *Sacred Cow*

Myth 3: Red meat causes chronic disease

As red meat consumption has declined in America, heart disease, type 2 diabetes, and cancer rates have all continued to increase at an alarming rate. According to the authors of *Sacred Cow*, "A systematic review of the current research against beef published in the *Annals of Internal Medicine* surprisingly concluded that the evidence against meat is of low quality, and we don't have the evidence to make public health recommendations to limit red and processed meat consumption." Red meat and a variety of animal proteins have been a human dietary staple for tens of thousands of years, which provides more time-tested evidence that this food is a nourishing piece that belongs in the human diet.

Download referenced infographics of these facts at *www.sacredcow.info/
helpful-resources*

You probably need to eat more animal protein than you're eating now. You
won't die sooner if you're a meat eater. Meat itself doesn't give you cancer.
Meat itself doesn't give you diabetes or any of the other crap you hear out
there. It's the quality of the meat, the preparation, processing, and preservation, and the cooking methods, as well as the combination of other foods/
drinks in your diet, that most influence a favorable or unfavorable health
span linked to your dietary choices.

If you eat charred steaks, chicken nuggets, fried fish, and cheap deli meats
every day—especially without 6–8 servings of colorful vegetables to combat
those toxins—your health will suffer. And especially when eaten in combination with other high-carb, highly inflammatory foods. Eat a variety of
slow-cooked meats from a regenerative farm, low-toxin seafood, and uncured
deli meats every day, and your health may flourish (or at least be better
maintained as you age). You'll experience less hunger and more satisfaction
from your diet, too.

Myth 4: Meat eating isn't environmentally sustainable

This could possibly be the biggest misunderstanding of all. We won't save the
environment if our families, or the entire neighborhood, stop eating meat.
The first thing to consider is that fake meat products like Beyond Burger
use far more natural resources and contribute more to greenhouse gasses
compared to regeneratively raised animal protein. In fact, experts have the
numbers to prove you'd have to eat a grass-fed burger from a regenerative
farm to "…offset the emissions created from eating one Beyond Burger or
Impossible Burger." I'll help you understand how that can be possible in the
next few paragraphs to follow.

Secondly, beef requires less water to produce per pound compared to avocados, walnuts, and sugar, which need copious amounts of irrigated water to

grow effectively for harvest, profit, and consumption. Furthermore, 94–97 percent of the water used for raising cattle is supplied by rainfall.

Thirdly, cow farts aren't actually ruining the environment or contributing to greenhouse gas emissions at 18–51 percent, as anti-beef proponents claim. According to the EPA (Environmental Protection Agency), if we include all livestock, not just cows, they only contribute 3.9 percent of those emissions. Agricultural plant crops create 4.7 percent. Transportation is the largest contributor, as well as electricity generation and the industry sector. Together, they create over 78 percent of the toxic emissions in our atmosphere.

Finally, cows raised on a regenerative farm—where they graze on fields of grass, and the herds are rotated onto new pasture frequently to mimic natural migration patterns—don't increase greenhouse gasses. In fact, these well-managed cattle help to sequester carbon from the atmosphere, resulting in an overall *reduction* of carbon. This is called a carbon sink. Pasture-raised cattle that are rotationally grazed in this way help absorb more carbon dioxide from the atmosphere than they release. It equals negative carbon and improves the atmosphere. Not only that, but regenerative cattle farms also help increase wildlife habitats, microbial diversity in the soil and surrounding plants, and the absorption of rainfall (thanks to the plush pastures they cycle on and off of). How cool is that. Nature didn't create herding, grass-grazing animals for nothing. They serve a purpose that nourishes us and Mother Earth!

When you consider the nutrient density of meat and how many areas of the world in which the land is unfit to farm plant crops (due to rocky, icy, desert-dry, or steep range land), sustainably raised cattle are more the answer than the problem for decreasing world hunger, improving nutrition accessibility and equity, as well as improving the earth's resources and diversity.

There's a lot more than that in the incredible documentary film *Sacred Cow* and the companion book. You can also gather a collection of these facts and associated scientific references from *www.sacredcow.info/helpful-resources*

Protein-Related Confusion Regarding Glucose and Insulin

As you've been learning throughout this book, it's important to minimize insulin production throughout the day to achieve healthy metabolic function and to effectively burn body fat. Fasting helps you do that. Low-carb dieting helps you do that. Together, they're even more effective. There's something about protein that creates some confusion on this very topic, however.

Spend some time in many of the plant-based or vegan interwebs, and you'll hear that protein causes type 2 diabetes because protein requires too much insulin and leads to insulin resistance. At first, I thought these claims were a bunch of bullshit dogma relied upon in the plant-based community as a way of getting people to stop eating meat.

To my surprise, turns out there's some truth to those claims, but it's tricky and too nuanced to put as simply as that. Even though protein causes an insulin response—and, in some cases, the insulin response to protein can be greater than insulin caused by carbs—endless scientific studies[32] have shown that the possible weight-promoting effects of it are counteracted by the slowed gastric emptying or *incretin effect* of protein consumption that results in longer lasting fullness and increased weight loss, not weight gain.

Regardless, in most cases, protein stimulates far less insulin compared to carbohydrates when we're talking about ingesting carbs or proteins alone. In the absence of carbs, protein consumption stimulates about two-thirds less insulin compared to if that person ate only carbs in the absence of protein. In the presence of carbs, especially when consuming whey protein, post-prandial blood glucose levels (tested 3 hours after eating) reduce below baseline, even in type 2 diabetics. This means the increased insulin from protein *with* your carbs helps to improve post-prandial glucose levels, especially when whey protein is consumed or when the protein is consumed in the afternoon or evening when glucose tolerance is reduced. [33]

Time and time again, research shows that a higher protein intake leads to improved metabolic markers in obese, insulin-resistant individuals (both men and women), even when compared to a Mediterranean diet. So don't worry about those alarm bells many plant-based enthusiasts are ringing. The science is there. Increased protein consumption leads to improved health outcomes in almost every case.

Protein's Role in Fullness and Staving Off Hunger

One of the things that usually sucks the most about 'dieting' is the fact that you're hungry or thinking about food all the time. Decades of eating crappy processed food and a high-carb diet have thrown our hunger and fullness cues out of whack. Ghrelin—the hormone that makes you hungry or easily allured by food—isn't working properly as a result. And neither is leptin, the hormone that tells your brain you don't need any more food. Food is always on the brain.

Well, not only will carb reduction and fasting help with that—ironically, fasting and low-carb living help to reduce hunger so you think *less* often about food. But one more thing we haven't discussed much yet is how effective *protein* is at helping you feel full from a meal. Protein keeps you full for hours after eating.

How great would it be if you could stay full for hours after a meal? That's what protein does for you. That's one of the top reasons to prioritize protein if you want healthy fat-loss and sustainable, healthy weight maintenance. The protein-fullness effect has been proven dozens, if not hundreds, of times in scientific research and human studies.

If you recall from Chapter 4: *Breakfast Myths*, I emphasized the importance of a lower carb, higher protein breakfast (or break-fast, your first meal of the day). When people consume more protein at breakfast, they feel more satisfied and report fewer hunger signals, which is explained in part by an increase in the satiety hormone leptin.[34,35]

When you learned about regulating hunger, I shared this fascinating quote, and it's worth sharing again:

> "…people will continue to eat food in order to satisfy their protein needs…protein is the most satiating of the macronutrients, and intake of 15–30 percent of total calories can be quite helpful in regulating appetite…inducing weight loss and blood sugar control."
>
> - Diana Rodgers and Robb Wolf

Protein-Sparing Effect, Autophagy, and Age-Related Concerns

I'd be remiss if I concluded this portion without mentioning a few concerns related to aging. Fasting has a protein-sparing effect, meaning when we trigger fasting pathways in the body simply by fasting, the body naturally preserves lean muscle tissue thanks to the increase in human growth hormone and intelligent autophagy systems. Autophagy is your body's cellular recycling system that clears out problematic or useless cells to build newer, more resilient cells.

In the case of a carb-dependent diet, classic low-calorie dieting, and as seen in runners or chronic cardio exercisers—muscle tissue can be broken down and turned into glucose (the undesirable version of *gluconeogenesis*) when glycogen stores are depleted and more energy is needed.

The good news is that fasting prevents this type of muscle tissue breakdown when a person is fasting appropriately for their circumstances. Problems can arise, however, in cases where the individual is fasting too much, particularly in persons over sixty years old or those without adequate body fat, sufficient sleep, or sufficient protein intake.

One of the reasons people become enthusiastic about fasting for their health is because fasting accelerates a process known as autophagy. Autophagy means, literally, *self-eating*. It is a normal series of complex processes that allow a cell to eradicate damaged parts of itself or recycle them for more useful applications. I like to think of autophagy like a recycling process. It's necessary so junk doesn't build up over time, leaving the cell, and therefore the human, more susceptible to diseases like alzheimer's, dementia, cancer, heart disease—really any age-related or chronic disease. In a fairly healthy individual, autophagy is occurring to some degree at all times as it is a critical process by which cells maintain balance in response to changing external conditions. However, autophagic processes accelerate when cells are starved of nutrients, especially proteins and amino acids, and in response to various stressors as the cell works tirelessly to promote its survival.

Two important things about autophagy must be accepted at this time. First, autophagy declines with age. Second, autophagy is extremely complex and can easily become dysregulated. This means, it's not always beneficial. You can stimulate too much autophagy which can cause it to be harmful—such as resulting in premature cell death or abnormal cell growth, as in the case with certain tumors.

Very few human studies have been conducted in the matter of autophagy, and many claims regarding how and why to stimulate autophagy for our health are based on animal studies and limited scientific data. Various factors influence how much autophagy occurs and whether or not it will be beneficial to the host in the bigger picture. Such factors include a person's age, individual gene expression, nutrient deficiencies, disease-related condition of specific cells, mitochondrial health, immune system impairment and infections, metabolic efficiency, and more.

In a November 2019 article, *Agephagy – Adapting Autophagy for Health During Aging*, published in the journal, *Frontiers for Cell and Development Biology*, researchers concluded that, *"The more evidence we gather for improvement of health during aging by targeting autophagy, the more complexities we are uncovering."*[36]

Fasting is one of the greatest inducers of autophagy; however the process should not be abused until we have a much deeper understanding in the scientific literature. The autophagy achieved with daily intermittent fasts combined with a nutrient-dense, moderate protein diet should be a safe and effective lifestyle choice for anti-aging benefits of autophagy without risking maladaptation that can occur.

If you're over sixty, be sure to consume enough complete protein in your daily diet, and it's critical you have adequate body fat to spare if you'll be fasting as part of your lifestyle. We need more protein as we age because muscle tissue naturally wastes as we get older. This can lead to the more-common-than-you'd-think condition, sarcopenia. It's therefore also vitally important to practice resistance training—like with resistance bands, weights, or bodyweight resistance exercises.

> *"As people advance into their seventies, they can lose half their muscle mass, which renders them frail and susceptible to falling and fracture."*
> - Robert Lustig, *Metabolical*

Building Your Plate with Protein:

Aim for a minimum of 25 g of animal-sourced protein (or *complete* proteins) per meal to supply adequate amino acids for muscle-protein synthesis and the prevention of muscle loss. Especially in pregnant or lactating women, underweight adults, and on days you exercise, 25 g for women and 30 g for men seems to be the minimum you want to reach to turn on anabolic signaling. In other words, if you want to help your body heal, repair, grow in general, or increase your muscle mass, you should aim for this minimum per sitting, and maybe more. Same goes for when you consume a protein shake or protein bar to supply your protein for that meal—25 g of animal-sourced or complete protein is your target. The more you fast, the more your protein per meal needs to increase.

"Muscle? I don't want more muscle."

Building muscle isn't as easy as some people think. So even if you don't want to build or get bulky (which you won't unless that's your intention), you should still increase or optimize your muscle mass. Why? This helps you live longer and stronger. *And, guess what?* It helps you achieve all the other things you long for. More space to store your carbs instead of storing them as fat—yup, your muscles are your biggest set of luggage to pack those excess carbs in instead of turning them into body fat, and more metabolic flexibility, less insulin resistance, and far less hunger and fewer cravings ruling your world.

Total Protein in a 6-oz Serving of Animal Proteins

- 6 oz top sirloin steak = 35 g protein

- 6 oz ground beef chuck (80/20) = 22 g to 28 g protein

- 6 oz beef ribeye steak = 27 g to 33 g protein

- 6 oz ground lamb = 35 g to 42 g protein

- 6 oz pork tenderloin = 34 g to 44 g protein

- 6 oz ground turkey = 34 g protein

- 6 oz sliced deli turkey = 22 g to 30 g protein

- 6 oz chicken breast = 34 g to 50 g protein

- 6 oz Italian sausage = 30 g protein

- 6 oz shrimp = 40 g protein

- 6 oz cod fish or salmon = 35 g protein

- 3 large eggs (approx 6 oz) = 18 g protein

In my work over the years as a health coach, the most common determiners of someone who needs more adequate protein in their diet are if they're hungry between meals, have increased their physical activity, are healing from an injury or serious infection, are fasting over 18 hours per day, or if they're over sixty years old and eat less than 5 oz of animal protein per meal. Start with a 6-oz serving of protein per meal, and let hunger be your guide.

CHAPTER 29

Train Your Tastebuds

This chapter is dedicated to individuals who are particular about which foods they enjoy eating. If you're a foodie who loves all variety of vegetables and proteins, you can move on to the next chapter.

At this stage in your life, 90 percent of the food you eat is probably food you *know* you're going to like. You rarely ever buy, cook, or eat foods that are unfamiliar to you. Am I right? Trouble with that is—well, if nothing changes, *nothing changes*. Eat the same foods, get the same results—or worse, develop food sensitivities due to repetitive consumption.

Do you want to see a change in your energy levels? Do you want to see a reduction in your waistline? Want to experience less of an appetite for junk and true enjoyment from healthy foods? I assume your answer is yes to at least one (or probably all) of those questions. And that means it's time to train your tastebuds!

Yes, it's entirely possible to train your tastebuds to enjoy more foods you once disliked and to reduce your cravings for foods you once craved regularly. The key way to influence your tastebuds is to increase or decrease exposure to a food you want to influence your taste for.

Let's take salad as an example. Maybe you're thinking salads suck. Salad is for rabbits. Well, since salads can be one of the simplest, most nutritious, most accessible foods you can eat, it would be advantageous for you to figure out how to start enjoying them! You might order a side salad every time it's available at a restaurant, for starters, if you eat out frequently. You might also try making salads at home using different types of lettuces and different types of dressings and toppings to help discover which elements you enjoy more or less than others.

It's not a race. This is something that happens over time because, hey, you're busy! Once you've experimented a few times, before you know it, you start enjoying salads. You start craving salads. Really! I've seen this happen with several clients before. You've trained your tastebuds, your brain, and your gut microbes to favor salads! How cool is that?

This also works in reverse by reducing your intake of addicting or unhealthy foods. Let's take peanut butter as our example here. Peanut butter lovers tend to think they're special. They think they have some exceptional love for peanut butter that can't be understood by other people who like peanut butter or by people who love peanut butter but only eat it once in a while. It makes me smile because, really, 98 percent of the population loves the taste of peanut butter. For the record, I love peanut butter, too.

The difference between people who generally love peanut butter and those who think they have an exceptional love for it comes down to one thing really: the frequency with which they consume peanut butter. The more often you consume it, the more you'll become addicted to it. The less often you consume peanut butter, the less often you'll crave it.

Peanut butter, coffee, wine, and beer are some of the most addicting substances that people become addicted to or obsessed with, and I hypothesize that their addictive qualities are primarily caused by the mold toxins we're exposed to in those particular foods/drinks. All four of those popular substances are highly prone to the development of mold toxins (known as mycotoxins, specifically aflatoxin in peanut butter). These have a strong influence on the population of microbes in your gut and, in turn, will have a strong influence on pleasure pathways in your brain. The more frequently you expose your gut to those toxins, the more you alter the composition of your microbiome and your preference for certain foods. Ahem. Those damn cravings.

Want to lose excess weight? The peanut butter's gotta go. The daily two-glasses-of-wine habit (or the daily bottle) has gotta go. You're sad. I know. You love it. You're sorta addicted, and it gives you something to look forward to each day. Well, I assure you, you don't have to give it up indefinitely (not unless that's what you decide to do down the line). You do, however, want to cut it out of your life for a few weeks or more to help change your taste for it.

You'll feel so much freer without the constricting grasp these foods and drinks have had on you before. Even if you decide to reintroduce it later, and your cravings come back in full effect, you'll be better off than you were when you started because you'll have more insight into the matter. You'll know what it feels like to live without those frequent cravings, and you know you can cut it out because you've done it before. That's empowering. That's how you make big changes in your life. Push yourself out of your comfort zone a little or a lot, pay attention to what comes from it, reflect back on what things were like without the challenge, and determine if it's worth it for you to continue or try again.

Let's get back to eating more nutritious foods.

Maybe right now you're like most Americans, and the only vegetables you normally eat are tomatoes (actually a fruit), avocados (again, a fruit), onions, potatoes (starchy carbs), corn (not a vegetable! It's a grain!), broccoli, cauliflower, and carrots. Maybe you eat the occasional asparagus, bell pepper, or green beans. That's it. And that's not enough. Sorry. It's not. It's important to eat more variety and more colors than you can get from that classic rotation.

Maybe you don't know where to start. It seems like every time you've tried to cook other vegetables in the past, they turned out bland or mushy, or your family hated them. So that's why you've stuck with your good 'ol rotation of those tried-n-true veggies you always buy.

Welp, baby steps are going to be oh-so worth it for you! Start small by trying something related to a food you know you like, such as broccolini instead of broccoli or snow peas instead of green beans. Buy one new vegetable each time you're at the store, and google *the best way to prepare____*, or *the easiest way to cook _____*.

Use spice blends, seasoning salts, freshly squeezed lemon, melted butter, and minced fresh garlic to add flavorful elements to any vegetable. Choose fresh veggies instead of frozen or canned because you simply cannot compare the two when it comes to the taste and texture of the finished dish (although, surprisingly, the nutrient content is quite comparable!). When it comes to mushrooms, don't buy canned or frozen mushrooms unless you already know you like those. Try fresh ones if they're new to you, and try stuffing them with a mixture of your favorite cooked ground meat, minced garlic, parmesan, and plenty of herbs.

When a person repeatedly exposes themselves to a particular food or a category of food, their brain begins to associate the food with positive feelings and experiences, changing the neurotransmitters that help them feel pleasure and reward. The more you consume the food or this category of food, the more it influences the populations of microbes in your gut and results in a modified preference for those particular foods. There's even more to it; the enzymes in your mouth will change over time because you're eating new and healthier foods. In summary, your taste preferences will change because of multiple factors involving your saliva, tastebuds, microbiome, neurotransmitters, and food memories in your brain. Foods that were once unappealing are now a source of enjoyment for you. How cool is that!

CHAPTER 30
Variety, Variety, Variety

Throughout history, humans typically consumed 150 different types of plant foods throughout the year and dozens of varied animals, seafood, and even insects. Today, the typical American eats the same six to twelve vegetables and fruits all year round, and it's even worse when it comes to protein (*chicken chicken chicken, anyone?*)

The most obvious reason you need more variety in your diet is that each food contains a unique profile of nutrients and a unique presentation of toxins. We humans require a vast profile of nutrients and have limits to our bio-individual thresholds for each toxin. To meet our nutrient requirements, we need to eat a diverse diet, or else we're exposed to too many of a certain nutrient, too few of another nutrient, and too much of a certain toxin. Over time, this takes a toll on our health, immunity, appetite, and quality of life.

The not-so-obvious reason we need to eat a diverse diet is that, just like with an exercise routine, too much repetition can result in reduced benefits and eventually negative outcomes. A good analogy for this is to think about how repetitive movement can result in chronic pain. Let's imagine a hairdresser and how, for six to twelve hours a day, five days a week, they have both arms raised to cut, comb, dye, and blow dry a client's hair. After months or sometimes years of repeating the same movements, keeping their arms raised for hours at a time, what starts to happen? The hairdresser has chronic pain in their shoulders and neck, and in their hands from gripping scissors, and even lower back pain from standing for so many hours every day. Instead of being able to adapt, the body suffers from maladaptation. *Mal* meaning *dangerous* adaptation. The result is a detrimental effect that's hard to catch and difficult to reverse without removing the root cause (like quitting that line of work or changing duties to avoid further repetition and maladaptation).

When you eat the same foods day in and day out, you're likely to suffer from gradual maladaptations in your health. Your metabolism, energy, and weight begin to suffer. Your hormones, neurotransmitters, and mood are affected at an increasingly noticeable rate. Your digestive health declines, and you begin to rack up several annoyances with your gut, and you even develop nutrient deficiencies and impaired immunity. Little do you realize this is all because you lack variety in your diet and daily habits.

Human bodies are meant to adapt to ever-changing circumstances and inputs. We've evolved with these sorts of expectations in our genes. The more your body and brain need to adapt—within reason—the more resilient you become. The less frequently you require your body and brain to adapt, the less healthy and resilient you'll become.

Ancestral health tells us a lot about the importance of variety in our diet. Historically, humans only had access to seasonal foods and foods that were native to their surroundings. Nowadays, we can eat whatever we want, whenever we want—and we can eat the same damn thing 365 days of the year (like a PB&J sandwich every day for lunch) if that's what we choose to do. The trouble is—well, there's a long list of concerns, really—to acquire different nutrients and encourage natural adaptation inside our bodies, we need to regularly cycle through different foods.

This isn't just about health, okay? This is also about that smaller pant size you hope to fit into. It's also about the better mood you wish you were in, the fewer colds you wish you caught throughout the year, and the bloating you wish would go away. By varying your diet, everything starts to work better.

Advantages of Increased Variety In Your Diet

- **Improved metabolic health** by providing enough diverse nutrients for your mitochondria to energize you and fight off disease

- **Accelerated weight-loss results**

- **Enhanced diversity in your gut microbiome:** healthier gut, digestive health, skin, dental health, immunity, mental health, and brain function

- **Enhanced nutrition:** different foods provide different nutrients (either entirely or in different combinations and quantities). Plants versus animals, land or sea, and nuances within each class. Cooked versus raw. Fermented, sprouted, seasonal, and colorful. All different nutrients in varied ratios

  o **Enhanced mood and/or mental health**

  o **Enhanced fertility**

  o **Enhanced immunity**

- **Reduced toxicity:** eating too much of one food leads to a build-up of certain toxins, nutrient imbalances, or an overload of irritants present in that food (even healthy foods like onions, tomatoes, etc.)

- **Improved palate for **different foods:** the more variety you eat, the less picky you become, and the more types of foods you'll enjoy

**This also applies to the foods you crave. The more vegetables you eat, the more you'll crave vegetables. The more processed carbs you eat, the more you'll crave processed carbs. The more nut butter you eat, the more you'll crave it. *Why?* Because you're changing the population of certain species in your gut microbiome, and those microbes send messages to the brain asking for *more, more, more!* [mind-blown emoji]

After teaching this for years in my coaching business, I fully realize this isn't the easiest thing to change. I understand you have reservations or limitations that make it difficult for you to commit to more variety in your diet....

Common Internal Conflicts About Variety In Your Diet

- You're friggin' busy, and you're stuck buying/eating/ordering routine foods to help save time or effort.

- It can be challenging at first when you don't know how to cook new foods or if you don't enjoy shopping for new foods.

- You might lack the willingness to deviate from your personal favorites or to confront a long-standing issue with the texture/taste/smell of certain foods.

- Your self-identity is intertwined with food restrictions. For instance, "I only like chicken. I haven't eaten beef or pork for years, and seafood grosses me out." Or, "I hate vegetables. Always have, since I was a kid."

- Members of your household don't enjoy variety and complain when you try to change things up.

- The last time you tried to eat more variety, like eating salads, you experienced undesirable symptoms in your gut because you took on those changes too fast, and your body didn't have enough time to adapt.

How to Increase Variety in Your Diet

- **Focus on variety in two categories:** 1) **Vegetables/Fruits/Herbs** and 2) **Meat/Seafood** (or a variety of plant-proteins if you're strictly plant-based).

- **Aim to eat different colored vegetables and fruits every day**: red, orange/yellow, green, blue, purple, and white.

- **Mix it up with raw, cooked, cultured/fermented versions daily**.

- **Eat *seasonal* vegetables and fruits**—or whatever is on sale (which is often seasonal foods and frozen foods). Here's a great list of seasonal fruits and vegetables if you're inspired to try eating more seasonally: www.seasonalfoodguide.org. Simply enter your state and the time of year to find what's growing in season.

- **Try picking out one new vegetable each time you grocery shop.** Then, while you're in the grocery line, google *best way to cook* _____, or *easiest way to cook* _____. Bonus points if you allow your kid to choose the new vegetable at the store, which increases the likelihood they'll eat it.

- **Try a delivery service like a *Butcher Box* meat/seafood subscription.** Many of our members like to subscribe to Butcher Box because the custom box allows you to choose your favorite cuts of beef, chicken, pork, and seafood, all combined in one box (they even have some bison and turkey options, pre-cooked grass-fed pot roast, and unbeatable rotating deals to add variety to your routine order!). Then, each month, you get a box of frozen meat/seafood delivered to your door. This helps you eat more variety without depending on self-discipline. The meat/seafood is all sustainably and humanely raised, there's organic and 100% grass-fed beef, and there are many admirable principles the company lives by.

2 More Ways To Incorporate Variety with Less Planning Required

1. **Try a meal delivery service** - Prepared meal delivery makes it so much easier to eat a nutritious diet. My *favorite* prepared meals are from *Balanced Bites,* although the price makes these meals inaccessible for many family budgets. I've tried so many prepared meal companies, and these are the best for clean ingredients, portion size, and restaurant-worthy taste.

2. **Join a vegetable CSA from a local farm.** CSA stands for *Community Supported Agriculture*, and if you like to cook or you're determined to cook more vegetables, you can get seasonal vegetables delivered to your door (or pick them up from a nearby farm) when you join the CSA of a farm near you. You pay upfront for the season, and that money helps support the farm to continue its practices. In turn, you get a box of freshly harvested, more nutritious, seasonal produce. This challenges you to figure out how to use new veggies—like rutabaga, squash, wild onions, and so much more! Prices range widely from farm to farm, but typically, you should be saving money buying direct like this. Find one near you: *www. csacoalition.org/farm-search*

A Simple Meal Prep Method for Variety and Ease

Do you like to meal prep and batch-cook food for the week ahead? If you do, here's a template you can use to ensure you eat a variety of foods throughout the week.

Meal prep on the weekend with my 10-4-3 Method:

Prep/Cook 10 Veggies

Prep/Cook 4 Sides

Prep/Cook 3 Proteins

Add diversity by changing 50 percent of the foods in each category, week to week.

Sample Meal Prep Plan using my 10-4-3 Method:

Prep/Cook 10 Veggies

- (3) Roast: broccoli, sweet potatoes, and red bell peppers
- (1) Prep zucchini noodles
- (1) Saute baby greens with fresh garlic, EVOO (extra virgin olive oil), and balsamic vinegar
- (5) Prep salads with five colorful ingredients like salad greens, shredded purple cabbage, diced tomato, diced cucumber, and avocado (refrigerate the *whole* avocado to stop it from over-ripening until you're ready to dice and add to a salad at mealtime)

Prep/Cook 4 Sides/Fillers:

- (1) Cook lentils
- (1) Finely shred green cabbage (makes a great substitute for rice when placed under a hot, saucy protein or stir fry)
- (1) Cook quinoa
- (1) Prep or cook cauliflower rice

Prep/Cook 3 Proteins:

- (1) Marinate chicken with one of Primal Kitchen's dressing/marinades or a simple combo of smashed garlic cloves, dried or fresh thyme and oregano, sea salt, black pepper, a dash of apple cider vinegar, and avocado oil

- (1) Marinate peeled raw shrimp with sea salt, chili powder, oregano, and EVOO.

- (1) Cube and season beef chuck roast and toss it in a slow cooker with water or broth, a halved onion, and two bay leaves

CHAPTER 31

Time or Money: Something's Gotta Give *(at first)*

If you want to do things right this time around, something's gotta give. I know you don't *want* to pay more money for healthy food. With rising food costs and inflation, maybe your budget is already spread so thin that you don't even have more money to spend on food.

I know you don't have much time to spare for meal planning, prepping fresh ingredients, and cooking everything related to eating healthy. I get it. But something's gotta give. Time or money. Or a little of both. You decide.

When you want to improve your diet so you eat more variety and more whole foods, it will either cost you more time or more money. It's a simple fact that can't be ignored, so let's dive in and examine your options.

Save Money, Spend Time:

To improve your diet without spending more money on food, you'll need to be more hands-on and self-sufficient. That means you dedicate a bit more time to sourcing and prepping healthy food at home.

Join a CSA from a local farm (refer to those CSAs I was telling you about in the previous chapter). You might join the CSA in April by paying $450 for the season, but then all of your produce is paid for for the next 5 months. It may seem like more money because you'll have to pay upfront, but it comes out to $25 a week on fresh, local, whole foods you don't need to shop for (get some time back here). They'll also be more nutritious (more nutritional bang for your buck) compared to grocery store produce.

It will require more time in the kitchen, planning, washing, prepping, cooking, and maybe even preserving fresh foods.

Or maybe you just stick with your usual weekly grocery run but add an extra stop each week to be sure you always have fresh vegetables in the fridge. Or maybe you use the extra trip to stop at a natural grocer to get a few specialty items that aren't available at your conventional grocer (like gluten-free keto bread, plantain chips made with coconut oil, or Primal Kitchen salad dressing).

You'll save money by shopping at multiple stores for the best prices and options, and you'll waste less food because you'll go more frequently to stock up, spending a bit more time making these extra trips and planning for what foods are running low or needing a quick cook to prevent spoilage. Try the *Flashfood* app, which locates groceries near you with a looming expiration date that can be purchased at a steeply discounted rate!

When you want to save money and eat healthy, you'll spend more time prepping lunch and/or dinner ingredients—say, about 4 days a week—so meals and snacks are always ready and you don't end up hitting the drive-thru due to a lack of planning. You'll spend more time doing the dishes because you're cooking more, but it's worth it because you and your family eat healthier, feel more energized, and spend more time together at the dinner table.

It's always more challenging at first because you don't have much experience or a good system to execute these new routines. Once you get a few months of experience under your belt, you'll be so efficient and routine with it all that you'll feel proud and entirely capable of turning this into a lasting commitment to your health.

Save Time, Spend Money:

Most of my clients opt for this one (but that's probably because the people who purchase health coaching programs can resource or save extra money for solutions to help them meet their health-related goals). They're willing and able to spend a bit more on food or resources to make healthy eating more convenient *and* save time in the process.

When you choose this route, you'll spend more money buying everything from the natural grocer versus stopping at multiple stores. You'll spend more money buying prepared meals or subscribing to meal kit delivery services. But you'll save oodles of time without the need to plan, prep, or even cook your meals, and healthy food is always ready and waiting for you.

You'll spend more money on other resources like buying supplements or working with a functional medicine doctor to figure out some underlying conditions and how that's been affecting your ability to reach your goals. You'll spend more money on services like a babysitter or hiring a virtual assistant to help delegate some of the excessive obligations and stressors in your life so you can more readily adopt and maintain a healthy lifestyle.

Hybrid Solutions:

Where can you reallocate your dollars so you can spend a bit more on pre-pared meal delivery while you get adapted to some of these new changes? Can you cut back on other subscriptions or streaming services or reduce the frequency of dining out at restaurants? Where can you reallocate your *time* so you don't get interrupted during work to drive your kid to practice. Instead, you can use that time to plan dinner or run to the store if needed.

A lot of these changes are only necessary in the beginning while you're trying to build a new habit. You want to standardize something before you optimize it. So maybe it's not ideal for you to spend money on a prepared meal service, but it's the essential move you can make to help kickstart a habit of healthy eating while breaking the habit of snacking all day, or eating frozen pizza, ordering fast food, or delivery.

Getting in your own way

I see this time and time again with my clients. They're ready to make the changes, and they want to start with what's ideal instead of first standardizing the changes. They'll say, "I just need to start meal prepping every Sunday." I ask, "Have you had some good experiences doing weekly meal prep in the past?"

They reply, "No. I'm terrible at meal prep. I always say I'm going to do it but never really have. Things always come up with the kids, and because I didn't plan the groceries, I just end up buying what's easy and routine."

Why would you expect to fundamentally change yourself to start a new habit? First, it's about standardizing a new action. Experimenting and getting a habit off the ground. *Then*, once it becomes more of a habit, you start to optimize it, shaping the new habit into what is ideal.

So maybe that client would, instead, temporarily start ordering a meal kit that sends pre-prepped ingredients so that they only need to make time for cooking and follow the recipe. That's already a change. Currently, they don't cook much at all. So if they use a pre-prepped meal kit and follow through with the action to cook the meal as planned, it's a win! It's a stepping stone toward the new, ideal habit of eventually cooking and prepping meals for the whole week.

Or what if this client goes to the grocery store and pays extra for those pre-chopped onions, zucchini noodles, and diced sweet potato from the produce section, as well as some pre-cooked frozen chicken breast and breakfast sausage? Even though they pay quite a bit for the pre-prepped stuff, they save time and effort as they get acclimated to the new responsibility of cooking real food. Then, once they get the hang of it, they'll buy whole produce and raw meats to save money and prep them at home.

Remember, fasting on its own is a time-and-money-saving endeavor. Once you're fasting more often, you'll see you spend less time thinking about food or preparing food. You save money by eating fewer meals during the week. You eat out less often. Over time, the daily practice of fasting means less pain and inflammation, less frequent medical visits, less need for medication, and less likelihood of developing chronic disease down the line.

Part 3 Action Step:
Try Building Your Plate Like This

To take action here and build a nutrient-dense meal for yourself, you'll need some healthy ingredients on hand and a plan of action. When will you next visit the grocery store? It's time to make a list. Or would it be easier to order your groceries online so you're more comfortable browsing new items and looking something up when you have a question? Use the Nutrient Dense Food List for inspiration (Chapter 22), and start small so you can follow through with confidence.

Next, what will you eat for your first meal of the day? Where will you order from, or when will you take time to prepare that meal? Planning ahead for *what* you'll eat makes it much more likely you'll be successful with intermittent fasting and reducing your intake of nutrient-poor foods throughout the week. Take it one day at a time because you're making changes, and habit change takes time.

If you decide to save time by using a meal delivery service, schedule some time upfront to find a service and place your first order. You'll need at least thirty minutes, probably more, to decide on which service and to set up that order. Picking out your meals is fun! Using your personal calendar, schedule a time to accomplish that within the next 48 hours. You want to take action now because there will be some lag time before your first delivery arrives. Don't let perfection or decision fatigue get in the way. Try one out as an experiment. You can easily cancel and try another if it's not right for you.

Action Step: Try Building Your Plate Like This

No matter where you're at on your IF journey, by following the general guidelines of this diagram, you'll eat a nutrient-dense, varied diet.

The Traditional Human Diet Plate

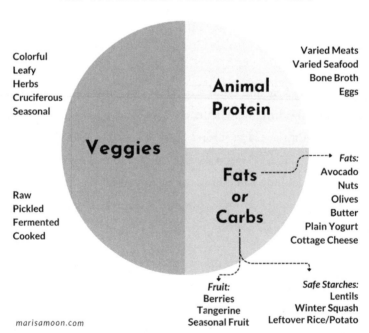

- **50% of your plate is comprised of vegetables**: a widely varied rotation of colorful, seasonal, leafy, and cruciferous veggies and plants, as well as raw, cooked, and fermented preparations.

- **25% of your plate (or more) is comprised of protein**: a varied rotation of clean meat, clean seafood, and/or nutrient-dense animal products like poultry, eggs, fish roe, wild game, canned sardines, bone broth, whey protein powder, etc., targeting 25 g or more of protein per meal.

- **25% of your plate (or less) is comprised of healthy fats or carbs (fruit or *safe starches*),** depending on your goals, your fasting routine, your daily activity level, and your individualized needs and preferences.

Some Healthy Fats to Consider:

- Avocado or Guacamole

- Nuts (variety)

- Olives

- Pumpkin Seeds (pepitas)

- Extra virgin olive oil

- MCT oil

- Plain full-fat yogurt or kefir

- Organic and/or raw milk cheese (if you tolerate dairy)

- Minimally-processed dairy-free cheese (typically nut-based)

Some Fruits and Safe Starches to Consider:

- Berries

- Tangerines

- Lentils

- Chickpeas

- Quinoa

- Mung beans

- Potato (especially eaten cold or as leftovers for the development of resistant starch)

- Sweet potato

- Winter squash

- Green plantain

- Yuca, taro, or malanga coco (preferably not mashed, pureed, or flour-based)

- White basmati rice (especially as leftovers for *resistant starch*)

- White glutinous rice (sweet/mochi rice) (especially as leftovers for resistant starch)

- Occasional (limited serving) paleo pasta, paleo tortillas, nixtamal-ized tortillas (corn tortillas made specifically with masa harina, which is corn processed with lime or calcium hydroxide to enhance digestibility and nutrition), paleo toast, etc....

To explore the many different ways you can start building your new, nutrient-dense meals, take a look at example meals at marisamoon.com/notsofast/resources or scan the resources QR code here:

PART 4

Extend Your Fasts

RESET

Reduce Carbs

Eat Nourishing Foods

Start with 12 Hours

Extend Your Fasts

Thoughtfully Adapt

CHAPTER 33

Not So Fast

Not So Fast.

This should be pretty simple. But it's not as simple as we wish it were. After coaching hundreds of people through my RESET method, I can see intermittent fasting isn't as simple as the fasting community makes it out to be. Popular advice usually suggests you start with 16:8 fasting and work your way up to 18-hour fasts in a matter of three weeks.

That advice tends to work only for healthy men, people on a keto-ish diet who are already fat-adapted, or people who already eat a nutrient-dense diet, are hormonally balanced and get adequate sleep. And guess what? That's a very small percentage of the population, like, less than 10 percent. That leaves us with 90 percent of our American population who are trying to follow dietary advice that ignores our common circumstances (chronic stress, hormonal imbalances, poor metabolic health, insufficient sleep, and a nutrient-poor diet).

Instead of hoping you're part of the lucky 10 percent who can just skip breakfast *and* lunch—because you'd rather sip on your coffee and not worry about preparing a healthy meal so you can keep working your ass off while praying for fat loss—I'll challenge you to extend your fasts in a more strategic way.

How to Extend Your Fasts

For individuals who are currently fasting < 18 hours per day

Step 1: Get clear about your current baseline fasting window. How many hours are you currently fasting most days of the week? 13 hours? 14.5 hours? Define that number by looking at your Life Fasting Tracker history so you're not guessing.

Step 2: Stick to your current baseline fast until it becomes seemingly effortless for ≥ 4 days in a row. *Because* weekends tend to disrupt your usual routine, I highly recommend you test this out by fasting the same length of time through the weekend, too, before increasing your fasting window.

Step 3: Assess how comfortable you've been for the past 4 days in your current fasting window. Once you're comfortable for a minimum of 4 days in a row, it may be time to increase your fasting window by 30–60 minutes. Repeat step two with this length of fast.

Step 4: Repeat Step 3.

Why stick with your current length of fasts for > 4 days in a row?

Because this strategy allows you time to experience the fasting window while situational variables change day to day. This serves as an essential wake-up call, gives your mindset time to adapt, and prevents you from having to rely on so much willpower to continue. It also gives your gut time to adapt so you don't have negative side effects like constipation that can occur from making abrupt changes to your diet.

Mary's story:

Mary is currently fasting for 13 hours consistently. On Monday, she decides to try a 14-hour window. Monday goes well as she fasts for 14 hours. It felt good, and when her window was up, she was happy to eat but didn't feel starving or out of control around food. She planned ahead for a healthy meal and made sure she could break away from work to eat around the 14-hour mark.

Since Monday went so well, Mary was inspired to try 16 hours on Tuesday because it's what she'd heard an ideal fasting schedule looks like. Tuesday rolled around, and she's watching the clock all afternoon. The voice in her head is saying, *One of those breakfast sandwiches from Dunkin sounds so good right now. What is wrong with you? Get back to work. It's not time to eat; you still have three hours to go. You're not going to lose that weight unless you show more willpower.* Mary can't believe how distracted she is by her appetite that day. Even at the 14-hour mark, she's glancing at the clock every fifteen minutes.

When I check in with Mary about her experience, I ask her a few questions: "Tell me more about Tuesday. Like, how was work? What was different about your work schedule and work tasks on Tuesday compared to Monday?"

We enjoy some back-and-forth conversation as we investigate the variables in her situation. More questions I ask include, "How was your morning on Tuesday? Anything different happen at home? What was your evening like on Monday? Did you have a relaxing evening or a stressful one? How did you sleep?"

Our conversation leads to some interesting discoveries. Mary explains, "I got in an argument with my teenage son Monday night because he wanted to stay at a friend's house on a school night, and I don't think that's appropriate, so I said no. Things spiraled, and he threatened to run away. It wasn't the first time. I cried myself to sleep. It was fine the morning after we'd both slept it off, though. And my workday was pretty normal. I had more meetings on Monday, but Tuesday was just easy stuff like updating spreadsheets and checking for errors. I also didn't bring my lunch that day, so I kept thinking, 'What should I order to eat? Will it be delivered in time before my 2 p.m. meeting?'"

Mary just listed three reasons that would explain why fasting for 14–16 hours on Tuesday was so much harder than fasting 14 hours on Monday. Can you spot the three reasons?

Reason #1. Mary had an emotionally charged evening that left her crying herself to sleep. That means she had unresolved stress and emotions lingering in her system the next day, which can result in increased cortisol and ghrelin, which means more urges to soothe unresolved emotions with food. Furthermore, it's reasonable to assume the stress and anxiety were enough to disrupt her quality of sleep. If Mary doesn't get as much restorative sleep as her body needs, her anxiety will be heightened, and hunger signals and food-reward systems will be heightened, too, making her more likely to think about food and feel hungry much earlier than usual.

Reason #2. On Monday, Mary had more meetings at work. Being at virtual meetings (or in-person meetings without food present) makes it easier to fast because you simply don't have the privacy to eat until the meeting has adjourned. Furthermore, Mary's work tasks on Tuesday were easy stuff, like updating spreadsheets and checking for errors. Those types of tasks can be passive or boring, which results in the brain looking for a hit of dopamine (which she'd get from behaviors like reaching for a snack, ordering food, or checking her Facebook notifications).

Reason #3. Mary didn't have food ready or planned for Tuesday. She was preoccupied with the possibilities of ordering food (dopamine hit!) and the urgency at which she should order so her food would arrive in time for her to eat before the 2 o'clock meeting.

So, what if, instead, Mary had stuck with 14-hour fasts according to my recommendations. From Monday through Thursday, or even longer so she could test it on the weekend, Mary's goal would be to stick with 14-hour fasts until it felt pretty effortless and natural for at least 4 days *in a row*. This gives her a chance, on days like that Tuesday, to become more aware of the changing variables each day and how that affects her hunger and ability to fast. She'll feel more capable of achieving the goal she set because she understands part of the accomplishment is to observe and be patient until her body and mind adapt. She'll stick with 14 hours until it feels pretty good on auto-pilot. That's why I call it a baseline fasting window.

I remind Mary that even if it takes a couple of weeks before she's ready to extend her fasting window, there are so many benefits to appreciate along the way. A slower approach means more practice at planning her meals in advance and building that habit so she's not preoccupied about what to eat when she breaks her fast, and she makes healthier choices at mealtime with much less willpower required. She'll feel more confident because fasting will become more effortless and routine before increasing the difficulty. Finally, she'll have more opportunities to experiment with non-food rewards to turn to while doing boring, passive tasks at work during the fasting window.

Remember, intermittent fasting should make you feel better, sharper, more energized, and healthier. If it's ever a nuisance, causing unwanted side effects, or just plain disruptive to your other responsibilities, that's a sign it's time to slow down and go back to a baseline fasting window that's comfortable for you at this time.

Hunger Pangs may occur when you shift your eating times or increase your fasting time, especially after being routine with your mealtimes. You experience that pit in your stomach when you try to switch your routine mealtime, and your stomach starts pumping out ghrelin as a result. Hunger pangs tend to fade within twenty minutes of onset. They're nothing to be alarmed about, although they can be quite distracting.

Experts suggest that, in a balanced person, the body can adapt to about a 45-minute shift per day when it comes to meal timing. Kind of like adjusting to a new time zone, your circadian clock and neural pathways need to adjust before you can expect to feel great eating at a new time. However, the ability to shift 45 minutes is only expected in individuals who are generally healthy and balanced. That's why it's important to take it slow. Most people aren't balanced, meaning they have hormonal imbalances, chronic stress, they're under-slept, etc.... Those imbalances suggest that even a 45-minute shift in your routine mealtime will result in feelings of hunger and discomfort. This brings us back to my recommendation that you aim to stick with a current fasting window (thus, a routine mealtime) for a minimum of 4 days, or until it becomes nearly effortless, before increasing your fast.

Fasting can be so beneficial because it provides a Goldilocks degree of stress on your system. This Goldilocks degree of stress triggers adaptation in your body, thanks to a system of reactions caused by *hormesis*. Once you understand a bit more about hormesis, you'll feel even more accepting of this slow and steady approach to fasting. Ready for more?

CHAPTER 34

Hormesis: A Beneficial Adaptation in Response to a Stressor

One key concept to familiarize yourself with when it comes to fasting is a term called *Hormesis*. Hormesis is a reaction that occurs in the body when our cells are adapting to a stressor. It's not just any stressor we're talking about here. *A hormetic stressor* is something you're exposed to that stresses your cells just enough to trigger a favorable, adaptive response, whereas being exposed to *too* much stress could cause an unfavorable, maladaptive response.

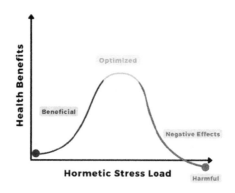

Figure 34.1 - Hormetic Stress Load

As you can see in Figure 34.1, hormetic stressors can provide you with many beneficial effects or even healthy optimization, but when hormesis is abused or overused in the wrong conditions, it can result in negative effects that are ultimately harmful to your system.

Exercise is a hormetic stressor, and so is fasting.

In the words of famous biohacker Dave Asprey, "Hormesis is a fancy word for 'What doesn't kill you or weaken you makes you stronger'."

It's easier to understand the adaptive benefits and potential downsides of hormesis when we use exercise as the example. You're well aware exercise can cause a range of positive reactions and benefits in your body and mind. The reactions and benefits range anywhere from feeling more energized, sleeping better, relieving mental stress, gaining stronger muscles, and increasing balance and agility to having stronger bones, increased circulation, clearer skin, and a better mood.

How is it that a certain degree of physical activity can stimulate all those seemingly unrelated benefits across your body and mind? Well, it's thanks to cellular reactions that are triggered by the stress induced by exercise. Those cellular reactions occur because we have programming built into our DNA that tells our cells they should learn and grow from this strenuous experience so next time it happens (AKA next time you exercise), you'll be able to handle it even better than before.

The simplest example of this is when you do strength training to help build more muscle. If you lift heavy weights or do enough repetitions, the stress will cause muscle tissue to break down, and energy will be depleted. Soon after the challenge has ended, muscle cells are prompted to regenerate and grow more muscle proteins (= bigger muscles) and to continuously take in more energy for hours after you've finished the exercise (AKA eagerly absorb the carbs and protein you ate after your workout). Your muscles adapt to a good workout by getting bigger, faster, stronger, and more efficient with how they utilize energy.

A parallel set of reactions occurs with fasting. You can think of it as if you're building your fasting muscles. When you're fasting, your DNA gets the message that it should handle the situation by optimizing energy usage, brain power, inflammatory processes, hormonal expression, and so much more. Your cells get chemical messages to prepare for food deprivation in the future by enhancing your ability to thrive in a state of such manageable stress.

When it comes to hormesis, *less is more*, so to speak. You train your body for increased hormesis, just like you train it for fasting, and thoughtfully adapt as your circumstances change.

Things That Stimulate Hormesis:

- Fasting
- Caloric restriction
- Diet-induced ketosis
- Exercise
- Sprinting
- Cold plunge, cold therapy, or ice bath
- Cryotherapy
- Infrared sauna or therapy
- Hot sauna
- Acupuncture
- Hypoxic breath work
- Intermittent hypoxic training (IHT)
- Blood-flow restriction training
- Ingesting certain plant compounds or supplements (such as resveratrol, curcumin/turmeric, and sulforaphane from broccoli sprouts)
- Learning something new and challenging
- Ozone therapy
- Hyperbaric oxygen therapy

I remember when I was hosting my podcast, The Foundation of Wellness, and interviewing someone about infrared light therapy. I asked my guest something I knew my audience was thinking: "How can this have so many wide-ranging benefits? And how is it that infrared light seems to have all these benefits, but so does exercise, and so does CBD oil, and the same goes for fasting?" I wish my guest had replied with the concept of hormesis because, at the time, that would've been pretty sweet for me and my listeners to consider.

As you can see from the list above, so many therapies and activities exist through which we can stimulate hormesis in the body. They each present our systems with a genetically-recognized stressor, in just the right amount, that triggers a cascade of beneficial adaptations and increased resilience. *Cool!*

It helps to become familiar with the concept of hormesis, so you understand how fasting can possibly have so many benefits across a seemingly endless array of health factors.

Then, when someone asks you how it's possible for fasting to reduce your high blood pressure, improve your arthritis, fibroid tumors, energy levels, appetite, metabolism, body fat, mood, and your ability to think more sharply—you can say "Because, just like exercise, it's a beneficial stressor that causes all these positive reactions to occur. Your body starts cleaning up messes and making you healthier on every level—as long as you don't abuse it."

"Hormesis is the ultimate natural pathway to anti-aging. Quite simply, it is THE only way to reverse aging and diminishing mitochondrial health."
- Energy expert Ari Whitten, Energy Blueprint Labs

Ari continues, "People who don't regularly engage in hormesis—which is over 90 percent of the Western world—are pretty much guaranteed to lose about half their potential to produce energy between the ages of twenty to forty…and again from ages forty to seventy. But this only happens to people who don't engage in hormesis."

*"When you indulge in endless modern comforts and conveniences—
like staying constantly warm and well-fed—and never stress the
organism to spur hormesis, your mind and body atrophy across the
board, and you become less resilient to all forms of stress."*
- Mark Sisson, *Keto For Life*

Note: if you're burned out, chronically under-slept, healing from injury, or if your body is under too much stress to a chronic degree, the safest forms of hormesis would be hypoxic breath work, hyperbaric oxygen therapy, some form of cold therapy, moderate use of an infrared sauna, and the ingestion of certain plant compounds and antioxidants. Most other hormetic stressors, including fasting, ketosis, and calorie restriction, cause too much stress when your body is already under a crippling amount. Same goes for high-intensity exercise or weight-lifting. Until sleep is improved and the body is more recovered, the risks far outweigh any possibility of benefits, and maladaptation is the most likely result.

～

Something I see with my clients quite often is this desire they have to push and push and *push* their bodies in hopes that more effort will yield better weight-loss results. I give plenty of warning, explaining the concept of hormesis in hopes we'll trust in the delicate nature of this pursuit. I then found a very helpful article on the SAFM (School of Applied Functional Medicine) website in which they advise practitioners on how to effectively support clients in their weight-loss goals. I found it to be validating and quite insightful.

Take a look at this excerpt:

"It is critical to teach people that the body views excess weight as an assurance against an uncertain future. The body will naturally increase adipose tissue if it feels our survival is being threatened. Weight loss will be natural (and sustainable) when sources of stress and inflammation are addressed. Forcing weight loss on its own, independent from addressing root causes, will not only be temporary but will likely cause new body weight reset points that are progressively higher. Setting proper expectations that weight loss is often the last perceived benefit of addressing the root causes of disease is, of course, critical for patient engagement, commitment, and persistence."

Let's go through that excerpt together, sentence by sentence, so you can really absorb the wisdom it provides.

- "It is critical to teach people that the body views excess weight as an assurance against an uncertain future."

As you learned in Chapter 15: *Carbohydrate Curve*, your body fat is designed to serve as a survival advantage, protecting against food scarcity and environmental threats and providing dependable energy needed to persevere through such challenges ahead.

- "The body will naturally increase adipose tissue if it feels our survival is being threatened."

When stressors become too chronic or threatening to your body (regardless of how serious you think the threat is), your body works hard to resist fat loss and to increase fat gain because, in doing so, it feels more prepared for future threats.

- "Weight loss will be natural (and sustainable) when sources of stress and inflammation are addressed."

It's an unfortunate fact of modern life that no matter how bad you want sustainable weight loss, in most cases, it won't be yours unless you get curious and become determined to reduce the chronic stress and inflammation in your body.

- "Forcing weight loss on its own, independent from addressing root causes, won't only be temporary but will likely cause new body weight reset points that are progressively higher."

You really want to lose weight for that beach vacation coming up, so you start some new fad diet like *Optivia*. Although you nearly reached your goal to lose weight before vacation, you feel defeated when, two months later, you've put all the weight back on. Then, things get even more disheartening when you're even heavier after six months have passed. What's happening here? Your body felt threatened by your drastic attempts to lose weight without addressing the root cause, such as an undiagnosed thyroid condition or unresolved PCOS, that it's now overcompensating to protect you from that weight-loss 'threat' in the future by making your baseline weight higher than ever before. This baseline weight is your new *weight set point*, and your body works hard to maintain it or increase it against your desperate attempts.

- "Setting proper expectations that weight loss is often the last perceived benefit of addressing the root causes of disease is, of course, critical for patient engagement, commitment, and persistence."

It's a tricky balance, really, for someone on a long-term weight-loss journey. When you first start intermittent fasting, and you follow the steps in this guidebook, you're usually pleased to see the weight coming off in those first few months of adaptation. Hormesis is working for you. But what happens when you continue to do the same thing, fasting the same length most days of the week, getting comfortable? Hormesis is no longer stimulated. Your body is used to the challenge, so it no longer needs to adapt. So, just like you'd need to change up your workout, you need to change up your fasts. Throw in a 24-hour fast. It sounds scarier than it is. Heck, throw in a 42-hour fast. That's the one that surprised me the most. I felt so dang good; my brain was unstoppable. Still, you don't want to abuse these longer fasts, or fasting in general, if your body is suffering from imbalanced foundational needs like emotional stress, sleep, hormonal dysfunction, chronic inflammation, or threats to your immune system.

CHAPTER 35

Stressed. Every. Day.

Earlier, in one of the very first chapters, I shared with you the 7 key factors that make or break progress with fasting. *Stress* is one of those key factors. Stress comes in many forms, including psychological or emotional stress—like the stress we all experienced when schools and offices closed during the 2020 pandemic lockdown, and we were forced to adapt to so many huge changes and endure those changes for an entire year.

There's also physical stress, which can even be caused by or exacerbated by those emotional stressors. Physical stress is like that chronic tension in your shoulders, the sharp pain in your stomach experienced after eating, the recurring arthritis pain in your knees and hands, or simply stubbing your toe on the corner of your bed frame. Then there's a wide range of biological stressors your body might be battling, such as infectious disease, chronic inflammation, autoimmune disease, lack of sleep, PMS and dysregulated menstrual cycles, chronic allergies, gut dysbiosis, and exposure to heavy metal toxins or mold in your environment.

Stress plays a major role in your ability to achieve results with intermittent fasting. One could say stress plays the largest role, and that's because fasting *is* a stressor. That's why fasting works—*or doesn't work*. It's a hormetic stressor, as you're now aware. If you try to fast too long for the current threshold of stress tolerance of your body and mind, you can see it backfire in the form of stalled weight loss, increased hunger, binge eating, forgetfulness, rebellion, self-sabotage, feelings of defeat or failure, and hormonal dysfunction (spotty periods, terrible PMS, thyroid dysfunction, infertility, etc.).

To ignore the stress piece is to ignore your ultimate goal of sustainable weight loss.

Stress is a normal and expected part of the human experience. We're designed to operate in stressful conditions and even improve as a result. But the degree and consistency at which we're being exposed to the stressor(s) is what takes this beyond what's tolerable and into destructive territory.

Acute stressors are sudden or targeted events that cause short-term stress. An acute stressor could be as short-lasting as a roller coaster ride or even as long as 3 days while you work your tail off trying to meet a deadline. An acute stressor could also be a sprained ankle or a few days of PMS before your period hits. The stress response caused by acute scenarios usually returns to normal levels once the original source of stress is over with–as long as you don't abuse your body while it's in a vulnerable state.

Here's the evolutionary mismatch we're now facing with acute stressors. Many of us are exposed to so many acute stressors so consistently (work deadline, asshole boss, teacher calls about problems at school again, financial problems, car problems, family illness, throwing your back out again, home renovations gone wrong, etc.). Together, the relentless stressors create chronic stress. *Chronic* is bad.

Maybe you try, but there's nothing you can do to get rid of those stressors. So, what can you do to prevent it from resulting in a state of chronic stress? You can learn to better cope in the state of stress, to manage or minimize the severity of the stressors, and to complete the stress cycle more regularly.

I first learned about completing the stress cycle from Emily and Amelia Nagoski, the authors of *Burnout: The Secret to Unlocking the Stress Cycle*. Right away, I recognized how much sense this made from an ancestral health perspective. The authors brought the concept to light by using a deer as their example of how and why to complete the stress cycle. A deer might be calmly eating grass when they suddenly hear a rustling in the surrounding woods. The deer's nervous system goes into high-alert, heartbeat raising, pupils dilating, ears waiting for just one more hint to dash, and bam! At alarming speed, the deer sprints away from harm and into safety. Minutes later, once the threat is no longer a concern, the deer shivers or shakes off the stress from head-to-toe. This full body shake helps the animal complete the stress cycle, signaling to the nervous system that it's time to shift out of the sympathetic fight-or-flight state and into a parasympathetic state—the relaxed mode in which the deer can calmly enjoy nibbling on grass again.

We modern-day humans don't complete the stress cycle, but we need to. Our coworker makes a snide remark about our ideas in the meeting, and our heart starts to race. When the meeting is over, we go back to our desk, our heart still pumping wildly, telling ourselves to just calm down and let it go. We try to stifle the stress and sweep it under our desk. We try to distract ourselves, watch a funny cat video and reach for a snack, but nothing works, and we're in a shit mood the rest of the afternoon. If, instead, we did something to complete the stress cycle, we'd feel like we'd hit the reset button. We'd shift our nervous system back to a state of calm, reminding the body it's no longer in danger.

There are very few instances in life where we instinctively *do* complete the stress cycle. One instance is when we ride a scary roller coaster at an amusement park (or insert any adrenaline-pumping activity such as bungee jumping or zip lining). What do we do when we're going down that scary roller coaster drop? We scream! We instinctively scream because it helps to move the explosive energy out of our bodies. When the ride ends, we're trembling. The whole body is shaking, and we let out a few more hoots, saying, "Woo!

That was crazy!" We laugh, we bounce our way off the ramp as we exit the ride, and we giggle at the thrill we just experienced. All of those reactions help reset the nervous system so you aren't trembling in fear the rest of the day walking around the amusement park (or even having trouble sleeping afterward).

11 Ideas to Help Complete The Stress Cycle

1. **Shake it off.** Literally shake your whole body like a dog coming out of a bath, shaking your arms and hips until you bust out in laughter or break a sweat (usually, this is just a matter of seconds). Let out a deep, sighing breath and smile. All is well.

2. **Punch a soft, inanimate object** like a mattress, couch, or punching bag. Punch, punch, punch like a maniac until you get it all out.

3. **Scream.** In your car, in your closet, in your pillow. Scream like you're starring in a horror movie if you have to. Get it out!

4. **Sob.** Cry your eyes out with careful attention paid to forbidding self-defeating thoughts. Instead, in your mind or out loud, repeat a mantra like, *Tears will help. You'll feel better soon.*

5. **Dance, dance, dance.** The music should be loud. Play a song that makes you move, and let it out (it's okay if you cry; it often triggers a cry in me, too).

6. **Sing out loud** to a favorite song with fortitude. Sing it like you mean it! Again, it's okay if you cry—maybe even better!

7. **Watch something hilariously funny,** like a stand-up comedy routine (preferably alongside another person since we laugh harder in the presence of others), for a minimum of twenty minutes. You'll feel refreshed and reminded that not everything in life needs to be so serious.

8. **Have sex or engage in self-pleasure** that leads to an orgasm. Afterward, remind yourself that life isn't all that bad.

9. **Do short, intense bursts of exercise,** like sprints, burpees, or hitting a round at the batting cages. Keep the intense bursts limited to between 30 and 60 seconds, depending on your current activity level. Take adequate breaks between bursts so your body can recover each time. Focus on the movement, not on the emotional stressor. Marvel in the ability of your body and finish with a few minutes of mindful gratitude.

10. **Do something that scares or thrills you** but results in the reassurance that you're safe: drive a speedy go-cart, go on a scary carnival ride, jump on a giant trampoline, ski down a mountain, play a game of tag, throw an axe, or watch a thriller and laugh at yourself when you scream!

11. **Take a 30–60-minute walk/jog/run** outdoors and in solitude (without music or listening to anything). It's imperative you resist ruminating thoughts about the stressor you're facing. Console your thoughts with glass-half-full perspectives and advice you'd give a friend in that situation. Remind yourself that even though things are hard, it will get easier or better with time. You can handle it. You will be okay.

CHAPTER 36

Mitochondrial Stress

W e can't talk about stress without talking about where energy metab-olism happens at the most important level: the mitochondria. You learned about mitochondria earlier in Part 3. They're those little energy factories, the powerhouses of the cells. Yes, but that's not all they are. There's a major function besides energy production that's not as widely known or mentioned. Mitochondria are also threat detectors and defenders. They detect threats to the cell's health—sensing danger, disease, inflammation—and determine whether the cell should use the energy to defend itself or to make new energy for you to thrive.

This threat-detecting function is called the *cell danger response* (CDR). "Persistent activation of CDR inhibits healing and leads to chronic illness. Mitochondria regulate CDR by monitoring and responding to the physical, chemical, and microbial conditions within and around the cell."

In some cases, this is called the *integrated stress response* (ISR). See the word *stress* in there? Yeah, the cell is stressed. Its survival is threatened, which means the mitochondria will switch over to optimizing survival instead of optimizing energy output.

Your mitochondria are partitioning energy in a teeter-totter-like fashion. The more stressed the body becomes, the more the mitochondria will prioritize cellular defense and neglect energy production. And the more it needs to prioritize defending itself, the harder it is to get back to energy metabolism for healthy living.

When you're chronically stressed, or your body is, it could mean you're at a crossroads with your health. A fork in the road. Stay straight, and you'll continue on the overly stressed cellular defense path that starts with tanked energy, leading to poorer health, chronic disease, and a shortened lifespan. Or, you can turn right, so to speak, taking the path toward wellness and start protecting your mitochondria from threats right now.

How do you protect your mitochondria from threats? By reducing your stress or getting better at coping with it, prioritizing sleep and optimizing it, reducing your chemical exposure, eating foods that agree with your body, eating foods that are nutrient-dense and antioxidant-rich, and engaging in appropriate degrees of hormesis—meeting your body where it's at. *Not so fast.*

Remember all that talk in Part 2 about chronic insulin (eating too often and eating too much in the way of sugar/carbs) and how years of that abuse leads to weight gain and insulin resistance? Well, Dr. Benjamin Bikman, a leading metabolic researcher, explains that scientists have identified **three primary causes of insulin resistance**:

1. Chronically elevated insulin

2. Chronically elevated stress hormones (primarily cortisol and adrenaline)

3. Elevated inflammatory proteins (known as *inflammatory cytokines*, which alert the immune system that it's under attack).

Number one, chronically elevated insulin, is the main reason you'll integrate fasting and reduce your sugar and carb intake in pursuit of greater health.

The last two causes, chronically elevated stress hormones, and elevated inflammatory proteins, are the reason for so much discussion on your stress hormones and the health of your mitochondria. Chronic stress and chronic inflammation are a recipe for insulin resistance, and it's time we get clear about how that's messing up your metabolism.

CHAPTER 37

Cortisol and Glucose

In his ground-breaking book, *The Obesity Code*, Dr. Jason Fung dedicates an entire chapter to Cortisol. Cortisol is our primary stress hormone and plays important roles in energy availability and carbohydrate metabolism. You may have heard of cortisol as the cause of visceral fat, the dangerous type of fat that accumulates around your belly and leads to a cascade of inflammation and systemic consequences that are best avoided.

This can become a vicious cycle between cortisol and visceral fat because the fat cells on your belly have four times as many cortisol receptors as the fat cells elsewhere in your body. Basically, your belly fat exploits cortisol and, as a result, uses it to build more belly fat.

Chronic stress = chronic cortisol pumping through your body. What's more, as Dr. Mindy Pelz says in *Fast Like A Girl*, "Cortisol can raise insulin as much as a piece of cake can."

When you live with chronic stress, you stimulate cortisol too consistently. You see, when you're stressed enough for the body to think you're in immediate danger, cortisol is released into your bloodstream, and a whole series of chemical reactions takes place so that, like the deer earlier, you're prepared and energized to fight or flee from whatever threat you're up against. This made sense for humans when we were pre-civilized beings living in nature with a wide range of predators and survival threats.

But nowadays, we don't need it as often. Our bodies don't realize that, though. The chronic anxiety, ruminating thoughts, rapid heart rate during meetings or presentations, rushing day to day trying to stay on top of your overbooked schedule—those experiences cause cortisol to rise too often and stay elevated. That means glucose is being dumped into your bloodstream whether you eat or not.

What's more is that cortisol and adrenaline inhibit insulin so that glucose remains available for fight-or-flight. Due to chronically-elevated cortisol and the complex interplay between hormones, this leads to elevated fasting glucose and insulin resistance. All the while, your brain sends hunger signals, demanding more nutrients, carbs, and junk for a whole slew of reasons I won't bore you with.

A sound explanation for why you become crazy hungry during high-stress periods is that today, we're living in a way that exceeds our genetic capacity for psychological stressors, especially without *completing the stress cycle*. Again, we're talking about another evolutionary mismatch. We're not built for that kind of chronic stress. Especially if you're a restrained eater—someone who consciously and consistently tries to restrict the amount of food you consume—you're far more likely to eat more when you're stressed, feeling out of control with your desire to eat, and bingeing out on sugar and starchy carbs.[37]

Unfortunately, that's not all that happens when our nervous system is so stressed. Because your body is preparing to fight or flee, it puts the breaks on other energy-intensive systems that aren't needed. This means the energy can be prioritized for the immediate threat. That means when you're highly stressed, digestion is stalled, your muscles and connective tissues no longer repair or rebuild, and you can even *lose* muscle tissue because your body starts to convert muscle proteins into glucose to help give you energy to fight or flee!

And if this happens every day for long enough, the consequences can range from high blood pressure and high triglycerides to chronic fatigue and Cushing's disease, or the accumulation of arterial plaque, excess belly fat, chronic inflammation, insulin resistance—of course, type 2 diabetes, and relentless weight gain.

So you can roll your eyes at me all you want when I talk about reducing your stress and improving your sleep, but the significance can't be denied. If you want to slim down, fight disease, and feel healthier, these are critical areas to prioritize and improve in your life. Somehow, someway, you can and you will. *Just don't give up.*

What to remember:

What happens when you're highly stressed? Your liver dumps stored glycogen into your bloodstream to prepare you for a fight. And for what? For you to just sit there and sweep that glucose under the proverbial rug? Thus, more insulin is required to direct that glucose out of your bloodstream and back into storage. So, next time you try to hold your stress in and bury it, go scream into a pillow instead. Run a quick lap, or do a round of burpees. Put that glucose to work, or it will work against you.

What to look out for:

The *I'm-too-busy-for-healthy-habits* trap

The cycle begins when you start getting busier—the kids get more activities, you get a new project at work, someone in your household is sick, etc. You need more time to deal with it all, but you're just too busy. So what do you do to find more time? First, you start cutting out sleep. You figure five hours will just have to cut it because you don't have time for squat. Soon, you realize there's still not enough time. You're so overwhelmed with responsibilities that you try to free yourself from other obligations. That's when you stop hanging out with friends, you say no to social invitations, and you stop cooking at home. You're not even thinking about what's for dinner because you'll go with whatever is the easiest and the fastest—even if it's pizza and fast food most nights of the week. You fast longer because *who has time to worry about food in a phase like this?* You stop taking those daily ten-minute walks; you're not cleaning or keeping up with household tasks. And then what happens after just a few weeks of this trend?

Your stress doesn't get any better. In fact, it seems to get worse once you realize all the bad habits that have crept back in—like snacking yourself to sleep and eating all the sugar all the time. Why? All the things you cut out are the very things that help your body cope with stress so you can actually accomplish and meet the demands of your busy life without sabotaging your health and mental fortitude. Ironically, the things we let go of—sleep, socializing, healthy eating, and low-level exercise—are part of the solution, not the problem. As a result, you've worsened your body's ability to cope with stress tenfold, and it's a recipe for burnout and worsened metabolic health.

Prevent this downward spiral by prioritizing basic human needs during times of high stress:

- Adequate sleep
- Proper nutrition
- Low-level activity (like walking or yoga)
- Love and connection

Restarting Fasts After Facing Chronic Stressors

Let's say your body is hit with a major stressor like a COVID-19 infection that had you bedridden for four full days. You feel better on day five, so you're already back to work. By day seven, you're thinking, "I really need to get back to my workouts and start fasting again." *Not so fast.* Your body needs wayyyy more time and resources to fully recover from the infection and the lingering effects it's had on your mitochondria, metabolism, and immune system. When you're coming back from a major stressor like COVID-19, you need to ease your way into exercise and fasting. Slowly, over a much longer stretch of time than you'd think.

When I say slowly, I mean you start with yoga and casual walks for the first couple of weeks. Then, you might add some twenty-minute resistance training for another few weeks. Then, if things are going well, you might return to higher-intensity workouts twice a week for another few weeks. All the while, you're eating nutrient-dense meals two or three times a day. Then, months later, you're back to your usual workout routine.

And what about fasting? You'd further impair your mitochondria, your metabolism, and your immune system if you tried going back to your former fasting schedule only a week after having COVID. After deviations like that, you need to restart with the RESET method. This brings us back to a 12-hour fasting window with a gradual increase every 4–7 days once the current window feels effortless again. Otherwise, you'll end up crossing that stress threshold too quickly, all over again.

Yes, you're restarting. You stick with a fasting length that's nearly effortless for you because, if you're like most people today, your body is already under so much stress. You want to trigger hormesis to see benefits, but be cautious not to overwhelm the body with another chronic stressor. Doing it a little each day is the perfect way to train or retrain your body and mind without this practice backfiring on you. Besides, it's important to flood your mitochondria with nutrients so you can adequately recover from the infection and bounce back to the abundant level of energy you depend upon.

CHAPTER 38
Essential Fasting Safeguards

I came up with the term *fasting safeguards* to identify which habits or behaviors help prevent a maladaptive response to one's fasting habits. *Fasting safeguards* not only protect against undesirable consequences such as plateaus, but they're also quite supportive. These habits and behaviors enhance your experience, giving you better results with fasting.

Fasting Safeguards:

- *Getting adequate deep sleep (and using a sleep tracker)

- Strategically cycling low-carb and moderate-carb foods

- *Eating a variety of nutrient-dense foods

- *Managing Stress

- *Cycling fasts with 3-Meal Days

- *Using the RESET method to start a fasting practice or return to one

- Taking Electrolytes

- Using a fasting tracker

- *Period tracking (AKA cycle syncing)

- Engaging in moderate activity with *adequate rest days

- Doing hypoxic breath work
  (or IHT: intermittent hypoxic
  training)

The safeguards with an asterisk are those I view as essential.

Notice the RESET method is one of the safeguards. Parts 1–5 of this book walk you through an in-depth understanding of the RESET method. By now, you've likely implemented the first four phases of the method: reduce your carbs, eat nourishing foods, start with 12 hours, and extend your fasts. The RESET method is designed to help anyone start and succeed with intermittent fasting or restart with intermittent fasting in a way that increases the likelihood of long-term success and a sustainable fasting lifestyle.

Depending on where you're currently at with this method, it may be time to explore the final phase of the RESET method and thoughtfully adapt, or it may be time to *restart* and revisit some of the earlier phases….

Maybe you've deviated from your nutritious diet since you went on vacation or behaved a little rebelliously when you were short on sleep and highly stressed. Do you need to RESET altogether? The RESET method is a fasting safeguard. It can be essential after a drastic change to your lifestyle. This might mean getting back to a nutrient-dense diet, reducing your carbs and sugar, and starting with 12-hour fasts (or your current, lowest comfortable fasting window) until you *retrain* your body and mind for this metabolic challenge.

It was only recently that I personally needed to restart with the RESET method. I was slapped with a dose of my own medicine in September of 2022 when I had a COVID-19 infection that took me down for five or six days. What I learned after my bout with COVID was that this infection causes the immune system and mitochondria to gobble up nutrients like never before. The body is using every last vitamin, mineral, amino acid, and antioxidant to fight and recover from the infection. *And I felt it.*

You feel it in the form of unmerciful fatigue. Even when you seem to have cleared the infection, you have a hard time readjusting to the way you were before having COVID—whether that's your appetite, fasting routine, workout intensity, sleep schedule, and/or the foods you eat.

That's why, over the next few months, I was only fasting for 12–14 hours, and I felt a little surprised that, several months later, I still wasn't easily fasting 16–24 hours like I used to. That's when it hit me. *Duh, Marisa! You need to RESET!* So I started back at my lowest comfortable fasting length, 14 hours, and stayed there until I experienced 7 days in a row where the fasting window felt practically effortless before I increased my daily fasts to 14.5 or 15 hours. I needed to retrain my body and mind for longer fasts.

At some point in your journey, that may be what you need to do, too (like after a vacation, after a stressful time in your life, or after having COVID). If you rush to another phase without building or rebuilding the foundation, it gets harder and harder to do, and your metabolism can start to work against you.

In Part 5, coming up, you'll learn about one of the most avoided but essential fasting safeguards you need to succeed with a long-term fasting lifestyle: 3-Meal Days. That fasting safeguard is part of the final phase in the RESET method, Thoughtfully Adapt, and it makes this into a long-term, effective strategy for achieving and maintaining a healthy weight with intermittent fasting.

CHAPTER 39
Mistakes Everyone Makes Here

CHAPTER 39.1
Grazing, Snacking, Undereating

O ne of the biggest mistakes I see people make when they start intermittent fasting is that they graze and snack throughout the eating window. It's not just beginners who fall into this habit but also fasters who've been doing it for a long time. When they go through an especially busy or unfulfilling time in their lives, they default to shortcuts. This habit can quickly turn into undereating or overeating, plus chronic insulin production.

So, how can that be?

Well, first of all, undereating is really common in the beginning. When you're new to intermittent fasting, you might be impressed once it's time to break your fast and you realize you're not really hungry. You might think to yourself, *I'm supposed to break my fast, but I'm not really that hungry. And I'm busy. So I'm just gonna break my fast with this protein bar. I want to watch what I eat anyway because I'm trying to lose weight, and less food must be better.*

It's easier to skip the meal and just grab a protein bar, right? You don't want to prepare food, you haven't thought that far ahead, you don't have a healthy meal planned or ready to eat, so you're not quite sure what to do. So many factors lead to that decision.

And so you undereat because you're afraid to have too many calories, or you're afraid you'll eat too many carbs, or you don't have the motivation to figure out *what* to eat. Or you're not sure how you'll find the time to finish your work if you stop too long to order food and eat.

What happens next is that you find yourself snacking again the next hour, and then you find yourself snacking again and again. By the time you're home from work, it's about six o'clock, and you're headfirst in your kids' bag of Doritos. You go to the fast food drive-thru because you don't know what to feed them tonight, and all the while, you've lost all sense of discipline and willpower after having starved yourself through low-calorie snacking for the entire day. You snack yourself to sleep and say, "I'll start my diet again tomorrow."

It's interesting how undereating can turn into *overeating* because what started this grazing habit in the first place is that you simply did not plan ahead for mealtime. You didn't prioritize or put in the five minutes of pre-planning needed to have food ready once it's time to break your fast and eat *an actual meal*.

I realize you don't want to prepare a nutrient-dense meal because you've got a lot of shit to do, and you want something easy. You wish you could just get it from a drive-thru or from a shelf in your pantry. You want to grab the chips and hummus. A granola bar, slices of cheese, and some pickles.

But the more you do that, the more you'll mimic a low-calorie diet, and your body will wonder, *Am I gonna get enough food? I'm not sure I'll get enough nutrients, so I'm gonna slow down the metabolism and increase hunger to protect myself. I'll increase the body weight set-point, too, so we always have more fat for emergencies like this.*

Your snacking and grazing habit backfires on you. You get the reverse of what you desire. The body fat won't come off. Fasting isn't working. And here's the other thing. The grazing and snacking will turn into a habit so fast and so hard it will stand in the way of your confidence and make you second-guess your abilities altogether. This isn't only because you undereat or overeat, but because snacking is a habit that instantly returns, like someone who relapses. It's as if you're an addict who quit drinking alcohol, and all of a sudden, after just one beer, you're drinking beers again every day.

That's what happens with snacking. You don't acknowledge or predict that a snacking habit will come back with a vengeance, even after two measly days of grazing through the eating window. You wind up facing the fact that it may be even harder to quit this habit again (and again and again) than it would've been to avoid it in the first place.

What to do? Take some time to get to know yourself. Practice being self-compassionate.

What does it mean to be self-compassionate? I'll tell you what it doesn't mean. It doesn't mean you respond to your actions as if everything is fine or acceptable. It means you practice patience with yourself as you work through something. Your snacking habit will sneak up. It does, for all of us at one time or another. But, if you're determined to prioritize healthy eating and to eliminate that snacking habit so you can reach your goals, you can eliminate it as soon as you recognize it—as long as you're patient with yourself.

Imagine yourself in this scenario:

You successfully plan ahead and prep a meal to bring to lunch at work tomorrow. Tomorrow comes, and you forget to bring that meal to work. When it comes time to break your fast, you think *I'm not really that hungry.*

I have my protein powder here, so I'll just make a protein shake and get back to work.

Later, your colleagues offer you some strawberries and homemade brownies. You thank them for the offer and eat the strawberries, foregoing the brownies (win!). By the time it's 3 o'clock, you have a break, and you think to yourself, *I haven't really eaten yet today. Since I have a break now and really don't want to work through it, maybe I should have one of those brownies and treat myself.* Just knowing the brownies are there is taunting you. You respond to the pressure by agitatedly rummaging through your desk drawers to find an old granola bar you forgot about. You eat the granola bar, assuring yourself you don't need that brownie. *I'll be good with this granola bar. Once I get home, I can heat up the lunch I forgot to bring.*

What happens when you leave the office that day? Things come up. You get a call from your Mom, who talks your ear off, and you pick up the kids who are arguing over who gets to sit in the front seat, which leaves your youngest sobbing in tears at an infuriating volume. Oh, and you forgot company is coming over tomorrow, so you still need to clean up the house!

You finally get home and dump the kids on your spouse while you clean and straighten up. Your spouse soon asks, "What're we doing for dinner? Should I order pizza?" You respond like, "I really don't care right now. I don't have time, sorry, just get whatever you want. I can eat my lunch I forgot to bring today."

The pizza arrives. It's hot and ready, and it smells intoxicating. What happens next? You grab one slice, swearing you'll eat the healthy, prepared lunch once you finish this last cleaning task. Next thing you know, you collapse at the dining table, eating all the pizza that remains because you feel sorry for yourself that you had such a crazy day. You start beating yourself up about it. That voice in your head says *You're never going to lose weight. You're too busy, and you don't have enough willpower to stick with it.*

Can you relate? First things first. Don't be so hard on yourself—or, I should say, don't let that voice in your head be so hard on you. Self-compassion. All you need to do is, with curiosity and empathy, acknowledge what happened. What happened was a *chain of events* that led you to the series of choices you made. And each choice you faced, or event that occurred is a distinctive opportunity to improve upon next time.

The Chain of Events:

1. Prepped lunch for yourself

2. Forgot to bring lunch to work

3. It's time to break your fast (you chose a protein shake)

4. You're offered strawberries and brownies (you chose strawberries)

5. 3 p.m. break (tempted to treat yourself to a brownie. Instead, you ate a granola bar and planned to eat your lunch when you got home)

6. You finally arrive home frazzled, stressed, and overwhelmed

7. Spouse asks if you want pizza

8. Pizza arrives (you eat it)

9. Voice in your head reprimands you for your choices

That's at least nine different opportunities to make a decision that aligns with your ultimate goal to maintain a healthy lifestyle.

Each choice you make along the way should be looked at as a singular opportunity. The further you look back into the chain of events (like back to number 2 or number 3), the easier it is to course-correct, and the sooner you can interrupt the pattern before it sweeps you up in its current. You'll have a better chance of preventing it next time, so you can really turn things around for yourself in the long run.

So, what would you do if you interrupted that chain of events early on? Once you were at work and you realized you forgot your lunch, what if, instead, you logged in to Grubhub and thought, *What can I get that's somewhat healthy. Can I get a stir fry? Can I get some fajitas from the Mexican place? I'll tell them to skip the tortillas and skip the rice. I can ask a colleague to order together and split the delivery costs, too.* Would those have been better options for you? Yes, absolutely. You can even order from a local diner, get yourself an omelet, and even enjoy that side of potatoes. It's still better than snacking your way through your eating window.

Snacking is a habit that comes back so fast. It can lead to binges, overeating, and quitting on your goals altogether. All of a sudden, you may find yourself snacking every single day. Sure, it takes diligence and planning. But your life will be forever transformed when you cherish mealtime. Because the more you fast, the more precious that mealtime is, and it deserves your attention and *intention*. Besides, you'll be cooking a lot less often and eating a lot less often since you're fasting now. Take your time building this lifestyle. You might as well experiment to find a system that works for you, so having healthy meals prepared ahead of time becomes a priority that's second nature. A foundational habit you wouldn't give up for anything.

CHAPTER 39.2

Fasting Window vs. Eating Window

In the fasting community, most people use the terms fasting window and eating window to describe the timespan during which to fast or eat. The grazing/snacking mistake I just explained is one of the main reasons I rarely talk about the eating window when I teach intermittent fasting. I also avoid using the term time-restricted eating because, either way, the focus is all on the eating part.

When we do this, that emphasis subtly influences your mindset to think predominantly about eating. Let's walk through the story of a client whose frame of mind is focused on the eating window.

Marsha's eating window is from 12 p.m.–6 p.m. She broke her fast at 12 p.m. with cheese sticks, pickles, sliced deli ham, and a keto protein bar. *I'm not that hungry,* she thought to herself. *I just want a little something that's quick, easy, and low-carb.*

She finished eating around 12:45 p.m. and now it's about 2 p.m. Marsha thinks to herself, *Well, this is my eating window, so I can eat whenever I want.* So she mindlessly turns to snacking, and she grazes through the eating window. As the 6 p.m. cut-off time looms into sight, she develops a scarcity mindset. This focus on the eating window, combined with the scarcity of the approaching fast, results in a habit of nervously eating throughout the eating window. It starts with breaking her fast with snacks. Every hour, she wanders to the fridge and pantry, trying to fill a recurring void and put as little effort as possible into mealtime. As the weeks pass, Marsha wonders *How come I'm not seeing results anymore? I'm hungry all the time during my eating window, and I can't stop thinking about food.* The eating window mindset is a big reason why.

Emotional Eating

Most of the time, you're not eating due to physical hunger; you're eating because of one or more of the following conditions:

- **Your brain is bored,** and it craves stimulation.

- **You dislike the task you're working on,** and you crave a reward.

- **You feel powerless** in your day, your life, or your current circumstance. This frustration or resentment makes you want to eat because it's one of the only things you can do to cope or demonstrate your freedom.

- **You use food to procrastinate** starting or continuing a task that's unpleasant or intimidating (guilty over here!).

- **You eat to demonstrate self-compassion**, comforting yourself in response to the hurtful self-criticism running through your mind.

- **You don't like the feeling of certain emotions,** so you eat to distract yourself from them.

- There's a saying in the world of emotional eating that suggests (whenever you feel out of control with your hunger or eating habits) asking yourself, *What's eating you?* What relational or emotional issues are unresolved? Deciding to keep your feelings in and bury them causes you to turn to food for comfort.

- **You rarely ever release your emotions**: you don't cry, scream, punch or kick things, have sex, or achieve orgasm; you don't sing aloud, dance, or laugh so hard your belly hurts. You lack a physical release for the emotional energy that's trapped inside you. (Your body turns to food to help in a desperate attempt to shift from the sympathetic fight-or-flight state to the calming parasympathetic state, but food is an insufficient solution, and eating in a stressed state has other negative impacts on your health.

- **You received a visual cue that triggered a desire to eat:** you saw a commercial for Chick-fil-A, you drove past your favorite drive-thru, you saw those golden arches, you saw someone on TV eating chocolate, etc. So, now you want that food, too.

- **Someone around you is eating,** and it's so distracting you decide you might as well just eat, too.

- **Any of the above reasons have led to this becoming such an ingrained habit**. You eat because that's simply what you've always done at this time or place or whenever you feel such a way.

A lot of us think eating or overeating is the problem we need to solve, but, really, eating or overeating is a *solution* we turn to out of habit. This solution is our effort to solve or cope with feelings of discomfort. I learned this from an interview with Marc David, the founder of the Institute for Psychology of Eating. Your problem isn't eating too much or overeating. Your problem is that you turn to eating to cope with other problems and discomforts in your daily life.

This is where self-compassion and curiosity pay off, big time. The more you get to know yourself and these patterns, the more power you have to change them.

Breaking your fast with a high-protein meal instead of snack foods is a great way to give you that control back. Once you feel more in control of your snacking habit, aim to take 2–4-hour breaks between meals and snacks so your blood sugar and insulin have time to resolve after eating. Your digestive system loves those intermittent breaks. This also helps ensure you're hungry enough to eat an actual meal once dinner time approaches.

Another reason I emphasize the *fasting window* over the eating window is because the fasting is where the magic is at! The number of hours you're fasting is what brings you the results, not the number of hours you're allowed to eat.

Think about it: it's more motivating to realize that you fasted 19 hours than it is to realize that your eating window was only 5 hours long. It's more motivating to ask yourself, *Can I do a 22-hour fast?* compared to, *Can I shrink my eating window down to just 2 hours?*

- Want to turbo-charge autophagy? Fast for ≥ 24 hours.

- Want to balance your thyroid hormone while doing some intermittent fasting? Fast for 12–14 hours

- Want to significantly boost stem cell production? Fast for 72 hours

- Want to get into *ketosis on a moderate carbohydrate diet? Fast 13–16 hours with exercise, or commit to 16–20-hour fasts when you're sedentary.

- Want to boost adaptation after consistently doing 16-hour fasts for the last two months? Increase your fasting window to 17 or 18 hours, most days of the week, and start adding in 3-Meal Days every 1–2 weeks. See Part 5 for more details about this under-appreciated fasting safeguard.

When you focus on the fasting window instead of the eating window, it feels more encouraging. It's science-backed and less likely to result in aimless eating behavior that's limited by nothing but the book-ends of your eating window.

You might only need 12 hours of fasting to get into ketosis if you're eating a low-carb diet, didn't eat many carbs in your meal the night before, exercise during your fasting window, do endurance training or cardio, and/or you're insulin sensitive and accustomed to intermittent fasting or keto dieting. Everyone is different, and every day is different. If you're eating like crap on vacation and want to get into ketosis when you return home, you might need to fast 18–24 hours to stimulate ketosis depending on how insulin sensitive you are, if you're active or sedentary, and if you eat low carb upon return.

CHAPTER 39.3

The 'More is Better' Mentality

I'd like to introduce you to the concept known as The Law of Diminishing Returns. Economists came up with this theory to explain why, beyond a certain point, extra effort or inputs result in lesser output or fewer benefits. Just like I explained in Chapter 34: *Hormesis: A Beneficial Adaptation in Response to a Stressor*, you can easily do too much, causing too much stress and resulting in a maladaptive response.

It's not just with hormesis that you can go overboard. It's in any pursuit of health. Let's consider the following list of strategies people might attempt, in any combination, in pursuit of weight loss.

- Increase aerobic exercise

- Increase weight training and resistance exercise

- Engage in high-intensity interval training (HIIT)

- Increase daily low-level activities like walking

- Reduce caloric intake

- Implement fasting

- Reduce portion sizes

- Reduce dietary fat intake

- Reduce carbohydrate intake

- Take weight-loss drugs

- Take weight-loss supplements

- Replace meals with diet shakes

Now, let's observe how a potential client fell into the 'more is better' trap by implementing too many weight-loss strategies at once.

Janet's Experience with More Is Better:

Struck with a sudden determination, Janet decides to change her body. She's sick of being overweight, and she wants to lose the weight this time. Nothing can stop her. Starting now, just four months before her brother's wedding, she decides to go big. Here's Janet's big plan:

- Weightlifting three times per week with a personal trainer

- Cardio kickboxing class twice per week

- Running/jogging for 1 hour every Sunday

- Swapping all her favorite snacks for low-fat, low-carb versions

- Committing to a keto low-carb diet for 60 days

- Fasting for 15 hours per day and working her way up to 18-hour fasts

- Counting calories to be sure not to exceed 1400 per day (because that's what the internet says she should do if she wants to reach her goal before the wedding)

- Start taking the following supplements and pills: pre-workout fat burner caffeine drink, metabolism-boosting herbal capsules, metformin to reduce her blood sugar

- Replacing her daily breakfast with a Shakeology meal replacement drink. Soon, she'll skip breakfast because she's fasting and replace her lunch with a Shakeology drink.

Not only are some of those ideas unwise and outdated, but trying to do so many of them at once would make things backfire due to the relentless self-discipline required to stay committed to all those changes at once. Even if we ignore the fact that it's likely to backfire, Janet is still likely to feel defeated along the way. Why? Because of the biggest factor; it's too much stress for her body to sustain and respond favorably to.

More is not better. More effort doesn't usually lead to more results—especially when it comes to weight loss. More effort can lead to more setbacks.

Stacking up too many interventions leads to more stress (psychologically and metabolically). And more stress means you're closer and closer to your personal threshold of hormetic stress. Your metabolism will see your efforts as a threat to its survival, and your body will initiate all efforts to defend itself.

More is not only not better, it's *abusive*.

If you want to see more returns on your effort, you need five things:

1. A timely, personalized strategy

2. Patience

3. Persistence

4. Continued, intermittent self-reflection

5. Thoughtful adaptation

I'll tell you a story about Lacey, and you'll see how the law of diminishing returns can get the best of you, too....

CHAPTER 39.3.1

Lacey's Story: More is Not More

Lacey booked one of my impromptu coaching calls because she's been trying to lose weight for several months now, combining IF and Keto, and has been frustrated with her progress.

When I got on the call with Lacey, she explained, "As I age, every time I start my cycle of getting in shape, it gets harder. Everyone says you need to make it a lifestyle, but I haven't been able to find a lifestyle that works for me. I'm very all in or all out. And when I let things go, I gain 20 lb very easily. I gain and lose about 20–30 lb what seems like every year, especially since having kids."

It was June 15th when she said, "In late March, I started IF and low carb with 16:8 fasting, then 18:6, then 20:4, and finally, a couple of weeks ago, I started OMAD." Lacey explained she'd lost 16 lb since starting in late March (that's in approximately 75 days). She decided to start OMAD and restrict calories to 1300 per day, with carbs down to 20–30 g per day. She kicked up her exercise routine at this time, too, exercising most days of the week doing dance, pilates, and yoga.

She then told me, "After a week or so of getting more strict with everything, I wanted to give up because I didn't see more results."

It was my turn to chime in and respond to what she'd shared about her current circumstances, and here's how it started:

"You've put in a lot of work to see changes in your body, Lacey, and you're feeling frustrated because you're no longer seeing results at this stage. I'm glad you didn't give up and you decided to reach out for support. What you're going through now is something I see regularly in my clients and followers. You try to do more of everything because if it works when you're giving it 75 percent of your effort, it must work better when you put in 100 percent of your effort, right? Unfortunately, that's not how it works with diet and weight loss. Especially with fasting…"

I then went on to explain how much stress she's putting on her body and how her history of repeat weight loss and regain is evidence that her body is hyper-vigilant in reaction to the stress she induces during these weight-loss efforts. I explained briefly what a hormetic stressor is and that her recent efforts to boost results have added too many stressors:

Increased fasting

Increased exercise

Decreased calories

Severely restricted carbs

Female hormones

Lack of sleep

Considering all the stressors she's added or combined lately, she's causing a reverse effect. *The Law of Diminishing Returns.* Instead of losing more weight, she plateaus because her metabolism is alarmed, slowing down to meet her forced lower-calorie intake and lower macronutrient intake and to meet her increased activity level. Her metabolism slows down, increases the size of her fat cells, and raises her body weight set point, all in an effort to ensure there's enough fat stored away for future stress loads like this.

I went on to explain that I'd guess with little kids and this type of dedication, she's not sleeping even 6 hours a night. She laughed, scoffed, and said, "No chance."

She then shared that she has a hard time understanding all this because she's read a lot of information on Reddit, and the 'experts' there strongly emphasize the importance of calories-in versus calories-out.

I empathized with her confusion regarding all the mixed messaging. I briefly explained that although we'd like for everything to be simply calculable like that (I ate X number of calories today, and I burned X number of calories in my pilates class), there are a few reasons it simply doesn't work that way. First, we know *calories* (or *kilocalories*) is a term used to quantify energy consumption and conversion in the body regardless of the various interplays that change how a calorie converts in the human body compared to in a laboratory.

I knew Lacey would agree when I said, "Your body would have a much different reaction to you eating 500 calories of broccoli with olive oil than it would from eating 500 calories of mini Snickers bars." Then I explained that even her smartwatch, her treadmill, or an online BMR calculator can't tell her how many calories she's burning throughout the day or how many calories she needs. I also explained that everything changes when you're fasting.

I challenged her to consider googling a counterargument for the claims she's reading on Reddit. "We need to be skeptical, informed internet browsers, and be open to opposing perspectives whenever we seek to find the truth about a polarizing topic such as calorie counting. Google *quality versus quantity of calories?* or *what's wrong with calorie counting?* or *the downsides of calorie counting.*

I also explained how lowering her carbs so much is too stressful with her female hormones and the major lack of sleep—not to mention the number of hours she's fasting.

One last thing she shared out of frustration was that she decided to kick things up a notch because she sees all these before/after pictures on Reddit where people share their 50-lb weight loss after just a few months of doing a keto-OMAD diet. I responded with empathy again, saying, "We don't know enough about that person to understand without making assumptions, but my assumption would be that this is the first time that person has gained and lost the weight," whereas Lacey has a history of yo-yo dieting and weight-loss-and-regain, which means it'll be a lot more challenging every single time she starts that cycle up again—because her metabolism is alarmed by the pattern, protecting itself from future threats. I explained that we also don't know the person's age, their state of health, how they ate before they started the diet, their genetics, their sleep habits, stress levels, and hormonal health.

She started to see that it was time to rethink her strategy.

To help Lacey feel encouraged to continue, I asked her what she's doing now that she actually enjoys or finds pretty easy to maintain. She loves exercise, and she's happy to be doing that again. She also likes doing 18:6 fasting because she can still eat dinner with her kids each night, compared to OMAD, where she's eating dinner alone or not at all. Lastly, I suggested she aim to keep meals around 20–30 g of carbs per meal if she's fasting 18 hours but to keep snacks lower carb.

I also suggested she consider the cycle of her period, increasing her intake of whole-food carbs during the week before she bleeds. That switch and fasting just 12 hours during the week before her period will help counter some of the stress her body's going through at that time.

Lastly, I acknowledged it's a lot and she's probably not feeling ready or interested in improving her sleep, but that her lack of sleep could be the single most influential factor in her body's ability to lose weight and get to her goal. It didn't have to be perfect, but even if she just aimed right now to get 6.5 hours of sleep most nights of the week, that would be a huge improvement. I explained that her cortisol, insulin, and glucose are all hyper-responsive when she's under-slept.

She was pretty quiet for most of the call once I started sharing my insights and concerns with her. That's understandable because it's like someone telling you everything you've been reading is sorta wrong, whatever you're doing is wrong, and you have to slow down to speed up the results—and you'll need to change something in your life that seems almost impossible and unappealing to change. Sleep!

About thirty minutes after our call, I received an email from Lacey saying how grateful she was for my honesty and challenging her to think differently about her approach to weight loss.

CHAPTER 39.4

8 More Common Mistakes

8 More Common Mistakes People Make When Extending Their Fasts

1. (Women) Ignoring their phase of the menstrual cycle

2. Ignoring sleep deprivation

3. Not allowing time for adaptation

4. Not fasting at all on weekends

5. Being too rigid: skipping 3-Meal Days

6. Expecting a linear journey

7. Fasting too long on exercise days

8. Comparing themselves to others

Mistake #1. Ignoring the menstrual cycle

For menstruating women, a common recipe for self-sabotage is to ignore your menstrual cycle when it comes to your diet, fasting routine, or exercise routine. When you track your period (and the approximate phases of your menstrual cycle), you're able to adjust your exercise, fasting, and dietary habits to work more cooperatively with your body so you minimize PMS, hunger and cravings, emotional instability, irritability, stress, insomnia, and weight-loss plateaus.

In Part 5, two entire chapters are dedicated to women and fasting. In those chapters, I'll help you understand why and how to start cycle syncing. This will help you to live more in concert with your menstrual cycle so you aren't working against what your biology needs during certain phases of the month.

Mistake #2. Ignoring sleep deprivation

I can't stress enough the importance of getting adequate sleep when you're on a journey to lose weight or optimize your health. Skimp on sleep, and your metabolism will fight against your efforts to lose weight. No amount of fasting will combat this, and it will only make things worse.

I have two sayings that really emphasize why you want to prioritize sleep:

"Lack of sleep makes you eat." Yes, you will be hungrier, you will be more rebellious, and you will have less willpower whenever you're short on sleep.

"Reduced sleep time plateaus your waistline." Yes, your body will fight your efforts to lose weight when you're short on sleep. You'll see weight-loss plateaus until you address this absolutely critical component of good health.

It takes some experimentation and genuine curiosity to fix your sleep, but I promise you that you do have time, and you can do it. And you'll be able to feel and see the difference, so it will be worth it.

You cannot achieve better mental or physical health without adequate sleep. It's a fundamental need in regard to every process and capability of your amazing body. Part 6 is dedicated entirely to the topic of sleep: a critical piece of the puzzle. Together, we'll explore exactly what you can experiment with to optimize your sleep, and your life will change dramatically when you do.

Mistake #3. Not allowing time for adaptation

This mistake underlies the primary premise of this book. *Not so fast.* My RESET method advises you to start with 12 hours and stick with your current fasting length for enough days or weeks in a row until it becomes effortless, which is a sure sign your body and mind have had enough time to adapt. Remember, you're training your fasting muscles. Just like with exercise, you need to work your way up to a longer fast—at the very least to avoid the unpleasant side effects—so you can drastically improve your likelihood of success. Push too hard, too fast, and your metabolism—or that voice in your head—will lash out, and you won't get the results you ultimately seek.

Same goes for when you've deviated from a fasting lifestyle after going on vacation or getting sick, or after the holidays, etc. Resist trying to return to your old fasting schedule so abruptly. When you take on *too much too fast,* your body and mind will suffer. You'll have better results if you RESET and retrain yourself for fasting, gradually working your way up to the level you formerly upheld.

Mistake #4. Abandoning the plan entirely on weekends

Weekends aren't cheat days. Weekends aren't a free-for-all during which fasting is irrelevant or impossible. You don't have to adhere to a 100 percent healthy lifestyle 7 days a week, but you do have to be reasonable about how often you deviate or make exceptions, especially when you've yet to enter maintenance mode. Abandoning the plan entirely on the weekends is like taking five steps forward during the week and two steps back on the weekend.

On Instagram, I recently saw a clever post by James DiNicolantonio, which said, "5 out of 7 is 71%. That's a C-. If you go off the rails every weekend eating like crap, don't expect 'A' results."

Great point, James!

To help quantify the magnitude of abandoning your diet on the weekends, I discovered a helpful analogy while in the process of writing my book. My daily writing habit was to hit at least 500 words a day. If I showed up every weekday to write 500 words, Monday through Friday, and I took the weekends off, then that meant I'd write 2,500 words a week, which yields about 10,000 words a month. What if I wrote 500 words on the weekends, too? How much of a difference would it make to write 7 days a week? That would help me write 3,500 words each week, or 14,000 words a month. In 6 months, I'd have made significant progress at 84,000 words writing on the weekends, compared to 60,000 if I took the weekends off.

Just like with fasting, however, there are advantages and disadvantages of writing on the weekend or taking the weekend off. It's advantageous to write 7 days a week because it helps me make more progress—*but that's only if I can stick with it.* On the other hand, taking the weekends off gives me time to recuperate and find that work-life balance. But then, come Monday, I'd have lost the momentum. Monday seems daunting, and I lack the motivation to reengage with my daily writing habit.

Maybe the solution is somewhere in between, like writing 500 words on Saturdays but taking Sundays off. That gives me a full day to reset and refresh for a Monday start.

Let's take this analogy a step further to help you see the significance of a person who stops fasting on the weekends and starts eating whatever they want. What if, on the weekends, I not only took the weekend off from writing but I also *deleted* 500 words from my draft on Saturday and *deleted* 500 words on Sunday. That would mean that after writing 2,500 words Monday through Friday, I'd end up with only 1,500 words on Sunday!

That sounds silly, you're thinking, but this is precisely what many people try with their fasting and healthy eating habits! They fast and eat healthy Monday through Friday, and then, not only do they skip fasting entirely on the weekends, but they also consider weekends cheat days on which they can eat whatever they want. They say yes to pancakes, french fries, mac n' cheese, pizza, beer, dessert, cookies, bagels, and sugary Starbucks coffee. *WHOA!* Now, we're not only deviating from the healthy habits, but we're self-sabotaging with destructive behavior that takes away a lot of the progress we've already made. And that's not all. Behaving this way on the weekends makes Mondays *wayyyy* harder to reengage in. Cravings return, and the negative cycle ensues.

Individuals who have this no-rules-on-the-weekends mentality experience a constant inner battle with themselves throughout this pattern of behavior. Trying to balance the tug-and-pull of healthy living with carefree *eat-whatever-and-whenever-the-hell-I-want* weekends leaves them wondering why dieting is *so hard* or if they'll ever have the willpower to achieve their goals.

If healthy eating remains a priority in your life, then maybe you're not fasting on the weekends because you're in maintenance mode. That's what it's like for me and many of my clients who've achieved a state of health they'd like to maintain. We eat a nutrient-dense diet, making exceptions that are timely or worth it. Sometimes we don't fast at all on the weekends. Most of us carry on with the baseline principle of 12-hour minimum fasts, but otherwise, we just go with the flow. We know what our baselines are for maintenance. It varies for each individual—some of us have a baseline of 12-hour fasts, while others have a baseline of 16-hour fasts (more common in people with a history of obesity, type 2 diabetes, or yo-yo weight loss and gain). All of us thoughtfully adapt the routine based on changes in our hormones or changes in our activity level. When we do a strenuous workout, we shorten the fast. When we have a lazy day, we prioritize some fasting or mindful food choices.

It's important to find a healthy balance that not only works with your lifestyle but also honors your primary goal to get healthy and stay healthy. Like I always say, it's about your willingness and persistent effort to sacrifice what you want *now* for what you want *most*. It's a lifestyle change. A shift in your priorities. An evolution in your self-identity. Are you ready to become someone who puts their health first?

Your health is your new hobby. How does that sound?

Mistake #5: Being too rigid: Skipping 3-Meal Days

You'll learn all about this in the Part 5 chapter dedicated to 3-Meal Days. Furthermore, throughout this entire book, I emphasize the downsides of being too rigid with your fasting lifestyle and dietary habits.

Mistake #6. Expecting a linear journey.

When you assume your path to better health will be a straight trajectory from start to finish, it's like you expect to win *big* the first time you play the lottery. The odds are terrible. That's simply not how it works.

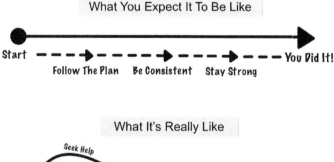

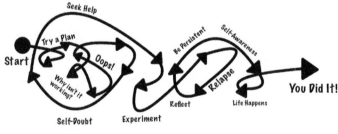

It's unrealistic to expect that your intermittent fasting journey for weight loss will be a straight trajectory. You probably don't even realize you're doing it. You plan out your goal, like, *My target is to lose 8 lb per month,* yet you don't consider the hundreds of possible obstacles and deviations that're likely to interfere. Life happens. Human biology is complicated. Your metabolism, your mind, your relationships, and competing responsibilities all complicate things. Your schedule changes, you get sick, you deal with unexpected emotional obstacles, your motivation comes and goes, you relapse into old habits—and then you start getting back on track, again. It's not a straight line from point A to point B. It's more like the jagged peaks and valleys you see on a hospital's heart rate monitor.

Unrealistic optimism leads you to underestimate the challenges and setbacks you're likely to face. And when outcomes don't match our expectations, we experience chemical reactions in the brain in response to what's called *dopamine-prediction error*. We experience it as disappointment, negative self-talk, and feelings of failure or even a decision to quit trying altogether.

There's a long-term commitment that's required of you. A commitment to your health and the unpaved road that will lead you there.

Mistake #7. Fasting too long on exercise days

Boy, do I see this more often than I expected. Fasting is somewhat addicting. Exercise can be quite addicting, too. And when you have a weight-loss mindset, you tend to view fasting and exercise as the solutions you can depend on. The thing is, they don't always work together. Evolutionarily, humans were more likely to feast on the days they worked really hard, and they'd conserve energy on the days when food was scarce. Our biology favors those input-output patterns and combinations. When you try to exercise more and fast more, it will ultimately impede your results. Now, this isn't to say there aren't benefits from engaging in fasted exercise. It makes complete evolutionary sense to exercise in a fasted state and is quite beneficial in most cases, but to continue a fast after engaging in intense exercise is unwise.

When your goal is to change your body composition (to lose fat or gain muscle), an essential part of the equation is to consume adequate protein after the exercise. Without post-workout sustenance, it's like riding a bike uphill with a flat tire. You're trying to achieve something that's already difficult, yet now you have a handicap that makes it even less likely that you'll reach the top.

Remember, adaptability comes in phases. You're training your body to favorably adapt to the increased challenges and changes you induce. In order for it to reward you with positive results, you must demonstrate patience and respect for the biology you were born with. All humans come with a genetic blueprint that no degree of grit or willpower can override because what you want and what your biology wants are often two opposing things.

Mistake # 8. Comparing Yourself to Others

At this point, most people come to intermittent fasting as a weight-loss strategy because they've seen some pretty compelling success stories online or because they've heard firsthand from a friend who's experienced incredible weight loss with fasting. Here's the problem: you're not that person. You're not the people you read about. Nearly everything about you is different from that person. Your health history, your hormonal health, your personality, your relationship with food, your schedule, your home life, your stress levels, your sleep quality, your mindset, your e-v-e-r-y-t-h-i-n-g.

Comparing yourself to others is a huge mistake. Just because Susan lost 40 lb in six months by doing 18:6 intermittent fasting doesn't mean you can or should do the same thing or expect the same results. I'm sorry, but it's just not that simple. Comparison is the thief of joy. Don't ask yourself, *Why is it working for Susan but not for me?* Instead, ask yourself, *What does my body need from me, and how can I start to provide it with that?* Honor the unique needs of your body and your self, and you will succeed in your own way. In your own time.

Part 4 Action Steps:
Incorporate Fasting Safeguards

You learned a lot in Part 4 about how to extend your fasts while still honoring your body's current threshold for stress. **When you fast too long for the current stress tolerance of your body or mind, it can backfire in the following ways:**

- Binge eating

- Plateaus and stalled weight loss

- Weight gain

- Increased hunger or cravings

- Emotional outbursts

- Insomnia

- Repeat infections or injuries

- Autoimmune flare-ups

- Light-headedness or dizziness

- Impulsive behavior

- Rebellious thoughts and behavior around junk food

- Relentless thoughts and distractions related to eating

- Repetitive self-sabotage patterns

- Apathy, demotivation, or disinterest in your health

- Feelings of defeat or failure

- Female hormonal dysfunction (spotty periods, terrible PMS, thyroid dysfunction, infertility, etc.)

To ignore the stress piece is to ignore your ultimate goal of sustainable weight loss.

Action Step 1:

Do the self-assessment below to determine if fasting or other hormetic stressors may be too much for your body right now.

Action Step 2:

Review the list of fasting safeguards that follows. Combine what you've learned to determine where your attention is needed to help your body respond more favorably to intermittent fasting.

Self-Assessment

6 Questions to Discover If Your Body Can Handle More Hormesis:

1. Do I regularly, or have I recently experienced two or more nights in a row with insufficient sleep? Sleeping under 6.5 hours per night is insufficient. Or four or more nights in the same week? Yes or No

2. Do I dread or feel overwhelmed by this hormetic stressor (fasting or exercise, for example) while engaging in it, approaching it, or starting it? Yes or No

3. Do I experience any negative symptoms while engaging in or after the engagement in fasting or exercise? Yes or No

4. Currently, is there a source of chronic, unrelenting stress in my life that's negatively affecting multiple aspects of my daily life? I.e., grief, working too much, or family issues at home making it difficult to concentrate, having no time for your personal needs or for eating healthfully, sleeping sufficiently, etc. Yes or No

5. Is my body fighting a chronic stressor that was either recently resolved or expected to have been remedied by now? Examples include repeat cold/flu/infections, autoimmune disease flareup, chronic injury, recovery from surgery, arthritis flareup, chronic digestive distress, insulin resistance, jet lag, or shift work. Yes or No

6. Does it seem like I've been doing everything right, trying hard to implement healthy habits and be consistent, yet I'm not seeing any results? Or have my results plateaued for more than three weeks straight? Yes or No

Count how many questions you answered *Yes* to.

If you answered yes to any one of these questions, it's time to seriously consider if your body is helped or hindered by your engagement with certain hormesis-inducing behaviors. You might try alternating them more often to see how different behaviors feel in different scenarios. Consider getting yourself a health tracking device that measures your HRV - heart rate variability. Your daily average HRV is a valuable indicator of how much stress your body is under and how well you're recovering from it. When your HRV is lower than usual, it's a clear sign to scale back on the stress load—catch a nap today, skip or reduce today's workout, and prioritize recovery—so you can make progress rather than face more unintended setbacks.

If you recall from the chapter on hormesis, the safest hormetic stressors to engage in even when the body is under tremendous stress include hypoxic breath work, hyperbaric oxygen therapy, some form of cold therapy, moderate use of an infrared sauna, and the ingestion of certain plant compounds and antioxidants. By engaging in those safer forms of hormesis, you can expect to eventually build up your body's stress tolerance and add more hormesis back into your plan.

If you answered yes to two or more of the questions, not only is it imperative that you consider the negative impact your fasting or exercise habits could be having on your life currently but it's probably time to start a habit of casually journaling your insights. As you add in a few more fasting safeguards (listed below and in Chapter 38) or other protective measures like working with a therapist, taking a targeted supplement, instilling personal boundaries, or using a quality sleep tracker, take regular notes about your experiences. You want to look for signs of improvement and signs of self-sabotage.

Meanwhile, scale back on your physical activity level. For example, instead of doing a 45-minute HIIT class twice a week, try it once every 7–10 days following a good night's sleep. Reduce the number of hormetic stressors you engage in until you've seen signs of improvement. If you can, integrate some of the low-stress hormetic activities like hypoxic breath work and infrared sauna sessions to help your body regain strength in the meantime.

How many fasting safeguards do you currently engage in?

Here's a list of what I consider to be fasting safeguards:

- *Adequate deep sleep, using a sleep tracker
- Strategically cycling low-carb and moderate-carb foods.
- *Eating a variety of nutrient-dense foods
- *Stress management
- *Cycling fasts with 3-Meal Days
- *Using the RESET method to start a fasting practice or return to one
- Consuming electrolytes
- Using a fasting tracker
- *Period tracking by women (AKA cycle syncing)
- Moderate activity level with *adequate rest days
- Hypoxic breath work, or IHT (intermittent hypoxic training)

*The safeguards marked with an asterisk are those I view as essential.

If you're engaged in at least three of the fasting safeguards listed above—especially those marked with an *asterisk*—then you could be ready for more challenging fasts. However, if you answered Yes to two or more questions in the self-assessment above, then I encourage you to consider adopting more fasting safeguards before you push the fasting any further. It might be best to take your fasts down to 12–14 hours *(gasp!)* per day and integrate regular 3-Meal Days until you've fully recovered and your body is ready for a deeper challenge.

PART 5

Thoughtfully Adapt

RESET

R educe Carbs

E at Nourishing Foods

S tart with 12 Hours

E xtend Your Fasts

T houghtfully Adapt

CHAPTER 41

Thoughtfully Adapting for Flexible Fasting and Better Results

There's something you should know about this phase of the RESET method: Thoughtfully Adapt. Years ago, when I first created this system, the T in RESET stood for Trust Your Instincts. I've changed it twice since then. First, I realized it's not our instincts that we should trust. Today, we're living with many evolutionary mismatches, like a propensity to favor sweets and carbohydrates, because, historically, it was advantageous whenever food was scarce. Body fat was a survival advantage, and carbs provided quick energy that also helped store fat for scarcity looming ahead. As a consequence of this mismatch, instincts can drive us to engage in unwise behaviors today.

That explains why I soon changed this phase to Trust Your Wisdom because it emphasized that your trust should be in the personal experience, knowledge, and self-awareness you accumulate over time. Underlying the entire purpose of this phase is the need to adapt your fasting lifestyle to fit with you and your body's ever-changing needs.

Finally, while writing this book, I realized the T in RESET should stand for Thoughtfully Adapt. That's what it's all about. Adapting your fasting practice, using the wisdom you've gained, and turning this into something that pays off for life.

Thoughtfully adapt. Both words, thoughtfully and adapt, have meaning that's essential to anyone who wants to succeed with fasting, or any other behavior change, for that matter.

What does it mean to be *thoughtful?*

Be careful	Be considerate
Be present	Be deliberate
Be attentive	Be reflective
Be mindful	Be wise
Be intentional	

Wow, all of that just from the word thoughtful? Yes, indeed. It's your responsibility to be present and intentional with the choices you make when fasting and eating.

Without your active attention, thoughtful consideration, and persistent effort, how will you change old habits? How will you override the voice in your head that tells you to just screw it and eat what you want? How will you thoughtfully reject the voice that thinks, *Who needs sleep? You need to wake up earlier and work out if you want to lose that weight.*

What does it mean to *Adapt?*

Adjust to changing circumstances.

Meet new challenges with curiosity.

Revise the plan.

Modify your actions to suit new conditions.

Accommodate your body's needs.

Reassess and alter your approach.

Adaptation is *the reason* you can depend on fasting to reach your goals. Without adaptation, there would be no weight loss. There would be no abundant energy, mental clarity, reduced inflammation, vitality, and improved metabolic health. It's the adaptation, the hormesis, that induces change.

> *"Remember, stretching your fasts out a little longer than you may be used to creates a hormetic response in your cells...lovingly encouraging our bodies to adapt to new stressors is a beautiful way to accelerate the healing process. Don't be shy to try some of the longer fasts; just make sure to do them at the right phase of your (menstrual) cycle."*

> \- Dr. Mindy Pelz, *Fast Like a Girl*

It's up to you to be thoughtful with your adaptation so the change you induce leads to favorable outcomes instead of detrimental ones. Instead of pushing into longer fasts, many of you may need to scale back.

Remember this graph?

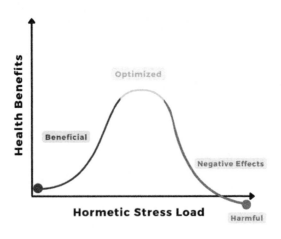

When you thoughtfully adapt, you stay in the green and yellow areas of the graph, where your health benefits are increased and even optimized. When you abuse fasting, eat like crap, or never adapt, you risk stagnation or negative outcomes that can actually make things worse than they were when you started.

Misconceptions about Thoughtful Adaptation and Planning Your Fasts

I often describe my style of fasting as "the most flexible fasting lifestyle." Really, though, it's the most adaptable fasting lifestyle. Either way, being flexible or adaptable doesn't imply your fasting lifestyle is unstructured or unplanned. You don't just go with the flow and ask yourself, *Do I feel like fasting today?* That's *intuitive fasting*, not adaptable fasting.

Adaptable fasting is:

- **Inspired.** It's a lifestyle inspired by what you know about yourself, your body, and what you really want.

- **Structured.** By setting a combination of personally-wise boundaries, you get more results with fewer obstacles along the way.

- **More automatic.** A thoughtful fasting plan takes the guesswork out of *when* to eat and *what* to eat once the time comes.

- **Experimental**. An experimental plan is one that you may not stick with, but it is a plan you test out and learn from; you grow wiser with each experience.

- **Ever-changing.** You often revise your plan to work with ever-changing circumstances and new self-discoveries.

- **Hindering self-sabotage.** A thoughtful fasting plan frees you from manipulative mental chatter and impulsive, self-sabotaging behavior.

What adaptable fasting is NOT:

- Impulsive

- Dependent on willpower

- Doing the same thing every day out of habit

- Resulting in regret

- A practice requiring mindfulness skills on par with a zen monk

- Changing your mind as soon as you have a craving, get pissed off, notice you have the house to yourself or want to escape the work you're doing

It's *not* flexible fasting when you back out last minute because you suddenly crave Chick-fil-A and you haven't thought about what's for dinner. Flexible, adaptable fasting is waking up with a headache and asking yourself, *Does my body need me to fast to feel better, or does my body need me to eat to feel better? Let's experiment and try to learn from this.* That's where the wisdom grows.

An adaptable fasting lifestyle depends on your unique wisdom, priorities, and current circumstances. Interestingly, *planning your fasts* helps you have a more adaptable fasting lifestyle because you'll *plan fasting around your life.*

Many sayings exist to remind us we can't have freedom without structure. Flexibility *sounds* so freeing, but when it lacks structure (or planning and self-awareness), it results in behavior patterns dictated by the voice in your head. That's the one that inevitably self-sabotages you because it always chooses the easy way out, the most well-worn path, or the most attractive option. So, unless you're a mindfulness master, you need structure to experience lasting freedom with intermittent fasting.

Let's compare unstructured flexible fasting with unstructured social media use. You've been there before, mindlessly scrolling TikTok in bed or whenever you glance at your phone to send a message or check the time. Especially with app notifications turned on, you unintentionally build this self-sabotaging habit of scrolling for hours every day when you could be spending that time on things that are more important and fulfilling to you.

Such an impulsive habit can result in enduring frustration. You feel enslaved by your TikTok habit, and you're hard on yourself as a result. You think the problem is you, and the solution is more willpower or self-control. In reality, the problem is a lack of structure (or boundaries). The solution is to create an *experimental plan*.

TikTok Problem: Lacking a plan or automated boundaries to prevent thoughtless TikTok use when you'd feel better using that time for something more fulfilling.

TikTok Experimental Plan: Go to *freedom.to/downloads* and download the Freedom app on any device or as a browser extension. Freedom lets you create a Blocklist of apps and websites you want to block during scheduled or spontaneous work sessions. Once it's activated, take a moment to create a quick list of things you might instead do with your time—and enjoy. Once it's activated, take a moment to create a quick list of things you might instead do with your time (things you'd enjoy doing).

See how much more effective this would be rather than expecting yourself to will your way around the impulse in the moment?

Trust the Process

Imagine it's five months from now. You didn't start this fasting method and decided to look for another quick fix because you were too impatient. The quick fix didn't work, and you're still 20 lbs heavier than you wanted to be five months ago. You wish you'd just started the process back then instead of trying another shortcut.

Time flies. You've gotta admit. I remember when I needed to find a new doctor for an annual exam I hadn't scheduled in many years. When I finally found one, they told me they couldn't fit me in for three months. I almost didn't schedule the appointment, thinking, *No way I'm going to wait this long because I'm already years behind schedule. I should find another doctor.* But then I realized I should schedule it anyways, just in case I couldn't find another doctor. Once I hung up the phone, I had no motivation to search for more doctors. Then, guess what? I blinked my eyes, and three months had passed! Time flies, and you know it. You will get there as long as you just don't quit and you keep a pace that's not too fast.

In the biographical film *King Richard,* Will Smith plays the tenaciously determined father of U.S. tennis stars Venus and Serena Williams. Every day at practice, since they were children, he hung a sign that read, "If You Fail to Plan, You Plan to Fail."

That's what we're talking about here. In the active pursuit of any goal, an unplanned day is a wasted day—especially when the number of planned days doesn't outnumber unplanned days by at least four to one. This means that for every five days of your fasting lifestyle, at least four of those were planned ahead of time (the fasts *and the food* make up the plan!).

You *will* need to thoughtfully adapt. Even with a plan, if you had a shitty night of sleep, it's very likely you'll need to adjust the plan accordingly. Thoughtful adaptation is an advanced skill you'll develop. You will advance to this phase if you want to continue experiencing the payoff intermittent fasting can have on your health.

~∽~

One of the absolute most important things about this phase, thoughtful adaptation, is you can't do the same thing every day for weeks or months on end and expect your body to continue showing results. The adaptation will stop. You'll get too comfortable, your metabolism will get too accustomed to your routine, and you won't continue to progress.

Just like with exercise, if you start with a workout routine doing bicep curls and pushups in an effort to build your arm muscles, it will work for a few weeks or so, but eventually, you'll need to change something in that workout to keep seeing muscle growth. You'll need to increase the weights or repetitions and eventually modify or expand upon the specific exercises you do.

Same goes for your fasting and your diet. Get too routine with it, and you'll stop seeing results. Plain and simple. Adaptation is the path to results. Your body's adaptation results from it enduring a new challenge you present it with.

At first, fasting from 8 p.m.–12 p.m. can help you get in the groove. This is called 16:8 fasting, where you fast for 16 hours and eat your food within an 8-hour window. It can boost your confidence, show you some early results, and help you overcome certain self-sabotaging habits around food and mealtimes. But, eventually, you'll need to change it up.

12 Ways to Change Up Your Fasting and Enhance Adaptation:

1. Increase your daily fasting window for up to 5 days a week.

2. Add a 45-minute walk during your fasting window, 2–5 days a week.

3. Add strength training at the end of your daily fast, and follow it with a high protein meal.

4. Women, practice cycle-syncing and change your fasts according to the hormonal phase you're in.

5. Fast longer on non-exercise days and shorter on exercise days.

6. Shift your fasting window to occur at different start and end times from day-to-day.

7. Once a week, after adequate sleep, add 8 hours onto the length of your routine fasts.

8. Once per month, toss in a fast that's double the length of your usual fasts.

9. Incorporate blood-flow restriction training, or other safe hormetic stressors like infrared sauna, cold therapy, or hypoxic breath work

10. Alter the macronutrient ratios in your diet by strategically cycling carbs, or reducing/increasing fiber, starches, fats, or protein.

11. Add significant variety to your diet by diversifying the plant and animal foods you eat, and by incorporating more fermented foods.

12. Increase your nutrient intake with 3-Meal Days, strategic supplementation, or a modified fast—fasting with food that's rapidly absorbed or clinically proven to keep the body in a state of ketosis (Chapter 57)

CHAPTER 42

Fasting Works Around Your Life

Thoughtful adaptation can be the very thing that separates those who ultimately succeed from those who stay stuck in the metabolic rut of gradual self-destruction. It's imperative we adapt our healthy habits over time. It's imperative we adapt our fasting. In fact, you want your fasts to be anything but a routine! Being too rigid and predictable with your eating habits will backfire or result in stagnation sooner or later.

As you've learned through this book, you'll need to adapt your diet so you can obtain a wider-range of nutrients, more diversity for your gut microbes, and a reduced toxin-load that would otherwise be a burden when eating a routine diet. Your eating habits need to adapt so they're sustainable. You adapt so it works with your changing hormonal status (women), your fitness habits, your schedule, your sleep quality and stress levels, your relationships, your state of health or disease, and all the huge things that will indeed change throughout the seasons of life.

Fasting works around your life

When you first commit to a new diet, you probably put some other obligations on hold or you move things around on your calendar so they don't interfere with your new commitment. That's a good way to prioritize and standardize your new habits and goals *at first!*

But.

If you want this to become the last diet you'll ever need, you'll need to make fasting fit around the other constants in your life. In other words, instead of trying to shape your life and daily routines around the diet and fasting schedule, you're looking for something sustainable. A sustainable fasting lifestyle is one where fasting works around your life and not the other way around.

That's right. Fasting shouldn't impede important plans or negatively impact your relationships. Why? Well, let's consider this example, shared mostly from a woman's POV, but men can experience similar obstacles. Check it out.

Let's say you're used to fasting for around 19 hours every day, and you've had some great results. You want to keep it going because you're not at your goal weight yet, and you want to make this stick (so that you don't gain the weight back once you get to your desired goal).

To help you progress to that point, you've postponed family vacations and scheduled work meetings to occur during your fasting window because it sure makes fasting easier when you have meetings to attend! When your kids eat dinner at 8 p.m. after getting home from their activities, you've been sipping on some tea instead of eating together because you're determined to close your fasting window at 6 p.m.

When your girlfriends asked to schedule an outing next month, they suggested a margarita night, and you convinced them to do a Zumba class together instead. You're watching your sugar and carbs, and there's no way you can do that at a Mexican restaurant.

When you attended a wedding this summer, you wanted to fast at 6 p.m., but you knew dinner wouldn't be served until later. You recall that when the invitation came, you felt so conflicted—like, you wanted to attend, but you had anxiety about it because it would screw up your fasting routine. The anxiety kept growing, and you even considered skipping the wedding, but your husband talked you into going. Thus, at the reception, you filled up on appetizers during cocktail hour and sat through dinner at the wedding sipping on decaf coffee, trying to hide in your chair as you awkwardly waved off each plate the server tried setting in front of you…. It was your fasting window, after all, and you couldn't possibly eat after 7 p.m.!

Some of those life changes might be sustainable, sure, but many of them are too restrictive and may ultimately be detrimental in some way. Over time, your decisions affect the other people in your life. And although, at first, they were patient with you on the new diet, they may lose patience when this continues for six months, a year, or longer.

Soon, your ten-year-old wants to skip dinners, too, because that's what Mom does. Or the kids ask, "Are you ever going to eat with us, Mom?" At work, your colleagues request that you move the morning meeting to the afternoon (during your eating window). Your girlfriends want to make up that margarita night in the fall, and your family wants finally to take that vacation.

What do you do in the face of such social pressure? If you're an all-or-nothing thinker, you might get trapped here, thinking you have to choose between your diet and your life. That's a surefire way to self-sabotage your efforts and throw the past few months out the window by bingeing on piña coladas, fried empanadas, and all the comfort foods you've been avoiding.

What if, instead, you experiment in each of the scenarios to discover how fasting can work more reasonably with the situation. Perfectly? No. Adequately? *Yes.*

As with all things related to habits and behavior change, patience and curiosity are required.

For several years, I co-coached a group of fifteen to thirty people through My6Method, a fat-loss program created by my friend and fitness nutrition coach Adrienne Hanover. When the registration period opens, newcomers contemplate whether to sign up due to potential conflicts in their schedules. We receive inquiries like, "I have a vacation coming up; will I still be able to do your program at the same time?" and "I'm getting married a month after your program; can I still do it if I need to go cake tasting and interviewing caterers for the wedding?" We always respond with something like this: "That's great! It may come as a surprise to you, but it's actually helpful to do our program when you have something like this (a vacation, a wedding) going on because you'll learn so much about how to adapt your diet or your habits to fit your life."

When you wait to do a diet until you can fit everything else around the changes, you end up with an unrealistic experience that you view as temporary. It's unrealistic because, when the diet 'ends', you abandon it entirely and default to your old ways because you didn't learn how to integrate these changes with your real-life circumstances.

Healthy habits have to become a *part of you*. You try them on, mold them, grow with them, and integrate them in ways that compliment your other priorities and become a part of your self-identity.

The question then becomes, how can we thoughtfully adapt in a realistic, sustainable way? An effective framework is what I call *Good, Better, Best*. It provides a methodical way to set tiered expectations and priorities. In the next chapter, we'll explore how applying *Good, Better, Best* enables the kind of thoughtful planning and self-compassion that makes fasting work long-term. It's a strategy to avoid rigid all-or-nothing thinking and instead set goals you can actually achieve. The *Good, Better, Best* mindset is essential for thoughtful adaptation.

CHAPTER 43

Thoughtfully Adapt with
Good, Better, Best

Thoughtful adaptation can require some planning, and it always requires experimentation. Imagine that, in an effort to lose some excess weight, you've been fully committed to fasting and eating a nutrient-dense diet for months now. You'd love it if you could achieve results in the shortest amount of time, but you realize it's different this time. You're playing the long game, and you want this to be the last diet you'll ever need.

Family vacation is coming up, and it's time to plan how you'll adapt. Vacation will make your fasting schedule difficult to maintain, so you look at it like an experiment. *What can I learn from this vacation that will help me continue a fasting lifestyle while still enjoying myself on this getaway?*

How I might coach you through this:

During our coaching call, I ask questions to get a feel for your initial expectations:

- How do you feel about your coming vacation?

- Have you thought about the habits you want to stick with and which habits you'll be more flexible with?

- If you were only able to stick with one healthy habit on this trip, which one do you feel most confident you can commit to?

- Imagine your vacation experience turned out pretty ideal. You returned home feeling proud of yourself because you stuck to several healthy habits throughout the trip. Describe to me the version of yourself that showed up to make this outcome possible.

- What are some things that might get in the way of your showing up in that way?

Notice there at the end, we wind up talking about what you feel an *ideal* outcome is and what barriers you can predict will get in your way. Automatically, most dieters only consider what is optimal. This sticks them in a limited frame of mind, with very little future empathy or consideration for how your future self might feel or act differently than you're projecting now. Instead, it's important to identify not only what is ideal but also what is *acceptable*.

That's where *Good, Better, Best* comes in handy.

- What's the *best* outcome you'll strive for? (Ideal)

- What's a *better* outcome that's not as great as the best but still pretty darn great? (Not quite optimal)

- What's a *good* outcome that's acceptable and still feels better than not trying at all? (Acceptable)

Hypothetically, let's say your ideal vacation outcome would be to fast every day for 16 hours, skip breakfast for a cup of black coffee, break your fast at 12 p.m., and close your eating window at 8 p.m. each night. You want to stay gluten-free on your trip and eat low-carb, too.

So your *best* plan is: 16-hour fasts (8 p.m.–12 p.m.), black coffee, low carb, and gluten-free every day.

Your *better* plan is: 14-hour fasts (flexible window of time), No alcohol after 9 p.m., black coffee (if the coffee is decent), and gluten-free every day.

Your *good* plan is: minimum 12-hour fasts, no fried food, dessert, or sugary drinks. *If my spouse orders ice cream, I might take a bite and savor it.*

This *Good, Better, Best* framework helps you consider not just what is ideal but what is reasonable, doable, and still worth the effort. We can then simplify the goals even further and create an at-a-glance list of your priorities:

- Fasting 12–16 hours daily
- Black coffee if the coffee is decent
- Low carb daily if possible
- Gluten-free daily if possible
- Skip the fried foods or sugary indulgences

Good, Better, Best helps my clients stay away from *all-or-nothing* thinking. It also helps them experiment with fasting and dietary habits that fit around their lives so that they can build sustainable habits and increase self-awareness, which means more control over their behaviors and a fulfilling degree of self-acceptance. In turn, they see increased confidence and progress that can last.

Good, Better, Best isn't just for unusual circumstances like a vacation. This strategy is also perfect for goal setting. When my client, Debrah, told me she wanted to work out four days a week, and she currently doesn't exercise much at all, I reminded her that *Good, Better, Best* can help us determine a range of progress toward that goal. Together, we agreed that the *Best* outcome would be to exercise four days next week, her *Better* outcome would be to exercise three days next week, and her *Good* outcome would be to exercise two days next week. Debrah ended up exercising three days that week, and she felt very proud of herself!

You can see how *Good Better Best* is valuable in a variety of situations when it comes to planning, experimenting, goal-setting, and adapting your fasts.

Next, let's explore how you can integrate more adaptation into your daily or weekly fasting lifestyle. That's where 3-Meal Days come into play. Humans are designed to fast and feast. Dipping in and out of both states helps ensure better metabolic health and optimal gene expression. If you want to achieve lasting benefits with fasting, this is one *fasting safeguard* you don't want to skip.

CHAPTER 44

3-Meal Days: Cycling Your Fasts with this Essential Fasting Safeguard

I know it may be hard to believe, but eating more meals in a cyclical fashion can help you get healthier and lose more weight. That's why this chapter is dedicated entirely to my favorite fasting safeguard: 3-Meal Days.

> *"If you maintain a constant reduced-calorie diet, the body will quickly adapt to it. Energy expenditure (metabolism) declines to match the reduced intake. Weight plateaus, and then it's regained... To prevent the body from adapting to the new weight-loss strategy and maintain weight loss requires an intermittent strategy, not a constant one. This is a crucial distinction...the difference between failure and success."*

- Jason Fung and Jimmy Moore, *The Complete Guide to Fasting*

If you recall, in Part 4, I introduced you to what I call fasting safeguards. Just as the name implies, safeguards are protective habits or behaviors that help to prevent undesirable outcomes commonly occurring with routine dieting. Safeguards are supportive, enhancing elements that promise you better results. Not only will your metabolism improve, but your overall health will improve, too. Refer back to Chapter 38 for the complete list of fasting safeguards.

Cycling Your Fasts with *3-Meal Days*

3-Meal Days are just as they sound. You intentionally eat more frequently, 3 meals in a day, once every 2 weeks—or as often as 7 days a month—depending on your situation.

When you've gotten used to intermittent fasting, you'll likely fall into a routine with it. You'll fast nearly every single day for around the same time. But here's the thing: fasting has always co-existed with *feasting*.

Humans would go days or weeks with severely restricted access to food, spending lots of time fasting. Intermittently, there would be opportunities to feast—eating everything in sight after a successful hunt because there wasn't a place for safe food storage or leftovers. Feasting also occurred when they found a fruit tree or bee hive dripping with honey because nature provides bounty in abundance. There was no way to save it during pre-civilized times when our human DNA blueprint was particularly evolving.

Today, we fast in an attempt to optimize our DNA—our gene expression— to promote better health, but we forget about the importance of an occasional *feast*. Most people in the fasting community call it a feast day, and some call it a *refeeding* day. I decided to call it a *3-Meal Day* because that, to me, sounds very clear. *It's not a cheat day. It's not an eat whatever-the-hell-you-want day.*

A 3-Meal Day is an intentional, strategic, nutritious breakfast-lunch-and-dinner day that floods your body with nutrients, prompts adaptation, and reassures your metabolism that it has everything you need to thrive.

Without a nutrient-dense 3-Meal Day, consistent intermittent fasting can eventually lead to chronic caloric restriction, insufficient nutrient intake, disordered eating thought-patterns, impaired healing, and hormonal imbalances that negatively affect your stress tolerance, metabolism, and immunity. Thus inhibiting your progress.

When should you consider cycling in a 3-Meal Day?

Many people will benefit from having a 3-Meal Day once every two or three weeks after they're fully fat-adapted. However, some groups of people, like the last four on the list below, would benefit from more frequent refueling days. Err on the side of caution if you fall into more than one category, and just start with the most frequent recommendation. You may actually lose more weight by eating more frequently if your metabolism has been too stressed for too long. Note that temporary weight regain is expected and a natural reaction to increasing your food intake. Don't be alarmed. Your body is distributing water weight and nutrients in an intelligently orchestrated fashion, not to mention your bowels are fuller than usual. Things will balance out in the bigger picture.

3-Meal Day Fasting Cycles

- Sedentary individuals with diagnosed insulin resistance, pre-diabetes, type 2 diabetes, or metabolic syndrome: Once every 21 days

- Beginner fasters who've been consistently fasting > 14 hours for less than 2 months: Once every 21 days

- Individuals without a history of significant weight loss and regain who have > 50 lb or 40 percent of body fat to lose: Once every 21 days

- Individuals with a history of yo-yo weight loss and regain cycles of > 20 lb in a 6-month timeframe, more than twice in the last five years: Once every 5–7 days

- Individuals who consistently practice OMAD or do prolonged fasts of > 36 hours more frequently than twice a month: Once every

7–10 days (For people who engage in extended fasts, the 3-Meal Day would ideally occur when you break the extended fast.)

- Individuals who regularly engage in endurance training or high-intensity training more than 3 days a week, or who exercise for 2 hours a day: Once per week, or on every intense/endurance training day

- Menstruating Women: 5–10 days per month, occurring during the week your period is approaching (the last week of your luteal phase—during PMS). Note that some women may need to incorporate 3-Meal Days during the ovulation phase of their cycle if enhanced fertility and hormonal regularity are the goal.

Tips For Incorporating 3-Meal Days:

- 3-Meal Days are focused on high nutrition + high satisfaction. Remember, eating a nutrient-dense, varied diet is another fasting safeguard. So, combining these two safeguards is essential in my mind. They work in harmony, making fasting easier and more effective.

- You'll need to plan ahead for your 3-Meal Days so you have a variety of nutritious options available to help prevent it from turning into a cheat day.

- It makes the most sense for a 3-Meal Day to occur on a day that includes physical activity or on a day when you break a longer fast (in the morning).

- When 3-Meal Days occur up to two times per month, and fat-loss is the primary goal, try increasing carb intake to 75 grams, or up to 130 grams of total *carbs on those days (*ideally from whole food sources)

- For 3-Meal Days that occur several days per month or more, especially when improved insulin sensitivity is the primary goal, aim to keep carbs under 50 grams of total carbs a majority of the time.

- The more hours you routinely fast, or the more aggressively you exercise, the higher you want to increase carbs and protein on 3-Meal Days.

- Eat your first meal before 10 a.m. or within two hours of waking, and ensure it contains a minimum of 25 g of complete protein.

- Strictly limit processed carbohydrates and sugar to avoid setbacks. Prioritize whole-food carbohydrate sources, a variety of nutrient-dense, colorful veggies, and adequate protein at every meal.

- Women may need to prioritize progesterone-boosting foods as described in Chapter 46 under *Fasting Guidelines for Women*

- Consider taking additional dietary supplements on these days, especially digestive enzymes and Betaine HCl (if advisable, see Chapter 27) with each meal. This helps increase your nutrient intake on a 3-Meal Day, revitalizing your cells. It also helps avoid potential discomfort due to increased food intake compared to your routine.

- You're not snacking; you're eating a meal. A smaller meal is fine, but your goal is to eat a quantity that doesn't feel restricted. Remember, meals = protein + veggies + healthy fats.

- If you're accustomed to intermittent fasting, it's normal to get super-full from eating a smaller meal compared to how much you used to be able to eat. You may not even be hungry in the morning when it comes time for your 3-Meal Day. That's okay. Eat anyway; just eat a smaller portion that leaves you physically full and satisfied.

One of the single most important reasons you'd need more frequent 3-Meal Days is if you're a woman in her reproductive years and perimenopause. It's incredible how female hormones impact our ability to fast and cope with stress, and it's time to dive into these undeniable differences.

CHAPTER 45

The Modern Woman:
The Interplay Between Female Hormones, Stress, and Fasting

Women and Men are biologically different. Plain and simple. Female bodies respond differently to lifestyle and environmental factors compared to men. It's empowering to familiarize yourself with the complexities of female hormones and how they influence your body, your mood, and your ability to set and achieve your goals.

This chapter and the next will cover two intertwined topics: women and fasting and how female hormones are affected by stress and behavior. I'll help you understand why fasting is plain easier for men (not just easier to do, but results come easier, too). I'll share what you need to know about stress and your sex hormones and how to eat and fast in concert with your monthly cycle. Some guidance will be provided for women in perimenopause and menopause so you can take the next steps to live more in harmony with your biology during those critical transitions.

You can take a deeper dive into this topic in the hormonally-centered book *Fast Like a Girl* by Dr. Mindy Pelz. For my perimenopausal women over forty, I highly recommend Dr. Mindy's latest book, *The Menopause Reset,* where she walks you through the specific fasting and dieting strategies that work to minimize the misery commonly experienced during perimenopause and make weight loss or weight maintenance a more effortless pursuit.

In this chapter, we'll also cover how your behaviors and obligations can positively or negatively influence your hormones and, in turn, affect your ability to pursue and obtain your health goals and experience more contentment in your life as a woman!

Human Biology Treats Females Differently

One hard fact about being a woman of reproductive age is that your biology has a number one priority to help you reproduce. Even if you don't care to be fertile, your body does, and it will initiate signs of dysfunction if it suspects that you're not fit to successfully grow a baby. This might be because you're under-nourished (i.e., too much fasting, too much caloric restriction, not enough nutrients) or that your body senses you're in danger (i.e., experiencing too much stress or anxiety, not getting adequate sleep, over-exercising). The most common signs of hormonal dysfunction show up as stubborn weight, missed periods, thyroid dysfunction, fibroids, endometriosis, low sex hormone levels, high stress hormones or adrenal burnout, infertility—of course—and so much more.

Fasting is just biologically easier for men. Looking at figure 45.1, notice the graph on the left, which measures the appetite hormone *ghrelin* throughout a 24-hour cycle. The black dots in the top line are for women, and the white dots are for men.

Do you see how high those ghrelin levels are for women compared to men? If you look at the bars on the right, the black bars are for women, and the white bars are for men. *Whoa.* Huge difference, right? You're biologically programmed to seek out food, so try not to be so hard on yourself.

Figure 45.1: Fasting and Ghrelin in male and female test subjects Source[38]

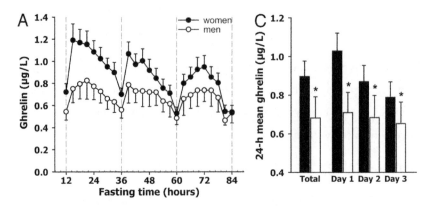

The production of ghrelin (the hormone that increases our appetite) varies widely based on a person's childhood experiences, dieting history, age, meal frequency, genetics, neurological factors, sleep, and much more. This can be a good thing because it means you may not need to worry about this, even if you're a woman. Maybe you're one of the women whose body doesn't make as much ghrelin, and you, therefore, can fast more comfortably, like a typical male. This small European study[39] and the graph of their findings, in figure 45.2, is a good example of that.

Figure 45.2: Ghrelin in male and female subjects over a 24-hour fasting period

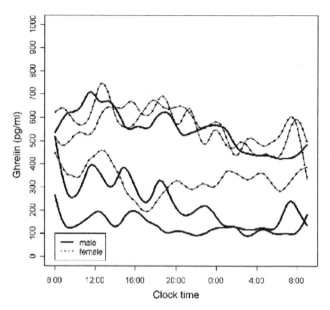

The three dotted lines represent three healthy twenty-five-year-old females. The three solid lines represent three healthy twenty-five-year-old males. Notice how two of the females had the highest levels of ghrelin, and there was one male up there with them. Then look at the lowest dotted line. One of the females had significantly lower ghrelin production during this 24-hour fast. That could be you, although, honestly, it's unlikely the case if you've been struggling with your weight, sleep, or chronic stress.

Even if a majority of us women do have higher ghrelin levels overall, don't allow this news to defeat you because what we also see on the first graph is that women experience a greater reduction in ghrelin as the 24-hour fast continues into an extended fast. The further they get into their fast, like around the 60-hour mark, their baseline ghrelin production is lower than when they started. This can help women completely reset their voracious appetites, and it helps us understand why, remarkably, people are actually less hungry during a long fast than they are during a shorter fast or when not fasting at all.

Fasting really is an effective way to lower your ghrelin and, therefore, your appetite overall. Fasting can also be quite powerful for improving female health, but it's absolutely essential that you learn to respect the differences in your biology and how your hormones require nuance in a fasting lifestyle so it doesn't backfire on you. It's not easy at first to coordinate your fasts with your fluctuating hormones, but it is definitely effective and worth it. Not to mention that the alternative could be slowing down your metabolism and bringing about the exact opposite results you seek.

Intro to Our Female Hormones

Most of us don't know squat about our key female sex hormones:

1. Estrogen

2. Progesterone

3. Oxytocin

It's worth clarifying that although these aren't exclusively female hormones, a woman's body requires and produces much higher levels of them compared to a man's body. What's interesting is most of us are completely unaware that, for many women, our modern way of life encourages the production of testosterone—yup, testosterone—and cortisol, which impede our ability to make those three essential female hormones that keep us feeling sane, healthy, and balanced.

Today, it's far less common for a woman to take a traditional housewife or stay-at-home role than it is for her to work a full-time job outside of the home. Scientists have been able to show, in the last few decades, that the things we do during the day and the roles we play have a hormonal effect on the body and brain. So, as we've shifted away from old-fashioned, traditional roles in society, we've shifted away from the evolutionary inputs our brain and body expect to produce balanced female hormones.

If you fit one of these descriptions or work one of the jobs listed below, it's time for you to learn about testosterone:

- The boss (or just plain bossy most of the day)

- A manager, team leader, or primary decision-maker at home or at work

- A single Mom (or you just feel like one)

- The primary income generator in your household

- A teacher of ages seven and up, professor, or adult instructor

- A lawyer

- An activist

- A feminist

- Self-reliant

- Building, constructing, or designing things

- Competitive at work

- Money-driven—money drives the work you do, and more effort equals more money

- Working at an impersonal or technical job

- Doing things all day that you don't want to do but have to do.

Those with the following lifestyles linked to the work they do *may be* exempt from the concerns about testosterone production because their daily activities may help produce more female-supportive hormones:

- Women whose days are *not* filled with doing things they don't want to do but have to do.

- Women who primarily work as nurses (not nursing directors), and it's important that the work feels fulfilling or natural rather than forced and accompanied by resentment.

- Women nursing an infant or caring for a toddler, especially when the obligations feel fulfilling.

- Female kindergarten or daycare teachers whos day-to-day work feels fulfilling.

- Female caregivers whos day-to-day work feels fulfilling.

- Stay-at-home wives.

- Women with a career they love doing, including the day-to-day tasks it involves, and which doesn't primarily involve managing others.

The Deal with Testosterone Production for Today's Modern Woman

Certain actions and behaviors, like being the decision-maker and leading a team, send signals to our biology to make more testosterone.[40] Even as women, when we engage in more historically traditional 'male' roles or activities, our bodies respond by making more testosterone. This is okay, actually. It's okay if we know how to shift back over to our female side after work so testosterone can go down and progesterone, estrogen, and oxytocin can rise. Then we feel rejuvenated. We feel balanced. We feel recovered. And then we can go back to work the next day and continue this dance as a way of life that's quite fulfilling and healthy.

Testosterone opposes the production of estrogen. When our testosterone is too high, we feel competitive, stressed, detached, sometimes resentful, and unfulfilled.

Notice, on that first bulleted list, the last entry is *Your days are filled with doing things you don't want to do but have to do. Sheesh, right?* Here's the kicker:

*"When a woman does something that she doesn't want to do but has
to, her testosterone levels rise, her estrogen levels begin to drop,
and she is unable to make oxytocin."*
- John Gray, *Beyond Mars & Venus*

It's pretty rare nowadays for an adult to have a day that's not filled with shit we don't want to do. But that's not all we're fighting against. We're also fighting against time. I can't tell you how many of my clients tell me they don't have time for anything. Nothing. No time. Zero. Can't take it anymore; there's no time!

Welp…. Feeling rushed in all areas of her life is the number one condition that contributes to a woman feeling stressed and overwhelmed," explains Dr. Gray. This way of life tends to create an overabundance of testosterone and detrimental inhibition of estrogen and progesterone.

Unfairly, men's bodies are designed to put up with this. They can feel rushed, they can have a day filled with too many things to do that they don't want to do, and the extra testosterone works in their favor. (Interestingly, however, if a man voices complaints about it frequently enough, he'll make estrogen and inhibit testosterone.) It hurts us women. It makes us feel stressed and overwhelmed. That's why this work-life balance pursuit we all dream of or strive for ends up being another burden. We feel it's another thing we have to do with time that simply doesn't exist.

Dr. Gray says, "Women can do it all, but when they do, they don't sleep well at night because they're so overwhelmed and stressed…women become overwhelmed with too much to do, feeling like there isn't enough time."— and I couldn't agree more. Turns out, it's biological.

At first, it's a bummer to learn this. But there are solutions you can implement for results you'll truly feel and appreciate.

How to decompress, reduce high testosterone, reduce stress, and refresh our hormones daily or cyclically

Female hormone experts often say all we need to do to reduce our stress from the day is engage in more oxytocin-promoting behaviors. Oxytocin is often considered the love and affection hormone because we can boost it with things like massage, cuddling, romance, petting an animal, hugging, kissing, etc. That's *not* going to work for most of us most of the time.

Oxytocin is tricky. Although it will help to reduce our testosterone, it won't always lower our stress unless we also engage in a behavior or role that also influences estrogen or progesterone. This is because we need those hormones to feel like ourselves. To feel balanced. The lowering of testosterone isn't enough. We need more of our female chemicals. (And yes, even if you're in menopause, this topic applies to you, too).

Most of the time, we can achieve an increase in oxytocin and other female hormones, especially estrogen, when we share our feelings with another person. But sharing our feelings doesn't include complaining (especially when the complaints involve the person you share your feelings with). Complaining makes us feel more drained and resentful. Sharing our feelings or a recap of our day's events with someone who will simply listen and not try to fix our situation helps us produce a significant amount of oxytocin and estrogen, which in turn helps us decompress and destress from the day. Once you're feeling relaxed and supported, you can then work toward finding a solution to problems or complaints that sustain your unmet needs.

There will be times when you don't feel like sharing your feelings, or when that's not enough—like the week leading up to your period, or when you're already at max-level resentment because you have to do so many things you don't want to do. This is when you need more social bonding or self-nurturing time.

I know you don't have *time* to spare, but hear me out.

If you can find a way to do something you enjoy (that's not evolutionarily masculine) without time pressure or pressure for it to turn out a certain way, you'll increase your female hormones and enable oxytocin to reduce your stress so you can feel rejuvenated. The cool thing is that with the right activities for you, you can do all of this at the same time: reduce testosterone, increase progesterone, increase estrogen, and reduce your stress and cortisol. Resetting for the following day.

Most women, at any age, can engage in the following oxytocin and estrogen-boosting activities or bonding relationships to effectively destress from the workday. (The exception is during the 7–10 days leading up to her period, during which she's less likely to feel like engaging in them and should instead see the second list. This includes things to help her produce progesterone, too.)

- Receiving support or services from others

- Anticipating support or appreciation from others (planning for a romantic date or planning to share good news with a friend)

- Praying

- Shopping in anticipation of wearing something new or gifting something to please or impress others

- Dressing or styling yourself in anticipation of being admired

- Nurturing others with whom you anticipate appreciation or affection in return

- Getting nails, hair, and skincare treatments done without feeling rushed; bonus points if you vent to your technician during the service

- Meeting with a therapist, coach, or religious authority with whom you primarily talk and feel heard

- Cuddling, hugging, being touched, or touching others in a sexual or non-sexual way

- Receiving flowers, affection, apologies, cards, notes, or respect

The following list is for women experiencing resentment or feeling overwhelmed with life's responsibilities and during the final two weeks leading up to their period, which is known as the luteal phase. This is especially needed during these 7–10 days when PMS symptoms are most likely to occur and/or women feel more resentment. This can also be effective during the first few days after the period has started.

Self-nurturing or social bonding activities that are stress-reducing and increase progesterone without time pressure or pressure to achieve a certain result. Many things on this list are adapted or inspired by the book *Beyond Mars & Venus*, which I can't recommend enough!

- Drawing, coloring, or painting
- Cross-stitching, weaving, crocheting, finger-looping, or sewing for pleasure
- Cooking for fun
- Journaling
- Practicing meditation
- Gardening
- Pursuing a passion or hobby that's driven by personal fulfillment
- Crafting, scrap-booking, organizing photos (if you find it enjoyable)
- Reading a novel, memoir, fantasy, or romance
- Spending time in nature or walking in solitude
- Listening to your favorite music, especially with head-phones, in solitude, and with your eyes closed
- Singing, dancing, or playing a musical instrument you enjoy
- Organizing or home designing (if you find it to be soothing)
- Taking a relaxing bath
- Engaging in a skincare ritual
- Experimenting with your makeup or hair (if you find that to be enjoyable)
- Caring for animals (if it's immersive and soothing to you)

- Learning something new (if it's soothing and fulfilling to you)
- Attending a group yoga or pilates class
- Playing cards or games with friends
- Bonding with a friend or external family member
- Having a girls' night out
- Joining women's support groups
- Sports or team activities

Getting these female hormones balanced throughout your life will help to drastically reduce your cortisol and help your body respond favorably to fasting, exercise, and other weight-loss and health pursuits.

Fasting Tips For Women Under 40, In Perimenopause, and Post-Menopause

Tracking Your Menstrual Cycle

Most women don't track their menstrual cycles. That's kinda crazy. And I'm not judging because I was one of these women for the first fifteen or twenty years of my menstruating life. To help you understand why it's kinda crazy not to track your period, let's compare it to something a little less complicated, like tracking the weather.

Let's say you're in college and you have to walk to school every day because it's too close to take the bus, but it's too costly to use a ride-share service like Uber while you're on a college student's budget.

You walk to class five days a week, sometimes in the early morning and sometimes in the afternoon, depending on what time your classes are each day. It rarely rains where you live, only a couple times a month, so you don't think about checking the weather—until you're getting poured on half-way through your walk to school. You get pissed off every time it happens because, of course, it happens when you just had a blow-out done on your hair, or the day you have an exam, or the day you're running late, feeling sick, on no sleep, etc.... You complain and complain, *I never catch a break,* or *Why don't I keep an umbrella in my bag?*

Years go by, and you continue to feel like unexpected rain is bad luck and has the potential to ruin your day instead of making a habit of checking the weather forecast once a day, which would decrease the likelihood of these bad luck incidents by 80 percent or more. Your life would be so much better. *Why aren't you tracking the weather?*

Hahaha, you can see what I mean now, can't you?

It's important to track your period using a smart tool like The MyFlo App so you can easily view and preview which phase of your cycle you'll be in at any given time. To my ladies on birth control or wearing an IUD, try the Clue Period Tracker App at *helloclue.com* to track your symptoms more closely to figure out which phase of your monthly cycle you're in. It's also helpful to look back to when you were acting out of character to see if the placement of your cycle helps explain why you felt or behaved the way you did.

If you want to dive deeper into the analysis of your current hormonal status, the DUTCH test is the most reliable comprehensive hormone panel for sex and stress hormones and will help you understand more about your current hormone imbalances.

Fasting with Your Female Hormones (for adult women of all ages)

It was in Part 4 that I dedicated entire chapters to stress and cortisol. I also introduced you to the important concept of hormesis, where stress can either help you achieve your health goals or be detrimental.

Some reasons stress and cortisol are such a big concern for modern-day women are that our cortisol is already high, in part because our testosterone is too high and oxytocin is too low, or because we are lonely or live stressful lives. That high cortisol counter-regulates the female hormones that would otherwise keep us balanced. Not only that, but when cortisol is in production, it sends a signal to release glycogen from your liver into your bloodstream to prepare you for the stress (in case you need to fight or run for your life).

This then leaves you with elevated blood glucose and cortisol if you don't complete the stress cycle (Chapter 35). Once your brain and body realize the perceived threat is gone, your pancreas will pump out insulin to help bring your blood glucose back to normal.

If you're insulin resistant, like most Americans today, insulin, glucose, and cortisol remain high, leaving the body in a negative feedback loop that promotes inflammation, hunger, fat storage, and metabolic dysfunction. This negative feedback loop explains why, no matter how hard you try, your biology can counteract your fasting efforts whenever you're under chronic stress. The only way to prevent such fruitless efforts and further damage is to practice lifestyle choices that respect the way your body is designed.

Simply with daily fasts of up to 24-hours,[41] cortisol levels increase regardless of gender, obesity or health status of human subjects. In a 2016 systematic review and meta-analysis, researchers Nakamura et al. concluded that "fasting showed a very strong effect in increasing serum cortisol."

In a 2021 review,[42] we learn that extended fasts exceeding 56 hours dramatically elevate cortisol levels. As you can see in the graph, figure 46.1, there's quite a difference in cortisol during a fasting day (dotted line) versus when those individuals were eating three meals a day (solid line). I hope these insights prove as further evidence to you that stress is a topic that cannot be ignored when it comes to your health.

Figure 46.1 Human cortisol levels while fasting versus eating 3 meals a day

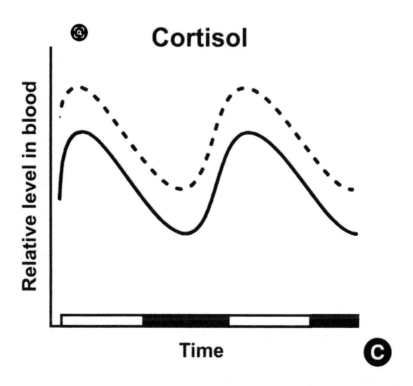

Estimated changes in cortisol after long-term intermittent fasting in humans (dashed line). Time is indicated by light box for daytime (6:00 AM–6:00 PM) and dark box for nighttime (6:00 PM–6:00 AM). Normal circadian rhythms of hormones were presented with solid line.

Fasting Guidelines for Women

Women can still fast, and they should—but only at the appropriate times, for the appropriate length, with their ever-changing circumstances.

For women with a monthly menstrual cycle:

During the last 14 days before your period, you're in what's known as the luteal phase. If you think of the luteal phase split into two parts, part 1 is when you might feel pretty fantastic. This time, immediately following ovulation, is when your progesterone and estrogen begin to climb, and progesterone peaks. It's not uncommon to feel game for some longer fasts during this time. Then, during part 2 of the luteal phase, all hormones begin to plummet, preparing for your period to arrive. This is a crucial time. A time when we must be particularly mindful of our biology, ladies!

During the 7–10 days before you bleed, your body needs nourishment. Your soul needs more self-regard. We're talking *less* fasting, more frequent meals, more nourishing foods, and more time for personal enjoyment. Ignore the needs of your biology during these 7–10 days before your period starts, and you can experience PMS, emotional instability, weakened immunity, exhaustion, erratic eating behavior, weight gain, self-blame, and lasting plateaus. We can't pretend this time of the month is like any other time of the month. It's not. Our behaviors must change; otherwise, the body is hit by the blunt forces of sinking progesterone, chronically high cortisol, and inadequate estrogen clearance.

Fasting too much during those 7–10 days before your period inhibits progesterone and sets you up for a whole mess of issues that include stubborn body fat and weight-loss plateaus. Instead, you can support your body once a month by adapting your fasting routine to work with your monthly cycle. *This adjustment is critically important for women who typically experience PMS, have hormonal disorders, lack sufficient sleep, or live a high-stress lifestyle, all of which leave them undernourished, insulin-resistant, and emotionally depleted.*

Cycling Fasts during the Luteal Phase—*for women who routinely intermittent fast ≥ 16 hours daily:*

- **Reduce your fasts to 12 hours for 7–10 days before your period arrives**

- **Incorporate several 3-Meal Days** to reduce cortisol and support social pleasure, increasing progesterone

o With your morning coffee, consider having a low-to-moderate carb breakfast with moderate protein, which helps reduce the stress on your adrenal glands.

- **Increase your intake of foods that facilitate progesterone** to reduce cortisol, detox estrogen, and make it to your period without *losing your shit.*

   o Foods to increase the week before your period include high-fiber foods like sprouted organic oats, cruciferous vegetables, cooked leafy greens, pumpkin/sunflower/sesame seeds, quinoa, and whole food starchy carbs like winter squash, lentils, beans, sweet potato, and moderate portions of white potato.

   o Satisfy a daily sweet-tooth with more progesterone-boosting foods like 80 percent dark chocolate, clementine tangerines, and moderate servings of tropical fruit.

   o Whole food carbohydrates should typically increase to 75-130 total grams per day in this timeframe leading up to your period, with more carbs on active days and fewer on inactive days.

- **Avoid high-intensity exercise or endurance training during this phase,** especially on days 25–30, to avoid excess cortisol and inhibited progesterone. Instead, go to a group yoga or low-intensity pilates class or engage in progesterone-boosting activities mentioned in the previous chapter.

- **Avoid any extended fasts during this critical hormonal phase of your cycle.**

Circumstantial Modifications:

If consumption of the progesterone-boosting foods listed above makes you feel out of control with your eating habits, return to your preferred number of daily carbs, but increase your intake of:

- Pasture-raised beef, bison, lamb, and goat to a serving per meal of ≥ 6 oz or 35 g protein. Whey protein powder is helpful here, especially on active days

- Salmon, shellfish, and bivalves (like oysters, mussels, clams)

- Beef or chicken liver, turkey-liverwurst, chicken liver mousse, pate, or organ meat/liver supplement capsules—all of which can help facilitate the production of progesterone

- Avocado, pumpkin/sunflower/sesame seeds, broccoli, cooked leafy greens, red bell pepper, lemon, lime, and sprouted oats and quinoa if tolerated.

Some of my clients who've been fasting for years really struggle with increasing their food intake as recommended. If you struggle with this, I suggest you **consider doing modified fasts** as a compromise during the week before your period. Drop fasts below 14 hours per day, prioritizing circadian fasting (eating in the morning, fasting longer in the evening), and supplement your fasting window with one or more of the following:

   o   Homemade Bone Broth

   o   *ProLon* Fast Bars

   o   *ProLon* Fasting Shake

   o   *Ample* meal shakes

   o   Chocolate whey protein smoothie made with water as the base + added collagen protein + berries + avocado or sesame/sunflower seeds/seed-butter

Summary for Menstruating Women:

Best times of the month for fasting are:

- Days 2–10 after your period starts

- Days 15–20 of your monthly cycle (This is after ovulating, in part 1 of the luteal phase.)

Time of the month when fasting is *not advisable:*

- Days 20–30 or 23–30 of your cycle. (This is part 2 of the luteal phase, which occurs during the last 7–10 days leading up to your period.)

During the last week to 10 days before your period, you'll reduce fasts to 12 hours. Consider eating a nutrient-dense breakfast with your morning coffee and incorporate 3-Meal Days to bring more joy and variety to your diet while nourishing your body during this stressful time in your monthly cycle. Prioritize whole foods and increase your daily carb intake with high fiber, mineral-rich foods like lentils, sesame seeds, quinoa, shellfish, and more from the list above. Keep carbs below 150 total grams per day, even with an active lifestyle, if weight loss is your goal.

For women who don't have a period and/or are in perimenopause:

Your focus is on optimizing your diet, and reducing your cortisol levels by way of stress reduction. Closely track your symptoms throughout the month (the Clue app is great for this, or a wearable tracker designed for women like the Basal Body Ring by Femtek). This will help you realize trends that suggest when your body needs more or less of carbs, fasting, exercise, and personal fulfillment. Many or all of the guidelines suggested for women who have periods still apply to you, but it requires more intention and tracking on your behalf since you can't rely on the onset of your period to guide you. I highly recommend Dr. Mindy Pelz's book, *Fast Like a Girl*, where you can learn her detailed protocol for a 30-day reset to help normalize your monthly cycle or assist in the transition through perimenopause. She also runs several group programs that will coach you through the cyclical fasting protocols she recommends.

Perimenopausal women would be well-advised to reduce their total carb intake to under 50 grams per day in order to optimize progesterone, estrogen, insulin, and adrenal function. In this stage, women typically need to increase progesterone and DHEA, a critical hormone precursor, in order to mitigate perimenopausal dysfunction. Many women will also need to optimize testosterone and thyroid hormones. A practitioner who specializes in endocrinology and functional medicine can be an invaluable resource here.

> *"If a woman is under significant stress—if she is overworked, if her diet fails to meet her body's needs, if she is physically ill, if she smokes and/or drinks, or if she's involved in relationships in which the energy isn't reciprocated—then she may find that her ability to keep up with the demands on her endocrine system is diminished. It will remain so until she's able to implement some changes in those areas of her life.... The result may otherwise be a tumultuous midlife transition, fraught with her unique combination of symptoms—from headaches, hot flashes, bloating, and fading libido to mood swings and sleep disturbances."*
> - Christiane Northrup, *The Wisdom of Menopause*

For Women in Menopause:

- Eat a nutrient-dense, low-to-moderate carb diet.

- Managing insulin is critical during menopause, and fasting works wonders for that.

- Incorporate 3-Meal Days once every 7–10 days to boost nutrient intake and remind your metabolism it has everything it needs.

  o On 3-Meal Days, add in more lentils, beans, edamame and sprouted tofu, quinoa, flax seeds, and single servings of tropical fruit. Omit the fruit if you're unable to control the portion size.

330

These foods will help encourage the production of estrogen and progesterone. Yes, you still make those hormones during menopause, just to a lesser degree.

Certain factors in your social life will greatly encourage the production of sex hormones in menopause. A particularly useful aspect will be to have a strong network of trusted individuals on whom you can depend. Having a community, a circle of trusted advisors (trusted doctors, therapist, etc.), friends and/or family who help you feel safe and supported has a tremendous impact on estrogen production. Having a social circle by whom you feel understood and doing things for your own enjoyment will stimulate more progesterone. Being too independent during your menopausal years only hinders sex hormone production, increases stress, and leads to more metabolic dysfunction, such as issues with stubborn weight and weight gain.

When a woman enters menopause, the ovaries pass the baton, so-to-speak, giving the sole responsibility of sex hormone production over to the adrenal glands. The adrenal glands already have a lot of work to do, regulating the metabolism and modulating the stress response, so the added responsibility of sex hormone regulation makes the adrenals particularly vulnerable during menopause. This is why special attention should be paid to menopausal women experiencing times of high chronic stress and who have trouble with insomnia. The hormone panel called the DUTCH test can be immensely valuable in assessing the disruptive impact stress is having on your ability to maintain hormonal balance.

Stressed-out menopausal women may need to drastically reduce fasting to reduce cortisol and relieve the adrenal glands, which work overtime during menopause. The most important thing your biology is asking of you during this time, post-menopause, is to do more of what you enjoy doing, to be heard, to be appreciated, and to follow your passions. This is the chapter of your life when you can finally be more selfish and think about what it is you truly want to be doing with your time and who you want to be doing it with. In turn, your hormones, your metabolism, will thank you.

CHAPTER 47

Weekly Fasting Plans for Enhanced Adaptation

Should You Switch Up Your Fasts? 10 Aspects of Your Lifestyle to Assess:

1. Your current hierarchy of goals

2. The length of your habitual fasts

3. The frequency at which you currently incorporate fasting

4. Your current level of chronic stress or anxiety

5. If you've had sufficient sleep

6. Your current exercise habits

7. Your unique nutritional needs

8. Current scheduling constraints

9. Current degree of hormonal imbalance (or phase of menstrual cycle)

10. Current state of immunity or inflammation

Below, you'll see two sample plans to boost adaptation and stimulate more results. If you don't currently fast at least 16 hours a day, then you'll continue training your body for intermittent fasting until you get to a place where 16 hours feels consistently effortless. The exception is during the week leading up to a woman's period when fasting isn't generally advisable.

Example #1) *Intermediate Weekly Fasting Plan for Enhanced Adaptation

*For people fasting effortlessly for around 16 hours a day

Monday 19-hour fast, Total Carbs < 50 g

- Fasting window: 6 p.m. Sunday–1 p.m. Monday

- Eating window: Monday 1 p.m.–6 p.m.

Tuesday 16-hour fast, Total Carbs < 50 g

- Fasting window: 6 p.m. Monday–10 a.m. Tuesday

- Eating window: Tuesday 10 a.m.–6 p.m.

Wednesday 16-hour fast, Total Carbs < 50 g

- Fasting window: 6 p.m. Tuesday–10 a.m. Wednesday

- Eating window: Wednesday 10 a.m.–6 p.m.

Thursday 23-hour fast, Total Carbs < 30 g

- Fasting window: 6 p.m. Wednesday–5 p.m. Thursday (drink high-sodium electrolytes like those from *drinklmnt.com*)

- Eating window: Thursday 5 p.m.–7:30 p.m.

This is a great day to schedule your errands, meetings at work, cleaning, decluttering, learning something new, outdoor activities, etc.

Friday *3-Meal Day* (13-hour fasting window), Total Carbs < 100 g

- Fasting window: 7:30 p.m. Thursday–8:30 a.m. Friday

- Eating window: Friday 8:30 a.m.–7:30 p.m.

Start the day with a protein-rich breakfast or a nutrient-dense smoothie with protein powder. This is a great day for high-intensity exercise or a minimum goal of 10,000 steps.

Saturday 14-hour fast, Total Carbs < 50 g

- Fasting window: 7:30 p.m. Friday–9:30 a.m. Saturday
- Eating window: Saturday 9:30 a.m.–7 p.m.

This is another good day for exercise or a minimum of 10,000 steps.

Sunday 15-hour fast, Total Carbs < 50 g

- Fasting window: Saturday 7 p.m.–10 a.m. Sunday
- Eating window: Sunday 10 a.m.–6 p.m.

This is a great day for exercise if your muscles aren't sore, or try active recovery like yoga, a pilates reformer class, home stretches, infrared sauna, swimming, bike ride, or leisurely walk.

Example #2) *Advanced Weekly Fasting Plan for Enhanced Adaptation

*For people with recent experience of 24-hour fasts.

This example is designed to incorporate alternate-day fasting and to facilitate increased fat-loss, autophagy, mental clarity, and insulin sensitivity.

Monday 16-hour fast, Total Carbs < 50 g

- Fasting window: 8 p.m. Sunday–12 p.m. Monday
- Eating window: Monday 12 p.m.–8 p.m.

Tuesday 36-hour fast (*no eating on Tuesday)

- Fasting window: 8 p.m. Monday–11 a.m. Wednesday
- Eating window: No eating on Tuesday (*or < 500 calories between 2 and 6 p.m. on Tuesday, choosing nutritious foods that are low in protein to facilitate autophagy. Drink high-sodium electrolytes like those from *drinklmnt.com*)

The only exercises recommended are walking or active recovery like yoga and stretching.

Wednesday *3-Meal Day* (12-hour eating window), Total Carbs < 100 g

- Fasting window: 8 p.m. Monday–8:30 a.m. Wednesday
- Eating window: Wednesday 8:30 a.m.–8:30 p.m.

Thursday 40-hour fast (*no eating on Thursday)

- Fasting window: 8:30 p.m. Wednesday–12 p.m. Friday
- Eating window: no eating on Tuesday (*or < 500 calories between 2 p.m. and 6 p.m. on Thursday, choosing nutritious foods that are low in protein to facilitate autophagy. Drink high-sodium electrolytes like those from *drinklmnt.com*)

This is a great day to schedule your errands, meetings at work, cleaning, decluttering, learning something new, outdoor activities, etc.

Friday *3-Meal Day* (8-hour eating window), Total Carbs < 50 g

- Fasting Window: 8:30 p.m. Wednesday to approx 12 p.m. Friday
- Eating Window: Friday 12 p.m.–8:00 p.m.

Start the day with a protein-rich breakfast or a nutrient-dense smoothie with protein powder. This is a great day for high-intensity exercise or a minimum goal of 10,000 steps.

Saturday *3-Meal Day* (10-hour eating window), Total Carbs < 50 g

- Fasting window: 8 p.m. Friday–10 a.m. Saturday

- Eating window: Saturday 10 a.m.–8 p.m.

Start the day with a protein-rich breakfast or a nutrient-dense smoothie with protein powder. This is another good day for exercise or a minimum of 10,000 steps.

Sunday 16-hour fast, Total Carbs < 50 g

- Fasting Window: Saturday 8 p.m.–12 p.m. Sunday
- Eating Window: Sunday 12 p.m.–8 p.m.

Engage in low-intensity exercise if your muscles aren't sore, or try active recovery like yoga, a pilates reformer class, home stretches, infrared sauna, swimming, bike ride, or a leisurely walk.

For any fasting plan, individuals with high cortisol levels from chronic stress would be wise to shift their eating window to occur earlier in the day. This means they'll accomplish most of the intermittent fast during the evening, prior to sleep, rather than during the day, after sleeping. This, as described in chapter six, is called early time-restricted eating (E-TRE) or circadian fasting. Daytime fasts cause a more dramatic elevation in cortisol levels, while evening meals also contribute to increased cortisol. That's why practicing circadian fasting can help remedy high cortisol levels. Remember, it's not all or nothing. Alternating between circadian fasting and intermittent fasting, which includes an evening meal, can benefit your adrenal health and stress-hormone balance.

For more sample fasting plans, like seasonal fasting and fasting with food, see the resources page on my site at marisamoon.com/notsofast/resources.

Part 5 Action Steps:

Review, Strategize, and Experiment

In Part 5, you learned plenty of ways to thoughtfully adapt your own fasting strategy. Let's keep the action steps simple, using this time to reflect and plan ahead.

Action Step #1:

Review the chapters in Part 5. Return to any bookmarks, notes, and dog-ears you've left. Which topic needs more of your attention? Where do you need to start? Choose one thing to experiment with.

Action Step #2:

Strategize. As I said earlier, whenever you're in active pursuit of a goal, days without a plan are wasted days—especially when your planned days don't outnumber unplanned days by at least 4:1. That means that for every 5 days of the week, 4 have a plan. For every 10 days, 8 have a plan.

When you strategize here, you'll need at least fifteen minutes to plan out your next actions. What reminders do you need to set? What dates do you need to add to your calendar for cooking, shopping, or fasting for success?

What day will you pause to reflect and revise your strategy? When will you revisit the other pages you've bookmarked in this section?

For women in their menstruating years, it's time to download the Clue app or the MyFlo app and start tracking your symptoms and/or your period if you have one. After just a few months of tracking, you'll be able to intentionally cycle your fasts and eating habits with the phases of your cycle so your body doesn't fight you on this. You'll see better results this way.

Action Step #3:

Experiment. Come at this with wide-eyed experimentation in mind. You're curious, observant, compassionate, and determined. Your health is your new hobby! You'll try something and tweak it when it doesn't go as planned. You'll reflect and learn each time, so you eventually figure out what works. Even then, something in life might throw a wrench in your plan. The wise response will always be to reflect, revise, and adapt again. Adaptation is key. It's a never-ending journey that rewards you every leap along the way.

Start by scheduling some 3-Meal Days that compliment your social life. Add in a scheduled date to try a more challenging fast on a low-activity day but one that's still busy. For menstruating women, schedule a more challenging fast during the first ten days after your period starts.

If you want a fasting buddy, hit me up! I offer a service called *Fast With Me*, where we can fast together (24–72 hours), and we'll keep each other accountable throughout the fast. Go to *marisamoon.com/services/fastwithme* to inquire about scheduling a fast together.

PART 6

Sleep: A Critical Piece of the Puzzle

CHAPTER 49

My Battle With Chronic Fatigue

I t wasn't until I could hardly stand under the weight of my body that I became curious about sleep quality and the stages of sleep. I'd just entered my thirties when I was crippled by chronic fatigue. When this happens, it creeps up so gradually as your thinking becomes more and more clouded by a dense fog, and it's difficult to conceive of the issue at hand. You aimlessly try to make it through the day, feeling you suck, life sucks, and basically, you are the problem.

A typical day in my life with chronic fatigue would go something like this:

I'd open my heavy-ass eyelids around 11 a.m. to the sound of my alarm—if I even set one; otherwise, I'd wake up around 1 p.m. After getting 12–13 hours of sleep, I'd still feel as though I'd taken tranquilizers and my body was filled with sand bags. I'd hit the snooze button three or four times, praying for a bit more alertness to draw on so my eyelids didn't feel like a pair of heavy black-out curtains.

I'd lie in bed looking at my missed texts and calls and browsing social media, desperate to give my brain some more time to function. I'd roll out of bed feeling so sorry for myself, but I'd feel guilty and ashamed at the same time.

I hated waking up in the afternoon at this point in my life. I felt like a loser or a college student ditching class to nurse a hangover.

I'd eventually make it downstairs, holding my body along the railing to nurse each step on my way to the kitchen. It was time for coffee. Time for hope. I'd drink my coffee, fantasizing about the vitality surging through my veins as the caffeine took me out of this walking coma. The fantasy never came true. I needed a bigger coffee mug because getting up two or three times to refill my mug was out of the question.

I'd look at the sink full of dishes, look at the clock, and try to imagine how I could fulfill my household responsibilities today, do a few hours of computer work, and still have time for a nap. Even though time seemed like one of my worst enemies, it was really the fatigue that plagued me. The thought of cleaning those dishes made it feel like I was being tasked with the assembly of a new dresser from Ikea. The task seemed insurmountable to me.

That's when the tears began to flow. *How can I possibly do the dishes? Why don't I have any energy? Am I dying? What the hell is wrong with me? Maybe I'm just the type of person who can't do mornings. I'm the type of person whose brain takes about two hours after waking up to snap back into functionality. I should just relax and kill time while I wait for my brain to wake up.*

Oops. I fell asleep on the couch, waiting for my brain to wake up, the dried tears crusting my eyelids together. *Get up. It's already 3 p.m. What is wrong with you?*

Tears. Anguish. Self-blame.

It's time to cook. Eric will be up in ninety minutes, and you haven't even cleaned the dishes or started packing his lunch.

More tears. Self-pity.

I should call Mom. She's been texting me, but she has no idea how f*ed up I am. I dial her on my cordless house phone, the weight of the phone so heavy I can't stand without holding myself up by my elbows on the kitchen counter. Mom answers my call. The sound of her voice makes me sob like a child. *Mom, I can't even hold the phone up. My arm is too heavy. I don't know what's wrong with me. I'm so f*ing tired, I can't stop crying. I feel like I've been hit with a tranquilizer dart or some shit.*

Mom suggests I go for a sleep study. I agree. I call around to different sleep centers and hospitals that offer sleep tests, and none of them will take me without a referral or accept my insurance, nor do any have openings for the next five months. I don't have a primary care physician yet since moving to a new state and getting new insurance. This makes me cry more and more. It's too much. It's too hard. I can't do this thing called life.

Now, imagine that day on repeat. Day after day. For weeks and months. In my suffocating state of self-pity, I managed to find a functional medicine doctor an hour away who accepted new patients and could see me in the next two weeks. *I'll pay out of pocket. I need help now!*

During my ninety-minute consultation (that's how functional medicine doctors are; it's amazing), the doctor decided to run all sorts of tests for my adrenal health (my stress hormones), oxidative stress, and a full lipid panel. She prescribed a bunch of supplements to help in the meantime with my debilitating PMS symptoms (premenstrual syndrome), my ADHD, and related depression. Our conversation helped me realize how many things I needed to consider when it came to my issue with fatigue. As soon as I got out of the appointment, I started learning about sleep hygiene, the stages of sleep, and what my body and brain are doing while I'm asleep.

First thing I changed was to use the sleep tracker on my Fitbit watch. The sleep tracker showed me that even though I was in bed for 12 hours, I woke up more than 20 times a night (which registers as restless sleep), adding up to 4–6 hours of the night. In reality, I got a total of 6 hours of sleep, hardly any of which was comprised of the essential stage called deep sleep (although my tracker at the time didn't measure deep sleep). Once I saw the evidence on my tracker, I realized how desperately I needed to improve my sleep. I needed to figure out how to stop the tossing and turning and fall into deep, restful sleep.

That's when I started sleeping with ear plugs. I was easily awakened whenever my dogs barked, or my husband entered the room (we slept on different schedules), when he got up to use the restroom, coughed, tossed and turned, etc. The ear plugs worked wonders for that! Wow, what a difference. I still use them to this day, eight years and counting.

Although the use of earplugs improved my restlessness by about 30 percent, I still hadn't figured out why I tossed and turned so much. One night, my husband realized it might be helpful to observe my sleep before falling asleep himself. What did he discover? I have sleep apnea. Even though I was a thirty-one-year-old woman and at a healthy weight (which made me less likely to develop sleep apnea), I still 'choked' on my own tongue when I slept on my back. This is common for people with narrow jaws because the tongue drops back, blocking the airway when sleeping in a horizontal position.

Eric, being a physician, decided to order me a CPAP machine, which is designed to help sleep apnea sufferers breathe better during sleep. The CPAP face mask didn't fit me, so I needed to special order a custom one. Meanwhile, I learned how to sleep on my side. It was not an easy change to make. I watched several youtube videos, read several articles online, and ordered special pillows to help me figure out how to comfortably sleep on my side. It took a lot of experimentation, pillows, and patience, but I finally figured it out, and my sleep apnea was gone!

My sleep improved dramatically. I only tossed and turned maybe five times per night. Soon, however, I noticed a disturbing trend. Although by that point, I felt rejuvenated most days of the week, my chronic fatigue symptoms would return every Sunday, Monday, and Tuesday. If my sleep tracker showed I was sleeping better, why did my fatigue hit again during that time of the week? On Friday nights, I worked a late shift and didn't get home from work until 4 a.m. My body and brain experienced jet lag from the whacky hours I worked—even though it was only one night a week at this stage! No matter how late I slept in or how early I woke up, I felt hungover and jet-lagged for days, even after consuming zero alcohol! That's when I knew it was time to put a stop to my Friday night shift work. It simply wasn't worth the three-day fatigue hangover I suffered every week.

Test results came back from the doctor, and my oxidative stress markers were in the red. How unusual for someone my age and weight. I was sick all the time, catching colds as often as once a month. My body was still under attack, and I knew my immune system would continue to suffer if I didn't get the issues under control. Over the next months and years, sleep quality was my number one priority. It paid off, and I never felt better.

It's not an exaggeration to say most of the clients in my health coaching practice suffer from insufficient sleep. At least half of those people don't feel 'ready' to do anything about it. And for all of them, insufficient sleep stands in the way of their health goals and robs them of the quality of life they truly deserve.

In the upcoming chapters in Part 6, I'll share with you the core concepts you need to know about sleep and precisely how I recommend you inch your way toward sufficient sleep. The information on the following pages could very well make the difference between succeeding or failing at any and every health goal you have in life from this day forward.

Sleep is an undeniable cornerstone of health and vitality. Without it, there's not a single facet of your life that won't be handicapped by this inadequacy.

CHAPTER 50
Critical Sleep Processes

7 Absolutely Critical Things That Happen While We Sleep

1. Liver detox

2. Brain detox

3. Cellular repair

4. Energy restoration

5. REM-related processes like memory consolidation, emotional processing, and sex-and-stress hormone regulation

6. Metabolic and appetite hormone regulation

7. Immune system regulation and optimization

It becomes glaringly obvious how critical sleep is for your waking life once you've suffered from chronic fatigue. However, there's another way to wake up to the importance of sleep without having to suffer first.

An Ancestral Health Perspective on Sleep

Our bodies have an ancient survival instinct that decides what functions are most important to keep us alive. This instinct comes from human evolution, and it dictates where they prioritize the use of energy and resources.

We're wired with this ancestral hierarchy of priorities. Your body is constantly using energy and resources to address whatever seems needed most urgently to stay alive—and rarely does that correlate with the things we'd like to use our energy for.

Keeping in mind that the body is programmed to prioritize threats to our immediate survival, how absolutely bonkers is it that we're designed to shut down for 6–9 hours every single night? It's shocking that we shut down like this because, for most of human history, people lived without the security of a roof, a warm bed, civilized communities, and Nest cameras or ADT alarms. Still, the body required 6–9 hours of partial paralyzation (did you know we're paralyzed during certain phases of sleep?) and unconscious rest every single night, during which the body is in its most vulnerable state! Not to mention that sleep occurs during the evening hours when new predators come out to hunt, and our sight and cognition are impaired! If that doesn't tell you how absolutely critical sleep is for human health, then you probably read through this paragraph too quickly. Read that again.

If you're short on sleep, the voice in your head says you're fine, but really, you're not. Human studies demonstrate that a sleep-deprived brain can't adequately conceive of the degree to which it's impaired. You think you're fine because your brain is unable to accurately compute, estimate, and assess its abilities in that sleep-deprived state. You tell yourself other things are more important to you than sleep, but a lot of the shit you're sick of living with could be improved or resolved entirely by optimizing your sleep.

Aren't you sick of the mounting anxiety, those angry outbursts, your stubborn weight, and your voracious sweet tooth? Don't you wish your nagging lower back pain would resolve? Don't you wish you had more energy each day? Don't you wish you made fewer mistakes, were more tolerant of stress, and had more self-control?

Lack of sleep sabotages your efforts to:

- Lose excess weight or keep the weight off
- Fix your metabolism
- Control yourself around food
- Experience life without sugar cravings
- Handle stress
- Be emotionally stable
- Be productive
- Think clearly
- Balance your hormones
- Follow through with a plan, especially at night
- Heal from pain or injuries
- Fight off cold/flu and prevent future infections

Sleep debt is a rising term for the cumulative effects of insufficient sleep. Sleep debt adds up quickly. Let's say your body needs about 7.5 hours of sleep to be well-rested. For the past 10 nights in a row, you only got 6.5 hours of sleep. According to sleep expert Jeff Kahn from risescience.com, even though you only shorted your sleep by one hour per night, doing that 10 nights in a row results in cognitive impairment that can be as severe as if you hadn't slept for 24 hours straight!

If this topic still annoys you, I get it. But let me just say this: it's detrimental and almost pointless to increase a fasting window beyond 14 hours if you're not getting adequate sleep.

"*Almost pointless?* How can you say that, Marisa?"

Welp, I say that because people who are chronically stressed and under-slept (especially women over forty and women in perimenopause) will find fasting much longer than 14 hours isn't only increasingly difficult, but that it will trigger the reverse of what they seek. Their metabolism slows down, weight stops coming off or creeps up again, they have less self-control around food, they rebel against their own needs and desires, and they have a hard time not saying *f* it!* to anything too challenging or inconvenient in the pursuit of health.

Two things I like to remind my clients:

- *Lack of sleep makes you eat.*
- *Reduced sleep time plateaus your waistline.*

It's okay. I'll help you. With enough frustration and enough exposure to enlightening information like this, you will take action eventually. You'll be empowered, and you won't give up on yourself.

Continue reading to discover how much power you really do have over your state of health, starting with your sleep. If you're not tracking your sleep, your head is in the sand. Let's start there.

CHAPTER 51

Sleep Tracking & Stages of Sleep

Have you used a sleep tracker before? Generally, sleep trackers provide a set of data that falls into one of two groups I distinguish.

The first only tracks when you fall asleep and when you wake up, calculating it into the total number of hours you slept through the night, and it may also tell you the number of times you woke during the night. These trackers are insufficient, in my opinion. It's simply not enough information to really change your life.

The trackers in the second group are much more legit because they provide more specific data. They not only monitor the total hours of sleep and how many times you wake up, but they also track the amount of time or the percentage you spend in each separate stage of sleep (light sleep, deep sleep, and REM sleep). When you know how much deep sleep and REM sleep you get each and every night, you have a massive advantage. This information is so valuable to have at your fingertips as it can help transform your mental and physical health and noticeably enhance your quality of life.

For years I used a dependable health and sleep tracker called the Oura Ring. Just weeks before publishing this book, I've switched to the newly released

Ring One by Muse Wearables (which does even more than the Oura Ring, like measuring blood pressure). I highly recommend one of these devices if you can afford it (they run around $300 USD). I love my health tracking rings for a number of reasons I won't cover here, but when it comes to sleep, I can view a total sleep score, time spent in each stage of sleep and how that compares to my usual. I can also track my average body temperature, heart rate, HRV (heart rate variability) and the associated recovery I accomplished during sleep.

A cost-free alternative to consider is the smartphone app called SleepScore, which works in airplane mode and, according to the developers, works even if you use a C-PAP machine. More trackers and apps to consider include SleepScore Max (a non-wearable device) and the AutoSleep app paired with the Apple Watch (by default, the Apple Watch doesn't track sleep until it's programmed to track with a sleep app). There are also specific Fitbit devices that track the time spent in each sleep stage (a premium subscription is required), the Polar Unite fitness watch and sleep tracker, the Whoop Strap fitness and sleep tracker, and the Rise Sleep App to enhance the insights gained from your existing sleep tracker.

No matter what your circumstances, it's worth tracking your sleep on a daily basis if possible. Build a habit of looking at your sleep data every morning when you wake up. At first, a low sleep score might discourage you and prompt your day to start off on the wrong foot. But, to me, this seems an essential part of the change process. Face the music enough times, and you'll soon be motivated to do something about it. You can't deny the facts for very long when they're consistently staring you in the face.

The 3 Stages of Sleep You Should Know About

- **Light Sleep**
    - o   Makes up around 50 percent of sleep per night.
    - o   It's not rejuvenating enough to live on.

- You're easily awakened during this stage. The more often you're awakened, the more light sleep you'll get, and the more you'll be robbed of the most critical sleep phases (REM and deep sleep)

- It still plays an important role in uploading information to your brain's long-term memory storage centers. However, memories and learning aren't adequately stored and retrievable without enough REM sleep and total sleep to finish the processes.

- **Deep Sleep**

  - Cellular repair occurs, including repairs in connective tissue, muscle, organs, and bones.

  - Muscle growth occurs.

  - Brain toxins are flushed away from the brain and metabolized for removal or recycling.

  - Physical energy is restored.

  - Adaptive hormones are optimized.

  - The immune system is replenished and optimized.

  - Anxiety is inhibited, and emotional tolerance is restored for the following day.

  - Memories and learning are optimized here, and the brain prepares for learning more the next day.

  - Deep sleep is greatly impaired by eating too much food before bedtime, drinking alcohol in the evening, drinking caffeine in the afternoon or evening, vigorous exercise too close to bedtime, staring at bright lights or digital screens in bed or immediately prior, stressful events or heightened anxiety before sleep, going to sleep after midnight, and certain prescription medications.

- **REM (Rapid Eye Movement) Sleep**

  - The sleep stage when dreams occur

o   Arm and leg muscles are paralyzed

o   The brain processes emotions and stressful events

o   Dopamine and serotonin levels are replenished

o   Long-term memory storage and learning are solidified

o   Creativity and visual/perceptual skills are optimized

o   REM sleep is optimized by regular sleep/wake times. It's reduced by consuming caffeine or stimulants in the afternoon and evenings, consuming alcohol, and engaging in vigorous exercise or stressful events before bed.

Percentage Goals Per Night for REM and Deep Sleep

• **REM Sleep** - Goal: 25 percent or more of your total sleep time.

o   REM sleep occurs cyclically through the night but increases in frequency and length *after* 3 a.m., typically between 3 a.m. and 7 a.m. in a typical sleep schedule.

o   25 percent or higher would equate to about 1.5 hours of REM sleep per night for optimal sleep and restoration.

• **Deep Sleep** - Goal: 20 percent or higher.

o   Deep Sleep occurs cyclically throughout the night, but the majority of deep sleep is accomplished *before* 3 a.m. This means that the later you go to sleep, the more robbed your body will be of the deep, replenishing sleep needed to thrive and provide energy you can feel.

o   When you achieve deep sleep of 20 percent or higher each night, it suggests you'll get at least 1 hour of deep sleep per night, even if you only slept 6.5 hours total. Most people feel much better throughout the day when they've had at least 1 full hour of deep sleep, but many people will need 1.5–2.5 hours of deep sleep to feel rejuvenated. The amount needed tends to decrease with age, but with today's stressful way of life, the majority of adults and seniors will only thrive when they hit that target most nights of the week.

"Oh, I sleep a lot!" New clients will brag, "I get 8 or 9 hours every night. I'm a good sleeper. I could sleep 10 hours if I didn't have to wake up for work." I've come to learn over the years that this is usually a bad sign. If we dig a little deeper, once the client starts tracking their sleep, we'll discover that they hardly ever go into the deep sleep stage. Most of their sleep time is spent in light sleep—making the occasional dip into deep sleep or REM sleep. Turns out they've been spending 75 percent of the night in the light sleep stage. That's why they're tired enough to sleep for ten hours a night.

I've been there myself, able to sleep so long that I thought I was a good sleeper. Before I started sleeping on my side, using ear plugs, and wearing a sleep mask, I was a terrible sleeper. My poor body and mind were being robbed of the deep, restorative sleep and dream sleep we so desperately need. This explains my poor stress tolerance, emotional instability, weakened immunity, and the alarmingly high oxidative stress markers shown in my lab work at the ripe young age of thirty-one.

Even if you achieve a high total of hours of sleep, human studies[43] have shown inadequate deep sleep results in an immediate decrease in insulin sensitivity and increased inflammation, both of which lead to reduced carb tolerance, increased blood glucose levels due to increased cortisol, and increased risk of developing type 2 diabetes, even in healthy young adults! Luckily, these outcomes can be reversed after achieving two consecutive, full nights of adequate sleep.[44]

Negative Effects Resulting from Insufficient Sleep

- Increased appetite

- Decreased willpower

- Reduced fat burning

- Decreased insulin sensitivity

- Mood instability

- Impaired emotional regulation

- Increased depression

- Increased anxiety

- Exacerbated inflammatory response

- Increased blood pressure

- Increased cortisol

- Impaired stress tolerance

- Reduced memory retention

- Inability to accurately self-assess one's degree of impairment

- Reduced productivity

- Reduced mental clarity and focus

- Reduced HRV (heart rate variability) and/or Irregular heartbeat

- Compromised gut health

- Weakened Immunity

Ready for some shocking stats? In the groundbreaking book *The Obesity Code* by Dr. Jason Fung, human studies show that after just one night of sleep deprivation, our cortisol levels increase by over 100 percent! The crazy thing is that the impact has long-lasting effects. Cortisol levels remain elevated around 40 percent through the following night. Next, we learn that when healthy volunteers restricted sleep to four hours, they experienced a 40 percent decrease in insulin sensitivity—after just one sleep-deprived night. Get just 4 hours of sleep per night for five nights straight, and the body pumps out 20 percent more insulin during the day; plus, cells are 25 percent less sensitive in response to the insulin! What a combo! Oh, and cortisol—that belly fat stress hormone—increases by 20 percent, too.[45]

CHAPTER 52

How Sleep Affects Anxiety, Hunger, and Fasting

Firstly, while you sleep, your brain and adrenals carry out the important job of calming the autonomic nervous system that rules your stress and anxiety levels throughout the day ahead. Researchers have proven that when people achieve a full night of sleep, anxiety levels decline significantly the next day. They've also been able to prove that a lack of sleep increases anxiety and emotional reactivity by up to 30 percent the following day.

In a Berkeley News article, author Yasmin Anwar points out these findings from sleep scientist Matthew Walker and his research team at UC Berkeley. "The results of their human studies showed that the amount and quality of sleep the participants got from one night to the next predicted how anxious they'd feel the next day. Even subtle nightly changes in sleep affected their anxiety levels."

If you have insomnia or trouble falling asleep due to chronic anxiety, I recommend you prioritize and address your anxiety first since sleep and anxiety have a negative feedback relationship, and anxiety can prevent you from falling asleep in the first place. For more support with decreasing your anxiety and sleeping more soundly, check out the work by Trudy Scott at *everywomanover29.com*, and explore the resources at *anxietynutritioninstitute. com* to learn more about balancing your neurotransmitters naturally through food and specific amino acid supplementation. If you haven't yet, remove alcohol consumption from your routine because it only exacerbates anxiety and insomnia, getting in the way of your recovery. In the U.S., check out the directory at *zocdoc.com* to find a therapist or other professional who's accepted by your insurance. It takes time and persistence to overcome anxiety, but you absolutely are capable of doing it, especially with a good support team on your side to talk you through it.

How Insufficient Sleep Affects Hunger and Eating Habits

I like to say lack of sleep makes you eat. Insufficient sleep contributes to obesity in many ways, but specifically, the lack of sleep increases feelings of hunger and susceptibility to the allures of food due to increased ghrelin hormone. Lack of sleep simultaneously reduces feelings of satiety, or the satisfaction and suppression of hunger, for which we depend on the hormone leptin and a gut hormone known as peptide YY.[46]

Adults snack more, especially in the evening, following a night of shortened sleep. And they don't just snack *more*; they impulsively snack on foods that are higher in carbohydrates. We straight-up make fewer healthy choices, and we've less self-control around food. We overeat as a result of being short on sleep. Forget about willpower. We're hungry, impulsive, rebellious, and more likely to self-sabotage. No doubt.

Part of the reason we make unhealthy choices when we're short on sleep is that our brain's reward systems are compromised. We're less aware of the ultimately negative outcomes or consequences of our actions; for example, *I should buy those cookies because they're on sale. What a great deal, and I deserve some cookies.* Whereas, if you were well-slept, you'd be more likely to see the cookies on sale and think, *Wow, what a deal! Usually, I'd fall for that, but not today. It's not worth the setback.*

Here's more. We humans always lack empathy for our future selves, but to an even greater degree when we're short on sleep. *What harm will a day of eating cookies do to me anyway? I'll go to the gym tomorrow and burn them off.* Tomorrow comes, and you don't want to go to the gym. Sure sounded like a good idea when tomorrow wasn't here yet!

Fasting is more challenging and less advantageous when you're short on sleep.

In case you haven't gathered this already, fasting is just plain harder and less effective when you lack adequate sleep. Lack of sleep makes everyone hungrier because the body senses sleep deprivation as a chronic stressor, which means our adrenals release more cortisol and our stomachs release more ghrelin, the hunger hormone.

Lack of sleep increases stress, and increased stress also raises cortisol, ghrelin, and fasting glucose levels.

Regardless of the physiological reasons above, we've got many more reasons to explain why people suddenly find it difficult to continue a fasting practice when they're short on sleep. Take, for instance, the reduced cognitive abilities and emotional stability needed to handle unexpected stressors and challenges throughout the day. Suddenly, fasting seems like less of a priority because you're trying to just make it through the day, and snacking or eating becomes more psychologically appealing when you have more stressors to deal with.

You might also be eating or feel hungrier because of trapped emotions you haven't allowed yourself to express or release. This is remarkably common and can eventually result in overeating, food addiction, depression, and panic attacks.

You *will* be short on sleep at times. That's inevitable in most of our lives today. So, when you wake up after an inadequate night of sleep, is it really a bad thing if your fast doesn't go according to plan? Nope. Whenever you're short on sleep, it's a wise choice to thoughtfully modify your plan. Shorten your fasting window and break your fast with a nutritious meal that satisfies you. It's often worse and more detrimental to your body if you force the fast. If you *still eat quality food and space out your meals*—so you're not eating crap food or snacking all hours of the day—it can be the smartest way to adapt.

Part 6 Action Steps:

10 Things to Stop & Start Doing For Sleep

Sleep Hygiene

Below, you'll discover dozens of effective ways to start improving your sleep.

Sleep hygiene is the term used to describe the practices you engage in to ensure routinely adequate sleep. When you practice good sleep hygiene, you prioritize quality sleep. You implement various tools and behaviors to get a healthy degree of sleep on a regular basis.

One of the most essential aspects of sleep hygiene is to wake up at the same time each day, give or take up to an hour, even on the weekends. You've probably ignored this advice any time you heard it in the past. You thought it couldn't make that big of a difference, or maybe that it doesn't work with your lifestyle. I'd argue that you've no idea what you're missing.

Waking up at a consistent hour each day is a game changer for your energy levels, your metabolism, and your immune system. Sure, having a routine bedtime is also important (especially if you struggle with sleep onset or late-night second winds), but your bedtime is where you can get some wiggle room. There's nothing quite as essential as getting up at the same time each day. It has the biggest impact on your circadian rhythm, your appetite, and your food choices throughout the day.

Make up sleep debt by going to sleep *earlier*.

Don't make up sleep debt by sleeping-in later.

A consistent wake time—with no more than an hour's variation—helps your body tremendously with orchestrating your stress hormones and wakeful hormones so your circadian rhythm remains aligned. You feel better and perform better in every way. Falling asleep and waking up become easier. Healthy eating and fasting are easier. Life is just plain easier when you stick to a consistent wake time. You won't even need an alarm clock anymore when you get this right. Oh, and the snooze button is your worst enemy. Trust me when I say you'll have wayyyy more energy in the mornings if you cut out that snooze button habit. Check out my podcast, The Foundation of Wellness, episode #72 about how Mel Robbin's 5-Second Rule helped me cut that snooze habit and get my ass outta bed when the alarm goes off.

Action Step #1a:

Review the following list of 10 things to *stop* doing so you can get better sleep and make strides with your health. As you read each item, circle those you have a habit of doing.

10 Things to STOP Doing (so you can get better sleep and make strides with your health)

1. Stop *eating within 2.5 hours of bedtime.

2. Stop drinking alcohol within 2.5 hours of bedtime, and stop using it as an excuse to help you relax or sleep because, in reality, it's making things worse.

3. Stop doing intense exercise, HIIT, or cardio within 3 hours of bedtime.

4. Stop **designing your evening routine around your family's evening/sleep habits (meaning, stop putting yourself last or acting as if your own needs are irrelevant).

5. Stop pushing your exercise, diet, or fasting routine without first improving your sleep.

6. Stop exposure to bright lights at least 1 hour before sleep. High mental or visual stimulation comes from doing stressful or exciting tasks, bright overhead lights, and looking at bright screens (TV, phone, laptop). Put screen brightness levels as low as possible, and avoid using these devices while lying in bed. User candlelight, dimer switches, or night lights for evening activities or midnight bathroom trips.

7. Stop using your pets as an excuse to get crappy sleep. What's more important, your health or your dog's preference to sleep on your bed?

8. Stop consuming excessive amounts of caffeine (> 150mg per day) or consuming caffeine within 8 hours of your bedtime.

9. Stop giving up after one failed attempt. Whether you try one brand of earplugs, one type of melatonin, or one night with no screens, it's not enough information. With determination and persistence, you'll soon discover which interventions can work for you.

10. Stop using the snooze button for longer than five minutes (or stop using the snooze button entirely).

* Eating too close to bedtime seems to make it more challenging to fast in the morning. Interestingly, you'll find that when you stop any snacks within 3 hours before sleep, you're able to fast more easily the next day. And that's not all….

"Eating late at night is not only bad for metabolism, it also affects sleep (falling asleep and maintaining deep sleep). In order to fall asleep, our core body temperature must cool down...but when we eat, our core body temperature actually goes up as blood rushes to the gut to help digest and absorb nutrients. So, eating late at night prevents us from getting into a deep sleep. To have a good night's sleep, we should have our last meal at least 2–4 hours before going to bed to ensure that the body is able to cool down."
- Satchin Panda, *The Circadian Code*

**You're limiting yourself with a narrative that says quality sleep is a luxury you can't have. Unless you're nursing a baby, working swing shifts, or sleep-training a toddler, there's no reason your needs should always come last. If you need help, delegate or arrange for more support. Change takes time, but it starts with initiative and a plan. Challenge yourself: when will you initiate, and what can help to ensure that you'll follow through?

Important Tip: The more stressed or sleep-deprived your body is, the more sensitive you are to things like excessive caffeine intake, bright lights/screen exposure before sleep, and even EMF exposure.[ii] Normally, these things might have little to no impact on you or your sleep. However, once your body is chronically stressed, it can become hyper-sensitive to these inputs.

---

ii   EMFs, or Electromagnetic Fields, are radiation signals emitted by mobile phones, Bluetooth devices, and Wi-Fi routers (among many others). Most wireless companies and authorities claim that EMF exposure is perfectly safe; however, a growing number of EMF scientists disagree. As a skeptic myself, I resisted putting my phone on airplane mode while sleeping. However, turns out my sleep tracker shows I sleep much better when airplane mode is activated (therefore disabling the cellular network, Wi-Fi, and Bluetooth signals). The more stressed your body is, the more likely EMF exposure is contributing to it.

Action Step #1b:

Go through the numbers you circled, one by one, categorizing them with one of the following symbols:

- E = Easy to stop
- C = Challenging to stop
- ✱ = 1–3 things you're willing to put a stop to, starting tonight.

Action Step #2:

Set reminders for the items you marked with a ✱. Use your phone's alarm or calendar to schedule a reminder, or hang a sticky note on the bathroom mirror as a reminder to put a stop to those sleep-wrecking habits starting tonight. Try the Rise Sleep app at *risescience.com* to schedule free text or email reminders to wear your sleep mask, reduce bright light exposure, or check your sleep environment.

Action Step #3a:

Review the following 12 things to start doing so you can get better sleep and feel fan-frickin-tastic! As you read each item, circle the ones you're willing to try or willing to learn more about.

12 Things to START Doing (so you can get better sleep and feel fan-frickin-tastic!)

1. Start using a sleep tracker that measures the percentage or total minutes/hours of *deep sleep* you achieve each night.

2. Start lowering the temperature of your house or bedroom at least thirty minutes before bed so your sleep environment is around 65 degrees Fahrenheit. If that's too cold for you or your family, gradually work your way down 1 or 2 degrees every week or so until you get there.

3. Start waking up at a consistent time every single day (within a forty-five-minute range and no more than an hour later on the weekends).

4. Start wearing a sleep mask every night. Try different styles to find one that's most comfortable for you.

5. Start using ear plugs or one of the following tools to block out surrounding sounds while you sleep. Try various types of ear plugs (and be patient while you practice proper ear plug application), use a white noise machine, a white noise app or playlist, or turn on a fan or air purifier to help drown out sounds that can easily wake you. Don't use the TV for background noise unless the screen is completely off.

6. Start listening to a guided *yoga nidra* meditation, or do some autonomic relaxation while trying to fall asleep. You can also listen to bedtime stories using Amazon's Alexa or a smartphone app like Aura. All these methods help turn off the chatter in your brain and allow you readily to fall into sleep.

7. Start turning your phone off, put it on airplane mode, and/or charge your phone in a different room while you're in bed.

8. Start seeking professional help for sleep apnea, snoring, or difficulty with nasal breathing if you suspect you have issues in those areas.

9. Start experimenting with a sleep ritual. A sleep ritual is a bedtime routine comprised of various predictable behaviors that the brain learns to recognize as a cue for sleep. Each time you engage in your sleep ritual—with behaviors like using lavender hand lotion, putting on your eye mask, saying a prayer, listening to yoga nidra, doing a bedside 'brain dump' onto paper, reading a non-stimulating book, soaking your feet in a magnesium foot bath, etc., your brain is being trained to readily surrender for the night.

10. Start enjoying your morning coffee outside during or after sunrise. You can even use an indoor sun lamp to expose your eyes and body to the proper light spectrum that regulates your circadian rhythm and energizes you for the day.[iii]

11. Start experimenting—relentlessly. Try different pillows or sleep positions, like incline versus lying flat. Try different supplements, habits, and anything else on this list, with experimentation as your goal. Over time, you'll learn what helps you sleep better and how to make it work for your situation. What worked before may not work now because what's affecting you emotionally, physiologically, or environmentally can change many times in your adult life.

12. Start taking a nap whenever you're short on sleep. A nap of ten to forty-five minutes is completely refreshing for a stressed and tired brain, and a nap of one-and-a-half to two hours is a full sleep cycle that rejuvenates the entire body and mind. If you can't nap, do a fifteen-minute guided meditation, which can be just as refreshing for a tired, stressed brain.

Circadian rhythm alignment "…involves more than buying the right mattress or avoiding caffeine prior to bedtime (though both are important). More than anything, it has a lot to do with your eyes detecting light and dark. When your eyes detect light, this tells your brain (the hypothalamus, in particular) to wake up and release cortisol and other hormones you need to increase your metabolism and get through your day."
- Dr. Anna Cabeca, *The Hormone Fix*

---

iii   The effects of morning light on serotonin, cortisol, and energy: when the sun rises, our brain responds to the onset of light by decreasing melatonin and raising serotonin levels so we wake up alert, refreshed, and ready to tackle the day. Light is registered first through the retina. The signal travels through the optic nerve to other regions of the brain, including the pineal gland that activates the release of serotonin. Levels of the stress hormone cortisol increase within the first thirty minutes of waking. This morning cortisol influx is a desirable genetic mechanism that prepares us for the demands of a busy day. The serotonin-cortisol effect is most powerful closest to dawn.

Action Step #3b:

Then, draw a ✷ next to one to three things you're willing to try this week.

Action Step #4:

Do you need to calendarize tasks related to the starred items you selected in action step #3b? Let's say you committed to using a sleep mask and getting help for possible sleep apnea or insomnia. When will you shop for a sleep mask? Who can you contact to schedule yourself for a sleep study, when should you get support for your insomnia, and who should you contact? Put these tasks on your personal calendar to help ensure that you prioritize them this week and follow through with the execution. Try the Rise Sleep app at *risescience.com* to schedule free text or email reminders to wear your sleep mask, reduce bright light exposure, or check your sleep environment.

PART 7

Crafting Your Unique Fasting Lifestyle

CHAPTER 54

Are You a Home or Away Faster?

Which approach to intermittent fasting works the best? It depends on your unique body and where you're at in your journey. The best approach, at first, is the one that makes you feel great and helps you be more intentional about your relationship with food. Sooner or later, the best approach becomes one you can easily commit to for the long term as a lifestyle. It's adaptable and sustainable. In your lifetime, you might try three, four, or ten different strategies because you change and your circumstances change. Your fasting lifestyle needs to change accordingly.

Later, in Part 7, I'll review the various fasting methods people adopt. Before you get into those examples, it's important that I challenge you to explore whether fasting is easier for you at home or at work. Knowing this about yourself will give you an advantage. It has a significant impact on your willingness to fast and your ability to follow through with your fasting plan.

Read the following two descriptions and ask yourself which person you're more like. The Home Faster or the Away Faster?

Home Faster: A home faster learns early on that fasting at work can be a real challenge. There's always a room full of donuts, cookies, and sweets, and meetings are often paired with pizza day. Whenever a home faster plans to fast all day at the office, they wind up feeling overwhelmed by the temptation and willpower required to stick to the plan and fast at work while everyone else is snacking, eating, and pressuring them to eat all the goodies. The home faster realizes that longer fasts are a better fit for them on days when they work from home because they know what it takes to follow through with the fasting plan. They intentionally stay away from the kitchen, keep busy, crush some productivity, and step outside for a walk whenever they need a rewarding distraction that has nothing to do with food. Fasting comes easier for the home faster when they're at home.

Away Faster: An away faster feels trapped in old behavior patterns at home. Maybe it started during the pandemic lockdowns of 2020, or maybe it's been ever since the kids were too cool to hang out at home. When an away faster is home, food is always on their mind. The voice in their head says, Eat, snack, eat! You deserve it! Once the lockdowns were lifted and their boss allowed flex work schedules, the away faster started going into the office twice a week. This is when it became obvious that fasting is so much easier when they're there! Their brain is always in work mode when they're at the office, and they're able to stick to a plan without needing so much willpower. No lunch, no snacks, no budging. It's easier because they feel more in control around food here. Maybe it's because they care what other people think and they prefer not to eat around them, or maybe it's just because eating at work never grew into an automatic habit like it has at home. Either way, an away faster knows they're better off planning longer fasts for the days when they're at the office.

Are you more of a home faster or away faster? Maybe you're a little of both. Or, maybe your circumstances don't even correlate with the examples I shared. Even knowing that will give you an advantage. I've seen people succeed in every kind of situation as long as they're willing to experiment and determined to find a solution.

CHAPTER 55

5 Types of Hunger

Humans are biologically hardwired to seek pleasure through food. Historically, that proved to be beneficial because it helped ancient humans prioritize finding food so they could thrive and propagate the species even in challenging conditions. However, we now live in modern society where food is available anytime, anywhere, so this hardwiring works against us in so many ways. It's another evolutionary mismatch that has us thinking about food all the time because it's the most pleasurable, easy-to-access 'drug' that's 100 percent socially acceptable and encouraged on a daily (or hourly) basis.

Are you eating because you're hungry? Are you eating because food sounds good? Are you eating because you're bored? To become wiser about the personal tendencies that lead you to eat more often than is necessary, you'll want to ask yourself:

Is it hunger or cravings? What type of hunger is it?

Try the following exercise to explore what I consider the 5 types of hunger. This tool helps whenever you find yourself questioning why you ate or why food was on your mind. With this understanding, you might be able to recognize why and do something differently the next time.

Exercise #1: What type of hunger is it?

Read the explanations below and try to specify the type or source of your hunger:

1. Head
2. Mouth
3. Heart
4. Stomach
5. Anticipatory

1. Head Hunger - I'm bored, I don't want to do this task, I'm stressed, or I saw/smelled/heard something that makes me want to eat now.

2. **Mouth Hunger** - I'd like to change the taste in my mouth right now, or I'm craving a certain texture or mouthfeel.

3. Heart Hunger - I have unmet emotional needs | I'm lonely | No one appreciates me | I need support | Life is hard | I wish I could tell that person what I really think.

4. Stomach Hunger - My stomach is growling or empty. I feel physically hungry in my gut.

5. Anticipatory Hunger - If I don't eat now, *when* (or what) will I eat?

Optional - Exercise #2: Cravings

Get curious about the meaning behind this craving.

Even once you determine your cravings stem from *head hunger*, you may still feel distracted by the urge to eat. In those cases, it can be helpful to explore the craving more deeply. Consider external factors that may be triggering the craving and try to identify patterns surrounding when and how intense the cravings arise. Analyzing the specifics of the craving and its greater meaning to you personally can provide useful insights to better address it moving forward.

Prompt #1: Is your craving driven by one of the following factors?

- You haven't slept well enough the past 1–3 nights

- Women, are you expecting your period in a week or currently bleeding?

- Was your craving triggered by something you saw, smelled, or heard about?

- Is the food you're craving something you've had a habit of eating regularly in the recent past (or ever)?

- Could there be an underlying nutrient deficiency such as magnesium, calcium, zinc, iron, healthy fats, or protein (or specific amino acids like tryptophan or glycine)?

If you answered "Yes" to any of the above, you can stop here and work on accepting this pattern, or you might seek out coaching or professional support to help address and improve the pattern.

Prompt #2: If you're still curious about the significance of the craving and want to challenge it, determine which most represents the type of craving you're having now:

A: I crave salty, crunchy snacks

B: I crave something sweet and refreshing

C: I crave comfort foods like mac n cheese

D: I crave chocolate, cheese, or peanut butter

Prompt #3: After deciding which describes your current craving, consider the challenge below that coincides with the letter you chose:

A: If salty pistachio nuts don't sound appetizing, you're probably not hungry

B: If crisp blueberries don't sound good to you, you're probably not hungry

C: If you're not hungry enough to eat a bowl of homemade chicken soup, you're probably not hungry

D: These cravings are mostly driven by former habits, hormonal imbalances, gut dysbiosis, or nutrient-deficiencies. It might be time to eliminate the food entirely for two weeks to help the craving disappear or to connect with a professional who can help you better assess and understand how to work with or resolve this craving.

Exercise #3: Reflect

What do you want to remember about these new insights? How can you further explore your insights so you eventually come to a place of greater freedom or acceptance with them?

Let this be a reminder that it takes time to break those patterns, but it absolutely does happen. My clients who persist in these efforts come out the other side, showing up each time like the version of themselves they'd always wanted to be around food.

CHAPTER 56

An Overview of Popular Fasting Methods

Here's a graduation-worthy overview of the various types of fasting that will help you reach your goals without having to read another book on fasting. What you're doing now, like 12–18-hour intermittent fasts, may be enough to help you achieve your goals over time. You might soon discover, however, reasons to try something different to trigger better adaptation or achieve greater results.

The following list is an overview of the many popular fasting methods out there. If you're already seeing results, congratulations! You may not need this information yet—or ever. If you feel a bit overloaded by new information now, consider skipping this chapter and coming back when you're ready for more.

#1) The 16:8 Method (including 18:6, 14:10, and 12:12 fasting)

This is what you've been working your way toward with the RESET method. The number *before* the colon is the number of hours you're fasting daily (your fasting window), and the number after the colon is the number of hours during which you can eat (your eating window).

When you first started the RESET method, you were doing 12:12 fasting. 12-hour daily fasts, with a 12-hour eating window. That's the bare minimum I think every adult should strive to do for optimal health, disease prevention, and effortless weight maintenance.

The 16:8 method is the most popular, perhaps because it doesn't disrupt a social life too much, and there's some good science to back up its effectiveness. This method also feels pretty natural to men and women alike.

In this category, I'd also include Bulletproof fasting. That's when you practice intermittent fasting that includes Bulletproof or fatty coffee during the fast. Without any carbs or protein in your coffee (or tea), you're technically still fasting and reaping the benefits. With only fats being ingested during the fast, you won't disrupt autophagy or prompt insulin secretion. Your mitochondria will have easier access to ketones, and you'll be quite satisfied. It's an effective long-term strategy that's rewarding and nourishing to sustain.

#2) 20–24-Hour Fasts, Warrior Diet, and OMAD (One Meal a Day)

24-hour fasts sound scary, but despite the name, you still eat every day. You're fasting for 24 hours, starting after dinner one night and breaking your fast at dinner the following night (or, it could be breakfast to breakfast or lunch to lunch).

Example:

- Finish dinner by 7 p.m. on Tuesday

- Fast the remainder of the evening

- Sleep until 7 a.m.

- Continue fasting all day Wednesday

- Eat dinner around 6 p.m. or 7 p.m. on Wednesday

In combination with an optimal diet that's low-to-moderate in carbohydrates, this range of fasting boosts ketones and autophagy in a big way. It helps the body get rid of damaged cells, repair DNA, and, basically, 'take out the trash'.

If you have serious weight to lose, and you've successfully tried 18-hour fasts, it's likely you should consider doing fasts ranging from 20–24 hours, 2–5 days per week for a month straight. Remember to incorporate one *3-Meal Day* per week to help flood your body with nutrients and reassure your metabolism. After a month, take a pause to reflect on how your appetite and relationship with food have changed. Some people do this type of fasting every day. Your stomach will shrink. You'll find it increasingly challenging to eat 3 meals a day, even when it's time to cycle your fasts to prevent plateaus. That's why I don't recommend doing 20–24-hour fasts so consistently. Check out #4 and #5 below to learn more ways to effectively cycle your fasts, and I encourage you to revisit the weekly fasting plans for adaptation in Part 5 of this book.

#3) Keto IF

Keto IF is very similar to what you've been doing so far, except you'd be cutting your daily carbohydrate intake down to < 50 g of total carbohydrates per day. So far, you've reduced your daily carb intake as part of the RESET Method. By the time you're extending your fasts, if fat-loss or increased insulin sensitivity is your goal, you'll simultaneously reduce your carbs even further in order to facilitate better results. Gradually work your way down, incorporate sodium electrolytes, and you'll mitigate any of the usual side effects people talk about in the keto community.

Individuals who are very insulin-resistant or sedentary may need to lower the carb limit even further (unless they incorporate extended or prolonged fasts). Intermittent Fasting for around 16 hours/day, combined with this low carb intake, is like a hack for the traditional *keto diet* which can require an even lower limit. Together, they have a synergistic effect where you enhance the benefits of IF *and* Keto because you stay in the fat-burning zone most of the time and more effortlessly.

For some people whose bodies thrive on a keto diet, this could be the single most effective and fastest way to reach your weight-loss goals. You'll keep the weight off for good if you turn lower carb eating into a lifestyle.

To keep the weight off, you don't have to stick with a keto diet indefinitely, either. In fact, it's most beneficial to practice *cyclical ketosis*. With cyclical keto fasting, you'd fast around 16–24 hours per day, eat < 50 g of total carbs during the eating window, do that consistently for a minimum of two weeks, and continue until it becomes effortless. Then, you can have a 3-Meal Day or carb cycle by eating 150 g of whole food carbs every 7–10 days while sticking to a keto IF plan for the remainder of the week. This is beneficial because it helps release water being held in your cells, release fat that's being reserved for your survival, and break through weight-loss plateaus by forcing the body to re-adapt. It also increases metabolic flexibility, which is a goal for us all!

Once you've reached your body composition goal, you'll be able to pull back from a strict keto IF lifestyle and modify it to meet your personal carbohydrate comfort zone. For some people, that's around 100 g of carbs per day for maintenance. For others, it's around 130–150 g per day. Still, others feel their best on a keto diet, and therefore, maintenance mode might be between 50–100 g of carbs per day with 12–14-hour intermittent fasts to keep your metabolism flexible and efficient.

Understanding Ketosis:

Humans possess an inherent capability to enter a metabolic state called ketosis, or ketogenesis—an innate process enabling our liver and mitochondria to produce and utilize energy derived from fat. Ketones are made when insulin and glycogen storage are low, which prompts the body to break down fat cells and convert the resulting fatty acids into ketone bodies in a process called ketogenesis. We humans were designed with this metabolic capability because it's a survival advantage. Ketosis helps humans go without food, or especially without carbohydrates while remaining strong, mentally sharp, energized, and healthy.

To enter a state of ketosis, where your body uses fat for fuel, you need to restrict carbohydrates and sugar, fast long enough, or do a combination of both to deplete your body's glycogen storage so it looks to your body fat for an alternate energy source.

Many people feel incredible while they're in ketosis. They're less hungry, their sweet tooth vanishes, they have abundant energy and mental clarity, and they usually like what it does for their body composition.

Benefits of Nutritional Ketosis:

- Provides Clean-Burning Energy
  - o Ketones allow mitochondria to create energy with less metabolic effort and oxidation compared to burning carbohydrates. This makes keto an effective anti-aging diet.

- Reduces Inflammation
  - o The cleaner burn of ketones lowers inflammation in cells and reduces disease risk.

- Enhances Cognitive Function
  - o Ketones are the brain's preferred fuel source and boost mitochondrial activity in the brain. This helps prevent conditions like Alzheimer's, dementia, epilepsy, and ADHD.

- Supports Cardiovascular Health
  - o Ketosis helps significantly reduce elevated blood pressure while providing steady energy for the heart.

- Increases Physical Energy

  o People often report feeling more energetic while in ketosis.

- Reduces Hunger

  o Ketosis suppresses appetite due to its hunger-reducing effects.

- Aids Weight Loss

  o Relying on fat stores for energy means ketosis helps shed excess body fat.

- Supports Hormonal Regulation for Perimenopause and PCOS

  o Chronic insulin shuts down estrogen and progesterone production. Ketosis reduces insulin, and improves insulin resistance, which is essential to prevent the negative side effects that commonly occur during transition into menopause, or while suffering from PCOS and related hormonal disorders.

#4) The 5-1-1 Strategy (or 4-2-1)

The 5-1-1 strategy is a weekly routine, as follows, in any order:

- 5 days of Keto IF

- 1 day with a 24-hour fast

- 1 day of feasting (which I prefer to call a *3-Meal Day*)

- (in any order)

This is a strategy I learned from Dr. Daniel Pompa. He designed it to help people cycle their fasts more frequently to encourage ongoing adaptation, adequate nutrition intake, and prevent plateaus. This strategy can progress to a 4-2-1 schedule, which implies you'd have 4 days of keto IF, 2 days of 24-hour fasts, and 1 day of feasting (a 3-Meal Day) each week.

#5) Alternate Day Fasting (ADF) or The 5:2 Diet

If you're stressed by the thought of restricting food on a regular basis, then ADF, or the 5:2 diet, might be a better fit for you. With these plans, you can eat more freely most of the week, and you throw in some 36-hour fasts during which you can eat up to 500 or 600 total calories. I think these fasting plans most closely mimic the feast/fast circumstances experienced by our ancient ancestors, which means they may be optimal for genetic expression and metabolic flexibility.

Although some people prefer this eating pattern because it allows them to eat more freely most days of the week, there are others (like me) who find it easier to fast without any food at all because having even a small amount of food triggers relentless thoughts about eating all day long. Take a look and try it out for yourself.

The 5:2 diet is a weekly plan as follows:

- 5 days of regular eating with daily intermittent fasts of around 12 hours

- 2 days of very reduced eating—under 500 calories per day for women and under 600 calories per day for men.

For some people, this increases compliance and satisfaction since you can eat something on your fasting days, and you still get many of the benefits of fasting (like the fasting-mimicking diet, which you'll learn about in the next chapter).

Alternate Day Fasting (ADF)

In this version, you fast every other day, and you're still able to consume some calories on the fasting days, just like the 5:2 diet. Men can eat under 600 calories per fasting day, and women can eat under 500 calories. The only difference between this and the 5:2 diet is that with ADF, you'll fast more days per week. ADF ends up equaling about 3–4 days of fasting each week.

Remember, if a plan like ADF says you eat one day and fast the next, the fasting day implies a 36-hour fast. The 36-hour fast comes from 8 hours of sleep the first night + 20 hours of fasting throughout the day + 8 hours of sleep the next night, after which you'll break your fast and resume normal eating on the second day.

Example:

- Wednesday night: eat dinner from 6 p.m.–7 p.m. Fasting window begins at 7 p.m.

- Sleep 8 hours (10 p.m.–6 a.m.).

- Thursday: Continue fasting all day and night (during which both men and women are allowed up to 500/600 calories).

- Sleep for 8 hours on Thursday night.

- Friday morning: gently break your fast and have a day of normal eating.

- Repeat, starting your next fast on Friday night.

#6) Extended or Prolonged Fasts (Fasts ≥ 36 hours, and Multi-Day Fasts)

It makes sense for all of us to try this at some point in our lifetimes since, without a doubt, our DNA expects to face this sort of challenge. Look at other fasting books or websites, and you'll encounter some heavy persuasion to fast ≥ 36 hours. Why is that?

Let's say you don't reduce your carbohydrate intake whatsoever, and you eat whatever you want. Even though you decide not to change the food in your diet and you rarely exercise, you want to experience the benefits of fasting. In this case, you'd have to fast for 36–72 hours to deplete glycogen stores and turn on the genetic switch that begins ketogenesis. The more metabolically challenged you are—insulin-resistant, type 2 diabetes, disproportionately large waist circumference—the longer you'd have to fast to force your body into ketosis.

Some people think that sounds better than trying to eat a more nutritious diet. The thing is, if you go that route, you set yourself up to suffer through a wide range of side effects that'll make you feel like shit and wonder why you ever thought it was a good idea in the first place. During those first 36–60 hours, you'll experience massive hunger, fatigue, headaches, irritability, lightheadedness or dizziness, mood swings, wild energy fluctuations, self-doubt, and obsessive thoughts about food. That sounds fun!

Enough with that hypothetical scenario (although it's a very real experience that millions of people have had because they jumped too fast into a keto diet or into a longer fast without first training their bodies for it. But, you? You're not doing that because you're using my RESET method.

Another big reason people do these longer fasts is because it's a faster way to reverse insulin resistance and recover from metabolic dysfunction. It really boosts anti-aging, healing, and disease prevention in a huge way.

Furthermore, once your fasts get to around 24 hours or more, you initiate a significant increase in autophagy (cellular recycling and repair) and mitophagy (mitochondrial recycling and repair). Once you get to that 72-hour mark, you'll be bursting with stem cells, revitalizing organs, growing new mitochondria (mitochondrial biogenesis), and replenishing immune cell activity.

Some people fast for 72 hours to help eliminate sagging skin they may deal with after achieving a significant degree of fat loss. Thanks to autophagy, old, useless skin proteins are recycled to feed and grow healthier, stronger cells. Learn more in Thomas DeLauer's YouTube video, *My 100lb Weight Loss & Loose Skin*. Other potential applications for prolonged fasts are to fight cancer and tumor growth and help with recovery after chemotherapy. The immune system optimization, autophagy, and stem cell production, achieved with longer fasts, are the main reasons they're growing in popularity in cancer-related therapy. Learn more about this topic in the book *Hacking Chemo* by Martha Tettenborn, and discuss it with a licensed medical professional before trying.

Safety

If you take prescription medication, you'll need to work with your doctor while incorporating fasting or a keto diet because your medication dose needs to be adjusted to this drastic change in your dietary intake. I see it all the time in my business, where a client's doctor needs to reduce their dose of blood pressure medication or diabetes medication because they're no longer eating as much food as they used to.

You should never stop taking your prescription medications without guidance and permission from your prescribing physician. Talk to your doctor about how intermittent fasting can indicate a reduced dose of certain medications you may be taking.

Your blood pressure and blood sugar should be monitored throughout the day when doing longer fasts. If you experience any symptoms of hypoglycemia, such as shaking or sweating, you should immediately check your blood sugar and ingest some quick-acting glucose like maple syrup mixed in water with lemon and salt. Fasting also lowers blood pressure, which can cause some individuals, especially those who take blood pressure-lowering medication, to experience dangerously low blood pressure and the associated dizzy, lightheaded feeling that results. Drink high sodium electrolytes or pickle juice, and consider breaking your fast right away in this case. Modified fasts or a fasting-mimicking diet might be best for you at such a time until you get help from your doctor to further understand how to keep your body in a healthy range of hormesis.

Discuss with your physician a plan for routine blood work that includes your sodium and magnesium levels, a standard lipid panel, HbA1C, and other relevant markers that correlate with your current state of health and disease.

Fasting should always make you feel better, not worse. Should you feel unwell for any reason, just break your fast immediately. Persistent nausea, vomiting, dizziness, fatigue, high or low blood sugar, and lethargy aren't normal with intermittent fasting and should raise a red flag. Hunger and constipation, however, are normal symptoms and can be managed. The most common causes I've seen behind those symptoms are low sodium, low magnesium, high potassium, chronic stress (with associated undereating and under-sleeping), and disproportionate doses of certain medications related to blood pressure and diabetes management.

If you have any specific questions about any medical matter, you should consult your doctor or other professional healthcare provider. If you think you may be suffering from any medical condition, you should seek immediate medical attention. You should never delay seeking medical advice, disregard medical advice, or discontinue medical treatment because of information in this book.

Personally, I feel incredible when I do 42-hour fasts. My brain is firing on all cylinders, and I have abundant physical energy. I'd like to do a 3-day water fast (or up to 200 calories per day) sometime soon. I imagine I'll feel unstoppable! Good news is, everything you're doing with my *Not So Fast* approach will prepare you to try them one day, too. If someone like me, who absolutely loves food and loves eating, loves the feeling of a longer fast, I bet you will, too. When the time is right for you.

CHAPTER 57

Fasting with Food?

One of the things I hope you realize by the end of this book is that you can rely more on your own personal wisdom and a discerning ear than you can on various claims you'll encounter along your journey to better health. When it comes to intermittent fasting, it's too easy to fall for hard and fast rules boasted by so-called experts, claiming that unless you adhere to them, you won't get the benefits.

By nature, fasting doesn't come with rules. Historically, it's something that happened to humans by circumstance. Today, when we want to mimic those circumstances to achieve the reported benefits, we get to be creative with it! Any break from eating that we grant to our digestive tract, our liver, and our entire body will initiate a revitalizing effect that, under the right circumstances, can stimulate long-lasting benefits to our physiology.

Some people might describe fasting literally as going without food. But to achieve a fasted state in which your cells perceive potential starvation doesn't actually require a person to go without any food or calories. Allow me to introduce you to some surprising alternatives.

Fasting Mimicking Diets and Modified Fasts

The Fasting Mimicking Diet and what I call Modified Fasts are eating plans designed to simulate fasting. These fasting alternatives give you a chance to achieve some or all of the same benefits of fasting but without as much restriction as required in a typical fast. These modified protocols allow you to still give your gut a break, reduce inflammation, reduce caloric intake, reduce insulin, and stimulate anti-aging pathways and cellular regeneration. The beauty of it is the opportunity to acquire more nutrients and experience a bit more pleasure while intentionally keeping your food intake low enough so your cells think you're still in a fasted state.[iv]

The Fasting Mimicking Diet and modified fasts are growing in popularity for many reasons. Firstly, even though the benefits of fasting are undeniable, many people are too intimidated to try it. Having some food makes it much less intimidating to try. That's exactly why the world's leading fasting researcher, Dr. Valter Longo, created the ProLon Fasting Mimicking Diet (FMD for short).

The 5-day FMD by ProLon gives you around 800 calories a day with bars, shakes, soups, teas, etc., all of which are formulated, packaged, and clinically validated by his company. As stated on the website *prolonfast.com*, "This 5-day meal program delivers scientifically researched micro- and macro-nutrients in precise quantities and combinations that nourish you but aren't recognized as food by your body and therefore mimic a fasting state."

As you might assume, eating 800 calories worth of prepared food makes it easier for some people to succeed with fasting rather than trying to go for 2–5 days without any food at all. I also appreciate the ability to acquire

---

iv   Dr. Valter Longo suggests that many people do better with some food during a fast because, without food in the GI tract for long enough, the body thinks, "Well, since we don't need this GI tract for digesting food or absorbing nutrients, we'll just recycle the cells of the gut-lining so we can conserve energy and use it for our essential bodily functions." That is why some people have worsened gut symptoms during or after extended fasts. Keep that in mind in case it's happening to you!

vitamins, minerals, and nutrients during the fast instead of missing out on nutrition altogether.

If you want to be entertained and get an inside peek, check out The Goop Lab series on Netflix, particularly the episode titled The Health Span Plan, where Gwyneth Paltrow tries ProLon's 5-day FMD. She was pretty miserable on it for the most part, and I think that's because she wasn't used to fasting at all, which means her body would struggle to get into ketosis. I also suspect she has a very low percentage of body fat and that she had a lot of stress, possibly even with insufficient sleep, given the pressures of recording the Netflix series.

In 2023, I tried the 5-day Prolon FMD myself. Since I'd already been fasting for years, it came pretty easy to me. I felt as if days one and two provided a lot of food. By day three, I was really cherishing the one or two bowls of soup I could enjoy. The serving sizes were very small, and I'm sure for a person larger than I am, this would be such a tease. I felt fantastic on days 3 through 5, and I also felt that if days 1 and 2 had started with smaller portions, I would've experienced that 'fasting high' much earlier in the span of things. My biggest takeaway is that it's not for everyone. While doing the FMD, I felt food was more frequently on my mind compared to when I fasted without any food. There's something about knowing you can eat sooner or later that makes some of us hungrier. That's ghrelin telling our brains to seek out food. I find it easier to fast without any food at all. Go figure!

Still, some of my clients have really enjoyed doing ProLon's FMD. It serves as a great reset and jumpstart to weight loss, reduced inflammation, abundant energy, and confidence. The ProLon company recommends doing the 5-day FMD at a maximum frequency of once a month. During the rest of the month, you eat as usual with some gentle intermittent fasting. That frequency is great for weight maintenance and anti-aging. However, I'm not convinced it's frequent enough to experience noticeable weight loss besides individuals who are technically obese and not ready to make more changes to their everyday diet. I believe their recommendation is modest to apply to a general audience and to prevent a slowed metabolism, which is an unfortunate consequence of consistent low-calorie dieting.

You also might wanna check out the DIY homemade versions that have surfaced online. Although the DIY versions aren't meticulously formulated or science-backed like ProLon's FMD is, it makes sense that you might be able to achieve many or all of the same benefits if you follow the specific guidelines (40 percent of calories come from fat, 10 percent from protein, and 50 percent from carbohydrates mostly from fiber-rich vegetables).

I first learned about modified fasts when I read the in-depth gut health recovery manual called *Healthy Gut, Healthy You* by Functional Gastroenterologist Dr. Michael Ruscio. In a clinical setting, modified fasts are a liquid-only diet that's intended to help people heal a severely compromised digestive system. When a person suffers from gastrointestinal issues, a liquid-modified fast known as an elemental diet can be incredibly reparative for the gut. It allows the GI tract a break so cells and mucosa can regrow in the gut lining, initiating balance in the microbiome and healing from a diet or environment that destroyed it. Elemental diet formulas are designed to provide easily assimilated macro- and micro-nutrients to ensure adequate nutritional intake without activating the stress response otherwise achieved with regular fasts.

Modified fasts aren't limited to this clinical version. You might notice the term modified fast being thrown around in all different ways, including the protein-sparing modified fast. This is a high-protein diet paired with short intermittent fasts with the intention of providing abundant protein during the eating window and, in turn, preventing potential muscle tissue wasting during the fasting window. I wish that version had a different name because it doesn't have much in common with other modified fasts. If you ask me, a modified fast describes an alternate fasting strategy used to address a person's circumstantial limitations with fasting and is designed for easy assimilation of nutrients during the fasting window without losing all benefits of the fast.

Versions of modified fasts I've encouraged in my coaching practice:

- Organic bone broth fast (1–5 days max, or replacing one meal per day for up to 30 days)

- Organic cold-pressed juice fast (1–5 days max, low-sugar juices only, predominately veggie juices and/or teas)

- Lemon-cayenne cleanse (1–5 days max)[47]

- Fasts supplemented with collagen powder, whey protein, or essential amino acids (EAA's, like the Aminos products from *getkion.com*)

- Fasts that include Ample meal replacement drinks (1–3 days max, or replacing one meal per day for up to 30 days)

- Fasts that include a Fast Bar, ProLon Fasting Shake, or ProLon's 1-day ReSet

Modified fasts will temporarily interrupt a fast, but the metabolic shift occurs so briefly that a person is typically in and out of a fasted state within 1–3 hours. The body readily returns to ketosis and fasting shortly thereafter because the nutrients don't require much digestion to assimilate. In some ways, this more closely mimics the fasted states our ancient ancestors would be in because they'd consume broth, scraps, herbal tea concoctions, and any stray food they could gather whenever food was scarce. The body doesn't necessarily turn off fasting pathways when we consume some nutrients during a fast because our cells' intelligence can detect that the nutrients aren't enough to fuel the body without fasting processes such as ketosis and autophagy still activated.

One more thing about doing extended fasts or modified fasts for longer than one day. Be aware that your brain might tell you to gorge when it's time to eat again, but *not so fast*. Gorging yourself is the last thing you want to do to break your fast. Take it slow and understand it can be a shock to your system to reintroduce solid foods or a large serving of food after giving it a day off. Don't indulge in a huge meal to celebrate the completion of a fast. Instead, break your fast with a handful of blueberries, for instance, letting the juicy berries stimulate your gastric juices and wake up your sleepy microbiome. Drink a little apple cider vinegar mixed with water to do the same. Eat smaller portions when you break this fast, and softer, slow-cooked foods that are easy to digest. If your gut has been impaired, don't break your long fasts with a salad. Raw vegetables (and grilled/seared/fried/blackened meats) are too tough to break down. Work your way up to a full-size meal over the next day or two to transition comfortably and prevent GI upset.

I do all sorts of modified fasts. It's freeing to vary your fasts based on your current needs or ever-changing priorities. I can *feel* the difference when I give myself the freedom. Our bodies expect a break, but that doesn't mean we need to follow a rulebook to provide it. Food isn't supposed to be so plentiful and frequently consumed. Our guts aren't supposed to be working so hard, so scaling back on the work required by your digestive system, your liver, and your metabolism—that's all that matters.

There are no rules, only principles. These need to become values of yours. Fasting, healthy living, nutritious eating. It's all part of your new identity. A lifestyle you cherish and honor. The moment you realize you've returned to a careless junk-food diet and constant insulin production is the moment you must again decide which life you want to live—one that burdens your body and erases your efforts or one that's supported by these life-giving principles. Then you can RESET.

CHAPTER 58

Gut Health Matters

Finally, we live in a time when health enthusiasts acknowledge the general importance of a healthy gut. It's incredible how much there is to learn about what makes up a healthy gut and how our cohabiting microbes impact our health in so many ways. Let me start by sharing that the number of bacteria and microbes in our bodies outnumber our human cells by 10–1. Most of the microbes live in our GI tract, and they work together in incredible ways to influence every aspect of our health and wellness.

The world of microorganisms living inside your gut is referred to as your gut microbiome, or microbiome for short. We have an oral microbiome in our mouths, a skin microbiome on the surface of our skin, and one within the deeper layers. We can consider the gut microbiome our second brain (or some would argue our first brain) because the connection between our gut and brain is a two-way street with exceptional functions that directly affect our mental health and cognition.

It's not a stretch to say that without a relatively balanced microbiome, you can't experience robust health and longevity.

Think of a lush rainforest with thousands of different species coexisting. Inside live thousands of different species of animals, insects, plants, and creatures that must live together in a way that benefits the success of the entire forest. Predator and prey balance each other, all with a significant role to play in maintaining overall harmony.

That's how it is in our gut microbiome. All the fungi, yeasts, pathogens, and probiotic microbes must coexist in a balanced way that promotes health in humans. Otherwise, certain species may be wiped out, and other invasive species take over. The balance is lost when this state, called *gut dysbiosis,* occurs. Massive shifts take place in your gut's ecosystem. These can be caused by various detriments like pesticides in your food, chemicals in your water, a nutrient-poor diet, smoking or drinking alcohol, and eating foods you're unable to digest. We see damage to the gut lining, or a leaky gut, which leads to an alarmed immune system, and all the while, certain microbes become invasive while others starve and dwindle to extinction. The result? A negative impact on your health that's more wide-ranging than you can imagine, from mental health dysfunction to chronic inflammation, cancer, obesity, infection, skin disorders, malnutrition, and autoimmune disease.

Have you ever wondered why, all of a sudden, it seems everyone has gut problems? Many different aspects of the way we live today and factors of our modern environment have massively screwed up the health of our microbiome, starting from the way we were birthed and continuing throughout our lives.

Major contributors to gut dysbiosis and compromised gut health:

- Delivered by Cesarean section rather than vaginal birth

- Being fed with baby formula instead of breast milk

- Antibiotic medications, especially during childhood and with repeat use

- Dental work with toxic chemicals and surgical procedures that directly affect the microbiome via the oral-gut axis

- Overuse of sanitation products in the home

- Reduced micro-exposures to immune-priming microbes throughout infancy and childhood.

- Diets lacking in live-cultured foods and various fermented foods and beverages

- Regular exposure to preservatives in the diet

- Regular exposure to artificial flavors and colors, food dyes, and synthetic ingredients in our diet

- Over-exposure to heavy metals such as mercury (primarily from seafood and silver cavity fillings), aluminum, and lead. All can be passed through the placenta trans-generationally

- Irresponsibly farmed food and soil doused in toxic pesticides

- Synthetic fertilizers used in farming

- Toxic weed killers, particularly Glyphosate (the active ingredient in Round-Up weed killer), a pervasive chemical used in farming around the world today. Humans are exposed everywhere, starting with the food we eat, the landscaping and grass we live around, the air we breathe, the water we shower in, the drinks we consume, and even the rain

- Frequent exposure to prescription medications and over-the-counter anti-inflammatories

- Chronic stress (yup, a major reason for compromised gut health)

- Massive agricultural and societal shifts toward using a modern dwarf wheat variety, which comprises an estimated 70–80 percent of global wheat production. In modern wheat, gluten proteins comprise around 80–85 percent of total protein, compared to only around 50 percent in ancient varieties. Modern gluten is more immune-reactive due to changes in the protein structure caused by hybridization

- Generational, cultural, and societal shifts toward a predominantly grain-based diet and heavy reliance on commodity crops (primarily corn, soy, and wheat)

- Socio-economic and cultural shifts to a processed food diet that's high in sugar and processed carbohydrates, lacking in food rotation and nutrient density, such as the Standard American Diet (SAD)

- Imbalanced ratio of Omega-6 to Omega-3. In the typical Western diet, this ranges from 10:1–30:1. This is due to excessive consumption of omega-6 fats from industrial seed oils, convenience foods, and reduced intake of seafood and omega-3-rich sources. Optimal omega-6 to omega-3 ratios are more like 2:1

Your gut microbiome and the integrity of your gut lining are responsible for over 70 percent of your immune system function. Your gut is also responsible for 90 percent of that serotonin feel-good brain chemical you need to stay sane and content in your daily life. The microbes in your gut ferment and break down food after it's left the stomach and help move the nutrients from your food through the gut barrier wall. Nutrients then enter your bloodstream to help meet your nutritional needs, while your gut barrier keeps foreign invaders in your GI tract safely eliminated or obliterated. Without an adequately functioning gut, nutrient deficiencies can develop, and your immune system can become impaired. Eventually, these outcomes can lead to a wide range of diseases and dysfunction.

If you suffer from obvious gut-related symptoms like discomfort after eating, bloating, gas, acid reflux, diarrhea, constipation, sharp pains in your abdomen, or not-so-obviously linked conditions like obesity, depression, and chronic anxiety or brain fog, skin disorders like eczema, acne, or rashes; or immune system impairment like frequently getting sick or suffering from repeat bouts of food poisoning or stomach bugs; or if you have an autoimmune disease, food sensitivities, relentless cravings, or any signs of chronic inflammation in your body—then you need to improve the health of your gut microbiome, where it all begins.

This isn't a book about gut health, so I'll keep it short and just give you what you need to get started and make significant improvements to your gut microbiome. It wouldn't be a stretch to assume your gut microbiome needs you to eat a more diverse diet and to reduce your exposure to harmful food toxins. It also wouldn't be a stretch to assume that now, or intermittently, your gut barrier is compromised and permeable, meaning you have a leaky gut. This means the foods you eat and pathogens and chemicals you're exposed to are causing inflammation, sneaking through your gut wall, and alarming your immune system. This means, like I did, you could suddenly develop new food sensitivities in adulthood. You can develop strange symptoms that seem unrelated to the gut, get sick all the time, or develop an autoimmune disease, not even realizing it all started with an imbalanced gut microbiome and associated leaky gut.

For some people, fasting can help restore balance to the microbiome and the integrity of the gut lining that's been damaged by years of unhealthy inputs. This damage might come from too much junk food and fried foods, foods that don't agree with your gut, binge drinking, chronic stress, environmental chemicals and toxins, or long-term use of medicines like antibiotics that disrupt your microbiome balance. Fasting gives your gut a break, a chance to rest and recover, just like resting a sprained ankle before pounding the pavement again helps it heal. However, for many folks, fasting alone isn't enough. Broader steps to actively nurture a healthier microbiome also need to be taken through diet, lifestyle, habits, and possibly supplementation. This multi-pronged approach is often required to rebuild gut health for the long run after extensive damage.

You can improve your gut health significantly by taking action with the steps described in the list below. As much as you might like to ignore the magnitude of this topic, just remember all disease begins in the gut. Even obesity. Even mental health disorders. Even heart disease. You need your gut to function well, and here's a great way to get started!

The top 10 things you can do to significantly improve your gut health:

1. Take digestive enzymes with every meal and increase your intake of enzyme-rich foods (a combination of raw, cultured, and fermented foods and drinks excluding alcohol).

2. Drink purified, chlorine-free water or spring water without plastic packaging.

3. Reduce processed food, specifically preservatives, seed oils, deep-fried foods, artificial ingredients, and high-fructose corn syrup.

4. Avoid antibiotic use whenever possible.

5. Reduce or eliminate the use of NSAID and anti-inflammatory OTC meds like Motrin, Tylenol, and Advil.

6. Buy non-GMO and organic foods to reduce exposure to synthetic fertilizers, glyphosate, and other pesticides and herbicides.

7. Avoid or greatly reduce the gluten in your diet, especially all-purpose flour and non-organic grains, and modern wheat from the US, and avoid any foods to which you have a sensitivity or intolerance.

8. Diversify your diet. Eat a variety of foods, rotating types within categories of food as well as the type of preparation, such as raw, cooked, fermented, cultured, and sprouted. Strive to eat ≥ 2 tablespoons of lacto-fermented veggies per day (like refrigerated sauerkraut or kimchi that contain live, active cultures and no preservatives). Rotate the brand or variation often.

9. Experiment with a variety of intermittent stress-coping strategies and prioritize daily stress reduction like it's your job.

10. Reduce alcohol consumption, especially beer, commercial wine, and straight hard alcohol.

If you weren't already aware, smoking cigarettes has been shown to damage gut health in several ways. The toxins in cigarette smoke can kill off beneficial microbes in the gut microbiome while allowing harmful pathogenic bacteria to thrive. This dysbiosis and inflammation caused by smoking impair the gut's ability to heal and function optimally. If you currently smoke, consider getting support to help you quit once and for all.

After reviewing the list above, are you surprised I didn't suggest you take probiotics and prebiotics? Well, although those are both beneficial (and could be 11. and 12. on the list), I consider them to be next-level solutions that won't necessarily improve gut health without first addressing the first-level problems. Besides, you'll consume more probiotics by eating fermented and cultured foods (8. on the list), and you'll increase the population of beneficial probiotics in your gut by increasing the variety in your diet and by reducing your exposure to offensive things listed. You'll get prebiotic fiber from eating fibrous and more diverse vegetables, too. Supplementing with probiotics can be just another thing to do, and without targeting what your unique body and gut specifically need, it can either be pointless or result in undesirable consequences like bacterial overgrowth, impaired digestion, and discomfort from gas and bloating.

So stick with the top 10 list above, and you'll be well on your way to an ancestrally, functionally appropriate gut microbiome that helps you thrive in the modern world.

CHAPTER 59

Advantages and Disadvantages of Combining Exercise with Fasting

W hether you currently exercise or not, this is an important topic to consider since the combination of fasting with exercise can either amplify your results or impair them. Out of necessity, humans have involuntarily combined exercise with fasting for tens of thousands of years under the circumstances of pre-civilized or destitute times.

Imagine a caveman living in the desert with his tribe without any food for two days and counting. They haven't found any plants to forage, and they've had bad luck with efforts to trap a wild hare or snake to eat. Luckily, by just being in a fasted state, the caveman's body will initiate a range of helpful processes to help him and his people thrive in these undesirable conditions. Our human DNA is pre-programmed to help us adapt and prevail in such distressing circumstances. If we were programmed without that ability, our species would've become extinct even before the first war occurred in human history.

While the caveman and his tribe go without food for days, they experience an increase in mental sharpness, which gives them the ability to think of a new plan to find food. They experience an increase in energy, so they have the agility to hunt and the fuel to endure migrating conditions on the way to new territory. That's not all. The cavepeople also experience the preservation of lean muscle so that their bodies don't rely on precious muscle tissue to convert into energy. Instead, the body activates autophagy and a protein-sparing version of gluconeogenesis (making new glucose) to make new glucose molecules from other substrates besides muscle tissue. Being in ketosis or a fasted state promotes a metabolic shift that allows the body to rely on fat and ketones for energy, sparing muscle tissue as much as possible. The human body has incredible presets, and that's what we want to tap into when it comes to fasting and exercise.

As with everything in health and wellness, there's a catch, though. These amazing adaptations aren't 100 percent dependable under 100 percent of circumstances. If doing exercise while fasting was guaranteed to give someone better results, every single athlete in the world would be doing exercise while fasting. But many of them aren't. Why not? It helps if we review the pros and cons of doing fasted exercise. Let's start with the cons—or disadvantages. This list will help you understand why exercising in a fasted state isn't always the best combo:

Potential Disadvantages Of Combining Exercise with Fasting

- If a person is carbohydrate-dependent and not yet fat-adapted

    o They may run out of energy during fasted exercise, and performance will noticeably suffer

    o They'll burn muscle tissue to make new glucose for energy for exercising in a fasted state

    o They'll experience an increased risk or occurrence of injury because the tissues don't have adequate building blocks to repair, strengthen, and rebuild

- o They'll experience reduced stamina during endurance training

- o They may risk hypoglycemia (dangerously low blood sugar levels)

- o They may risk severe dehydration or inadequate sodium and electrolytes

- If a person is fat-adapted and their body is accustomed to fat burning or fasting for energy

  - o They may lack adequate amino acids and building blocks to prevent the breakdown of muscle tissue needed to fuel the fasted workout

  - o If they don't eat after the workout, it's possible that post-workout muscle repair and growth will be impaired.

  - o If they work out too much and/or do too much fasting, they may experience a plateau, slowed metabolism, or stagnated performance.

  - o Without adequate nutrients, they may experience greater stress, fatigue, and likelihood of injury, as well as impaired immune system function.

  - o They may get caught in a reverse fasting/feasting cycle where they eat less on workout days and gorge themselves on non-workout days as the brain and body attempt to compensate for the high energy output and inadequate energy (nutrient) input.

Potential Advantages of Combining Exercise with Fasting

- When you do it right, stacking exercise with fasting is like doubling down on your results without doubling down on your effort, so you'll accomplish more in less time and with less exertion.

- The body becomes more efficient at partitioning glycogen, calories, amino acids, and ketones or fatty acids.

- The body relies mostly on fat burning and ketones for energy, which means dependable energy is readily available, energy burns cleaner (there's less oxidative stress), and more body fat is burned during and after the workout.

- One can burn 15–20 percent more body fat during a fasted workout.

- The body has more blood flow and oxygen and more time to meet the demands of the workout compared to working out while digestion is still underway.

- Exercising near the end of your fasting window can make the final hours of the fast easier to accomplish, and they can be perfectly timed with your post-exercise 'break fast' meal.

- Enhanced HGH, autophagy, and metabolic flexibility help ensure muscle tissue is preserved and recycled for growth and repair as needed.

As with many hormetic stressors, fasting and exercise have a lot in common. **When done responsibly, fasting and exercise are each known to:**

- Increase epinephrine or adrenaline in the body.

- Increase norepinephrine in the brain, which results in better mental sharpness.

- Increase human growth hormone (preserving muscle mass and helping build more muscle).

- Improve mood (by decreasing stress and increasing feel-good neurotransmitters).

- Increase energy you can feel.

- Increase stress tolerance.

- Increase BDNF (brain-derived neurotrophic factor) to help grow new brain cells and improve learning.

- Increase autophagy (recycling junky cell parts and improving healthier cells).

- Repair and grow new mitochondria (mitophagy and mitochondrial biogenesis).

- Increase fat burning and ketone production.

- Improve insulin sensitivity.

- Improve metabolic flexibility.

- Improve glucose uptake.

- Improve cardiovascular health.

- Improve immune function (and reduce disease risk).

- Increase longevity and healthspan.

- Decrease appetite or improved leptin sensitivity.

- Enhance detoxification .

- Improve physical capacity and resilience (in part thanks to increased muscle regulatory factors that help regenerate and protect muscle tissue).

The Biggest Issues I See In My Clients Who Engage In Fasted Exercise:

- Reduced appetite post-workout (and/or insufficient time or planning for a meal), which leads to longer fasts on workout days (which is the opposite of what your body needs from you) and can result in stalled fat-loss or stalled muscle growth

- Being chronically under-slept and stressed, meaning fasted exercise puts too much added stress on the body, leading to a myriad of consequences like slowed metabolism, suppressed thyroid function, chronically high cortisol, injury, illness, etc.

- Engaging in chronic over-exercising without adequate rest days and/ or without adequate nutrition or 3-Meal Days to strike the crucial balance required for optimal nutrition and recovery

- Under-consuming carbohydrates in the meal that precedes a fast and the fasted workout (especially in cardio/endurance training)

- Under-consuming enough complete protein or essential amino acids to support their exercise and fasting regime

- Under-consuming electrolytes, particularly sodium and magnesium

- Starting a new or more challenging exercise routine while acclimating to fasting (therefore undereating), which, at the very least, creates the perfect storm for a slowed metabolism or weight-loss plateau. Then they want to quit because they don't understand why the scale won't budge two weeks after starting their new exercise routine

Timing Exercise with Fasting

Doing a daytime workout while in a fasted state makes more sense than almost anything in life. I say that because, if you think about it, long before the times of civilized living, refrigerators, and breakfast cereal, humans had to find their food or catch something to eat nearly every day. It's a natural process for the body to exert energy to acquire food. It's like you *earn* that food after exerting such effort. At times, even, you'd exert all that energy and end up with nothing because your food got away or because someone or some animal stole it from you.

The best time to do a workout is during the last 1–3 hours of your intermittent fasting window. Working out toward the end of your fast has several advantages. First, you may already be in ketosis by this time, which means fat burning is already underway. Your body fat can be a dependable energy source for your workout.

A second advantage of timing workouts toward the end of your fast is that, at times, it can be a bit challenging to persevere through the final few hours of a fast. By that time, you might be thinking about food, looking at the clock, and debating whether or not you should just go ahead and break your fast. By engaging in exercise during that timeframe, you'd boost appetite-suppressing hormones and forget all about food as your body and brain use your own fat for food instead.

Finally, it's great to plan your workout at the tail end of your fasting window because it makes the most nutritional sense to 'feast' after you've exerted all that energy. Post-workout, your muscles are primed to suck up all the carbs and protein you eat and most efficiently put them to use. Your blood glucose levels will be in a healthier range or display a more optimal pattern, and your insulin sensitivity will have improved, too. The more muscle you have, the more storage you have for carbs since about 80 percent of the glycogen stores we have are in our muscle cells.

Is it critical to eat after a workout?

Sometimes yes, sometimes no. How do you feel? How hard did you push your muscles? How hard did you train? How long was your workout? What are your goals? If you want to build more muscle, consume ≥ 25 g of animal protein, whey protein powder, or EAAs (essential amino acids) within 30–120 minutes after a workout. Some studies show you can still benefit from the post-workout muscle-building effect for up to 3 hours after a workout.

If your goal is to burn fat and simply maintain your muscle, you can continue fasting post-workout. As long as you've consumed adequate protein in the meal(s) that precede your fast, fasting with resistance training will boost human growth hormone to remarkable levels. Because of that, lean muscle is preserved even if you fast for 2–3 days after working out! It's incredible, really.

This isn't license to exercise and fast all the time and try to rush the process. I see my workout enthusiasts and overweight female clients do this all the time. They're so busy and so eager to lose weight (and skip anything time-consuming, such as planning a healthy meal) that they end up doing fasted exercise almost every day and waiting to eat for 3–4 more hours after the workout! Abuse the combination of fasting and exercise enough, and over time, you'll see the metabolism slow down. You often see more infections like cold or flu and an increase in injuries as well. Perhaps it's because these individuals already have screwed-up metabolisms, because they don't sleep enough, or because they have too much chronic stress in their lives. But, no matter what, the combination of factors gets to be too much for their body, and the metabolism fights back. The immune system suffers. The body maladapts due to too much hormetic stress.

Fasting post-exercise only works in the long run for those who are willing to put in the work required to strategize how their workouts + fasting schedule + nutrition + meal timing all complement one another along with their ever-changing lifestyle conditions.

How to Hack Your Fasts

The key reason you should eat after a strength training workout is that your body probably needs more protein to rebuild and repair after the strain experienced during exercise. There's a fasting hack, however, that can help you sidestep the need to eat an actual meal post-workout and help your body return to a fasted state shortly after.

If you want to continue fasting immediately after strength training, you can consume a pure protein powder or supplement that will temporarily break your fast, allowing you not only to build new muscle and repair but also to return to a fasted state (specifically ketosis) within an hour or two afterward.

What I suggest to my clients is to drink a high-quality whey protein isolate mixed with water (≥ 25 g of protein per serving) or, more ideally, to supplement with essential amino acids (or EAAs for short). Specifically, it's ideal to supplement with a serving of around 6.5–10 g within 30–60 minutes of your workout. You can also sip on it as a drink during your workout. Because these protein sources are, literally, just the amino acids that make up the protein and are therefore in a highly-absorbable form, the body doesn't have to digest or work to break down the protein into those amino acid building blocks as it would if you consumed protein in the form of food. This means you get the amino acids in your bloodstream right away, less insulin is required, and you'll speedily return to ketosis shortly after. You won't risk compromised muscle growth and repair, or injury, and you'll still get most of the benefits of fasting: fat burning, mental clarity, energy, enhanced immunity, and a break for your digestive system.

I discovered an EAA powder and supplement from Ben Greenfield's high-performance brand, Kion, at *getkion.com*. Kion Aminos drink powder comes in various flavors, and there's an Aminos supplement sold in capsules (7 capsules are needed per serving, though). For decades, serious weight lifters relied on a supplement or powder made up of BCAAs (branched-chain amino acids), but it doesn't compare to EAAs like Kion Aminos. I'm not affiliated with this product; I'm just excited to have found it so my clients can get the best results with this fasting hack. BCAAs only provide three of the essential amino acids, while Kion Aminos contains all nine essential amino acids. What's more, is that Kion adds 40 percent more leucine (one of the three BCAAs) to provide the scientifically-backed ratios of amino acids needed to grow more muscle and achieve an adequate degree of recovery. Kion states muscle building (muscle protein synthesis) can increase upward of 300 percent when consuming Aminos in this formula compared to consuming whole food proteins after a workout.

Now you've got enough detail to move forward with confidence and combine your exercise with fasting in a way that compliments your health and fitness goals.

If you don't currently exercise, let it be known that simply by taking a walk after you eat, you'll give your body somewhere to put the glucose. Your walking muscles and your heart will happily use that glucose to meet the demands. This means your blood glucose and insulin response are both improved.

Want to get more of these advantages? Start doing some resistance training in an effort to build more muscle. Not only will you experience immediate benefits regarding glucose-insulin regulation, but over time, you'll create more safe storage space for the carbs you ingest since your muscle tissue is the primary place glucose is stored before the overflow is converted for storage as body fat. Exercise is a long-proven therapy to resolve and even reverse type 2 diabetes and insulin resistance. And the impact is immediate!

CHAPTER 60

Experimentation and Self-Reflection

Already, you've begun to implement some key changes in your life with the action steps I've shared throughout this book. Whether you're going at it alone or with the help of a coach, I've got a few self-help concepts to keep in mind so the change process goes more smoothly for you. Let's dive into the importance of experimentation, repetition, reflection, self-awareness, and self-regulation.

Experimentation

This could be the most important missing piece in anyone's journey for change. The importance of experimenting is to collect data, find out what works now, and grow more self-awareness.

> *"I don't know what to do; I know what not to do.*
> *What not to do is what I've been doing."*
> - Simon Sinek

The change process requires you to continuously change your strategy and learn from it. If nothing about your approach changes, nothing about your results will change. You know you want to experience a *change* in your life, your health, your body, and your habits, yet, most of the time, you keep trying the same things over and over, expecting yourself, your body, and your habits to magically change.

Instead, you'll need to experiment. Once you define a behavioral goal you want to change, such as *I want to cook three days a week*, experiment with just a few variables at once. Variables you might experiment with include the time of day, day of the week, location/setting, time allotted, frequency, effort required, with or without assistance, with or without tracking or account-ability, etc. Experimenting helps you incrementally change things through a lens of curiosity, so you're more likely to succeed at building a habit that's meaningful to you.

In most cases—other than the extreme circumstances when you're amped for a complete lifestyle overhaul (moving to a new town after a tough divorce or receiving a life-threatening diagnosis)—it's unwise to start experimenting with a full set of variables that match your ideal outcome. Instead, if you want to succeed, you start by experimenting with just one, two, or three vari-ables. You start with whatever gives you the least friction so you can figure out what *not* to do and inch yourself closer to knowing what works *for you*.

Thomas Edison famously said, "I haven't failed. I've just found 10,000 ways that don't work…." He added, "Every failure told me something to incorpo-rate into the next attempt…when I have eliminated the ways that will not work, I will find the way that will work."

Failure is *feedback*. Remember that.

I'll often remind my clients to standardize before they optimize when build-ing new habits. This tip comes from James Clear, the author of *Atomic Habits*, who says, "A habit must be established before it can be improved…. Make it the standard in your life, then worry about doing it better."

For instance, let's say your goal is to cook a homemade meal 3 days a week, but currently, you're not cooking at all. While 3 days is the ideal outcome you desire, I recommend first standardizing one day, like Mondays. This gives you a chance to experiment with variables like grocery shopping, time of day, making enough for leftovers, doing the dishes, and finding recipes to try. Once you've smoothed out the kinks, you're ready to add Wednesdays and/or Fridays.

You may be thinking, *Marisa, if I don't go all-in with 3 days right away, I won't gain enough momentum. I'll just forget to do it, or I won't take it as seriously.* Okay then, what if, instead of cooking full meals, you start by spending fifteen minutes on Monday, Wednesday, and Friday prepping simple healthy snacks or salads. The key here is to have less of a gap between the habit you have now (not cooking at all) and the experiment you start with (preparing a healthy snack). This initial change requires less time and effort, reducing the pressure and associated excuses while still challenging you to plan, shop, prep, and experiment to gradually build a new routine.

You're Not The Same Old You

One false assumption people make is *If it worked for me in the past, it will work for me now.*

My client, Jennifer, told me, "I used to cook every single day of the week, and I was in the best shape of my life! I need to start cooking again." I listen and return with some inquiry, "Tell me more about that time in your life, Jennifer. What was different at the time—like your job, your family situation, your schedule or routine, your age?"

She thinks about the complexity of my question and says, "Well, back then, I was going to the office. I had two kids in school full time, and I was maybe thirty-five years old. I got home from work at 4 p.m., an hour or so before the kids got home from activities. I'd use that time to start dinner prep right when I came through the door. I would exercise for twenty minutes or so while the food was in the oven or while I waited for the kids to come home. I remember getting pretty good at timing the meal for right when they returned. I had so much energy back then!"

I pointed out to Jennifer that a lot of things in her life were different at that time, which means we should think differently about how it can work in her life at *this time*. It's unreasonable to expect herself to adopt that old routine when her schedule, family life, and current habits don't complement it now.

I guided Jennifer to think of this as a series of experiments, changing a few variables at a time, working to reduce the friction and make it more effortless to get started. We'll build a habit as we simultaneously gather feedback. Along the way, she'll grow wiser to her changed circumstances and current needs. After a few months of trial and correction, we were able to develop a routine that works for her now: shopping on Sundays and batch cooking on Tuesday mornings (she has a late start at work on Tuesdays). She orders prepared meals for her own lunch on Thursdays and Fridays, and she makes fifteen-minute meals every Saturday morning (thanks to the list on her fridge of such meals she knows the family will eat).

Another way I encourage clients to experiment is to try a set of 'crutches' to help get a new habit off the ground. Jennifer's crutch was to try some prepared meals. She also experimented with cooking on Mondays, but time was scarce. We relied on some crutches here, too, like starting with a store-bought rotisserie chicken or cooking something she already knew how to make without a recipe. My favorite crutches are prepared meals from Balanced Bites, meal kits from Green Chef, and buying pre-cut veggies from the produce department—you know, those cubed sweet potatoes or pre-cut zucchini noodles that cost a painful $7 per container. That means fewer excuses running through your mind when you feel like abandoning the plan to cook because you're too busy.

I think you get the idea now. Experimentation is key!

Repetition

Let's have fun for a minute and imagine the world's most dependable fortune teller told you, "You'll fail at your diet forty-five times before you succeed. It will take three years, but you will succeed." How would that prediction affect your efforts? Would you quit on your dreams to succeed with healthy eating, or would you dig deep and get started knowing that a few years from now, you *will* eventually succeed?

I play around with similar predictions with my clients. I tell them what I know to be true: "Most of us need to repeat the same annoying mistake or bad habits a hundred times—and feel the ensuing remorse a hundred times—before we've finally built enough self-awareness to actually stop ourselves mid-sabotage and act differently next time."

I can't count how many times a client has told me something about needing to be more consistent. But really, I tell them, what they need is to be more *persistent*.

Being consistent is unrealistic for most of us. It's persistence that will help us reach our goals. When you're persistent, you know you'll figure it out eventually. Being open to repetition means you'll have time to recognize the patterns you're trapped in. You'll have enough time to grow tired of your self-identifying excuses. Repetition gives you a chance to become familiar with yourself and wake up to your current situation so you can finally grab hold of the reigns in the moment! Finally, you'll stop acting in pursuit of what you want right now (instant gratification) and start acting in pursuit of what you want the most.

It's part of the process to have patience with yourself. We coaches call that self-compassion.

Reflection

If only we could learn from our experiences more effortlessly. If only we could remember what we ate, felt, or did last Monday. All this health stuff would be so much easier! You've got a lot on your plate, though. You do a lot. Your brain works hard to store information you actually *need* to remember, and it makes room for that important stuff by releasing unnecessary clutter (like what you ate, felt, or did last Monday).

So, how can we learn from our experiences and stop wasting time and effort in the process of change? Build a practice of self-reflection. A recurring practice (nightly, weekly, bi-weekly, or monthly) helps you draw conclusions from your observations and data to reassess your plan or priorities and make the necessary adjustments. This doesn't even need to be a habit you build yourself *(another habit? Sheesh!)* because you can externalize it. A recurring coaching call with a health coach, life coach, accountability buddy, etc., works wonders for this. When you have a recurring appointment to discuss your goals, it comes along with a dedicated time for reflection. It's like automating your efforts to reflect and reassess the experiments you've been running. Through this, over time, you build more self-awareness and self-regulation. The result? You act more in alignment with what you really want—and that, right there, equals more self-efficacy (yes, I can!) and greater progress.

Self-regulation is your ability to act in accordance with your long-term best interest and ultimate values.

At one time or another, you probably thought to yourself, I just need more willpower so I can stick with these healthy habits. Sure, habit change can require a notable degree of self-discipline. But when it comes down to lasting change, what you really need to improve is your ability to self-regulate.

"Habit change is not achieved through an act of will. It requires development of self-regulation skills…neither intention or desire alone has much effect if people lack the capability for exercising influence over their own motivation and behavior."
- Bandura, 1998 (Bandura & Simon, 1977)

Being someone with ADHD and the associated neurochemistry that worsens self-regulation, I can't help but share that two of the greatest determiners of self-regulation are quality of sleep and the degree to which a person is able to regulate their emotions. Emotional regulation can be improved by learning to effectively cope with stress and uncomfortable emotions and instilling personal boundaries that help mitigate emotional disruptions in your day. Work on improving your sleep with the help of those lists in Part 6 of this book, and you'll greatly improve your ability to manage yourself and change your habits in pursuit of a goal.

Self-Sabotage and Revising Your Self-Image

Self Sabotage

Self-sabotage is a subconscious effort made by the inner voice in your head to stay in your comfort zone or take the path of least resistance—even when it will be detrimental to your well-being.

"If you want to have success in weight loss, work, or life in general, then you have to get out of your comfort zone and make sure self-sabotaging inner dialogue doesn't stand in your way."
- Jeremy Rolleston, Dual Olympian

An Outdated Self-Image Causes Self-Sabotage

The root of self-sabotage is your outdated self-image. Your subconscious mind holds on to old identities and patterns, aiming to sabotage your current and future self and prevent change.

For example, a mom may have long identified as putting her kids and household first, above all else. Now, with kids getting older, she decides to commit to healthier eating and losing weight. But soon, self-sabotaging behaviors emerge. *Why do I keep eating this junk food,* she wonders. *If I just cooked the veggies as planned, they wouldn't rot in the fridge.*

Her subconscious clings to the outdated self-image as a mom first. She's used to just eating whatever is easiest or whatever the kids didn't finish. The kids don't eat many vegetables, so she also stopped eating them at home. Her conscious mind makes her feel guilty about prioritizing her own needs and desires. Her subconscious mind sabotages efforts to put her health/self first, fearing that it proves she's not as good of a mom.

Build a New Self-Image

To overcome this, she can start revising the outdated self-image. Using her love for family as a driver for healthy choices, she intentionally ties her family values into a new self-image as a mom who prioritizes healthy living.

Affirmations for this new self-image:

- Making healthy choices means I'm an honorable example for my kids.

- Setting healthy boundaries means my kids will learn to do the same.

- Taking time for personal growth empowers my kids to adopt a growth mindset.

- Persevering through challenges models determination and self-efficacy for my kids, too.

You're actualizing your best self, which provides a life-giving example for the whole family. In summary, identifying and evolving outdated self-images can help overcome subconscious self-sabotage on the path to positive change.

Psychologically speaking, the process of self-reidentification can be a difficult pursuit for certain people. These individuals experience a sense of significant personal loss when they try to change the way they live. It's as if an important part of their personal history, personality, or tradition will be gone forever.

Revising your self-identity doesn't have to be so scary or formidable. You can start small. Let's say you want to cut back on sugar, but it overwhelms you to imagine yourself as someone who misses out on all the sweets you're used to enjoying. That's why you decide to start small with your habit of eating sweets with your morning coffee. Ever since childhood, the adults in your family start their day with a biscotti or coffee cake alongside their morning coffee. It's a cultural thing you adopted the moment you started drinking coffee, too. You've been doing it that way for decades now, and you can't believe you have to give it up.

First, let's acknowledge that your resistance to change is completely natural. Then, let's acknowledge that the association between your self-identity and a sweets-with-coffee habit is, in fact, standing in the way of what you want the most for your health. Finally, try revising the story you tell yourself. *It's not like I can't have biscotti with my coffee ever again. I enjoy it sometimes as a special treat. When it's a holiday, when I'm with my grandma, or when I have something to celebrate. I strive for balance now because it feels good to take care of my body in this new chapter.*

Have you ever been in a toxic relationship that you knew must come to an end? A relationship so meaningful to you that it was your *everything*? You were in denial for months or years because your identity was so intertwined with it. The only solution was to put an end to the relationship, but you fought that truth for a long time. You eventually made a courageous choice to end it once and for all, and even though it made you so sad to endure, you decided your life, your self, are better off without that person. Now, looking back, you feel good about the choice you made and the challenges you overcame to get here.

And so, I look at your beloved tradition of having sweets with your coffee as a positive experience from your past. It's something you once had, something so meaningful to you. Yet once it began to hold you back, it was time to move on. Here you are, now, choosing a life without it because it no longer serves you.

I don't expect you to read this and simply say goodbye to an old habit cold turkey. Just like when you first break up with someone you love, we all know you're going to slip up a few times, second-guessing the decision you made. In moments of doubt, that voice in your head tries to convince you there's still a modified version of that relationship that can make it work. Eventually, though, after enough of those lapses, you finally realize what you deeply and truly want—to be happy and healthy, which couldn't happen if you stayed in that relationship.

Embracing change and revising outdated self-images may be challenging, evoking a sense of loss and resistance, but it paves the way for personal growth and positive transformation. Just like ending a toxic relationship, it takes courage and determination to break free from self-sabotaging habits and create a healthier, more fulfilling life.

Remember, it's okay to stumble along the way; what truly matters is your unwavering commitment to grow through what you go through. Embrace the journey of self-discovery, and you open up a world of endless possibilities.

CHAPTER 62

This is a Way of Life

People often think of health as an outcome they seek. Something that is achieved someday. I invite you to think differently. Health is not an outcome. It's a lifelong pursuit. Just like spirituality, it's not a destination; it's an ongoing principle that guides you through your life choices. It's a core value you live by to whatever degree it resonates with you. The principles I've shared with you in this book are the same. Collectively, they offer you a healthy template as your guide.

Intermittent fasting and carb moderation are a way of life for me. What will it be like for you?

If we zero in on the word *diet*, all sorts of limiting beliefs and associations can arise. A diet isn't just something you go on and off in pursuit of better health. A diet is what you eat. For many of us, it changes like the seasons, but it's a constant in our lives. Even if you eat like shit (the Standard American Diet), that's still considered your diet. That's why I like to think of diets as part of a spectrum. At any given time in your life, you may fall more toward the far left of the spectrum, eating more freely and being careless with your diet. Other times, you may be quite restrictive, falling more toward the right side of the spectrum.

DIETING SPECTRUM

WHAT IS REALISTIC AND SUSTAINABLE FOR YOU?

MarisaMoon.com

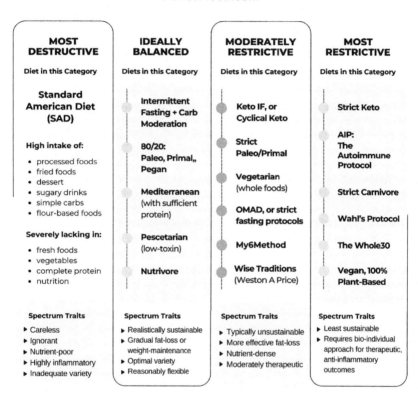

MOST DESTRUCTIVE	IDEALLY BALANCED	MODERATELY RESTRICTIVE	MOST RESTRICTIVE
Diet in this Category	Diets in this Category	Diets in this Category	Diets in this Category
Standard American Diet (SAD)	**Intermittent Fasting + Carb Moderation**	**Keto IF, or Cyclical Keto**	**Strict Keto**
High intake of:	**80:20: Paleo, Primal,, Pegan**	**Strict Paleo/Primal**	**AIP: The Autoimmune Protocol**
• processed foods			
• fried foods		**Vegetarian** (whole foods)	
• dessert	**Mediterranean** (with sufficient protein)		**Strict Carnivore**
• sugary drinks		**OMAD, or strict fasting protocols**	
• simple carbs			**Wahl's Protocol**
• flour-based foods	**Pescetarian** (low-toxin)	**My6Method**	
Severely lacking in:			**The Whole30**
• fresh foods	**Nutrivore**	**Wise Traditions** (Weston A Price)	**Vegan, 100% Plant-Based**
• vegetables			
• complete protein			
• nutrition			
Spectrum Traits	**Spectrum Traits**	**Spectrum Traits**	**Spectrum Traits**
▸ Careless	▸ Realistically sustainable	▸ Typically unsustainable	▸ Least sustainable
▸ Ignorant	▸ Gradual fat-loss or weight-maintenance	▸ More effective fat-loss	▸ Requires bio-individual approach for therapeutic, anti-inflammatory outcomes
▸ Nutrient-poor	▸ Optimal variety	▸ Nutrient-dense	
▸ Highly inflammatory	▸ Reasonably flexible	▸ Moderately therapeutic	
▸ Inadequate variety			

No matter where you're at, you won't stay there forever. You'll oscillate and grow, and you'll update your relationship with food throughout the years and chapters of your life. You'll moderate eating habits to fit the needs of your family or your job, and you'll restrict foods to fit the urgency of a new goal. You'll abandon ship sometimes when shit hits the fan, and then you'll meander back one day when you realize your health is still important to you.

I challenge you to consider how much you ask for from your body without asking what it needs in return. If this were a friendship, between you and your body, this friendship could look very one-sided. You want energy from your body, you want to stay youthful, to be free from injuries, to prevent getting sick or to get well with ease. You want to feel good, look good, and perform well, all of which requires your body to give, give, give. What does your body need from you in order to meet your expectations? Adequate nutrition, sleep, stress management, joy, connection. Your relationship with your body must be continuously reciprocal in order to experience and depend on those benefits you wish for.

Without health, what do we have, really? Without health, life feels a bit hopeless underneath it all, wouldn't you agree? Even if you're currently sick, fighting chronic illness, the hope lies in your pursuit of health. *That's* where the hope lies. You don't need good health in order for it to give you hope. You simply need to pursue it. It's your guiding principle—or at least, it's mine, and I hope you can also claim that for yourself.

Acknowledgements

You know that expression, "It takes a village to raise a child?" I have this voice in my head that often says, *It takes a village to raise me*. I depend on many people, systems, and resources to make everything happen in my life, big or small. I could never have written this book if it weren't for my husband, Eric, who encourages me to challenge myself and go for my dreams. He patiently supported me as I dragged my fingers across the keyboard, trying to write this book. Thank you, babe. You keep me grounded in reality, and I'd be all head-in-the-clouds without you. The moments you mentioned that you're proud of me served as the rocket fuel I needed to reach the finish line.

A special thanks goes out to my friend Adrienne Hanover for encouraging me to share my knowledge with her clients many years ago. Through our partnership, I was able to fine tune my fasting method for an even greater impact!

Two of my biggest cheerleaders in life are my mom and my dear friend Jessica. Throughout this entire process, they've looked at me with wide-eyed confidence and adoration that I can feel inside my bones. Gosh darn it, I'm brought to tears as I write this.

Thank you, Jessica, for having confidence in me that never wavers. For always seeing the positive and for encouraging me to be myself.

Thank you, Mom, for always believing in me. You've been along for the ride every year, starting in my teens when I flip-flopped around different ideas about what I wanted to do with my life. I never felt judged by you when I shared my new ideas. That's important, and I cherish that part of our relationship so much. Thank you for allowing me to take leaps, backpedal, change course, and come at life from all different angles.

And to my dad, who is one of the very reasons I turned out to be the nutrition enthusiast I am today. Since childhood, I didn't understand why he wouldn't let us buy *Fruit By the Foot* or why he read the ingredients on packaged foods before approving or rejecting them. He'd say, "Sorry, nope. You're not eating that crap. It's filled with artificial colors and flavors." I didn't appreciate it growing up, but it absolutely shaped me into the aspiring health coach I eventually became. It was because of him that everything clicked for me when I first discovered the Paleo Diet. Why is there so much crap in our food? Thank you, Dad, for being so persistent and for protecting our family from excessive junk food when it could've been so easy to cave and allow it, anyway. Your passion for real food, your talented family of cooks, our Italian heritage. What an impact it has made on me, and I'm here to pay it forward.

A sincere thank you to my skillful editor, Joy Sephton, who is not only lightning fast and efficient, but a kind and relatable human being. Joy, you made this whole process much less intimidating for me, and you absolutely amaze me with your skills. I am so grateful for you.

Finally, I want to thank the Self-Publishing School, my coaches Kerk and Andrew, and my morning writing buddies. Because of this program and this network of friends I've made, I had the confidence to finish something I started...something way bigger than my ADHD brain would've been willing to see through on its own. Thank you, SPS, for helping me become a published author and spread the *Not So Fast* word about prioritizing our health for a life worth living longer!

Author Bio

Marisa Moon is a National Board Certified Health and Wellness Coach, Master Primal Health Coach, and the intermittent fasting coach behind MarisaMoon.com. Ranked as Google's #1 Intermittent Fasting Coach since 2018, Marisa is recognized as a leading expert in the fasting community, especially when it comes to flexible intermittent fasting strategies that work for real life.

She's been recognized as one of the nation's top health coaches by Coachfoundation.com and Chicago Entrepreneurs Magazine. Marisa also dedicated years to a collaboration with LifeOmic's *Life Fasting Tracker* app as a timely integration of her coaching methodology into the digital space.

In addition to her successful 1-on-1 and group coaching programs, Marisa is a dynamic, sought-after speaker, presenting at virtual summits, including Fasting for Freedom and The Fasting Reset Summit. She's written blog articles for the Primal Health Coach Institute and serves as a mentor coach for Flowell.co, guiding new health coaches in their early development.

Through her relatable coaching style and podcast *Not So Fast* (formerly *The Foundation of Wellness*), Marisa helps frustrated dieters put an end to the confusion about what's healthy and finally experience results that last.

Follow Marisa's Podcast

Work with Marisa

Thank You!
I am thrilled to have you as a reader!

What did you find most helpful,
and how did this book stand out to you?

PLEASE take two minutes now to leave a helpful review on
Amazon letting me know what you thought of the book. Your review
helps get more eyes on my book so we can help more people:

MarisaMoon.com/notsofast/review

Scan this QR code for direct links to leave your review:

Thank you so much!

- Marisa

Want to Become a Health Coach?

If you're inspired by my journey and wondering if health coaching can be a career for you, I'd love to share this free resource from the Primal Health Coach Institute.

How to Become a Health Coach:
5 Steps To Embarking On a Career You'll Love

In this free guidebook you'll learn...

- How to find the best healthy coaching program for you

- How a coach differs from an "expert"

- What it takes to get a coaching business up and running

- If you need the credentials, *and much more!*

Download this free guidebook with my ambassador referral link here:

Endnotes

1 Qian J, Morris CJ, Caputo R, Garaulet M, Scheer FAJL. Ghrelin is impacted by the endogenous circadian system and by circadian misalignment in humans. Int J Obes (Lond). 2019 Aug;43(8):1644-1649

2 Spiegel, Karine et al. "Twenty-four-hour profiles of acylated and total ghrelin: relationship with glucose levels and impact of time of day and sleep." The Journal of clinical endocrinology and metabolism vol. 96,2 (2011): 486-93

3 https://en.wikipedia.org/wiki/Medieval_cuisine#Meals

4 Papakonstantinou, Emilia et al. "Effects of Diet, Lifestyle, Chrononutrition and Alternative Dietary Interventions on Postprandial Glycemia and Insulin Resistance." Nutrients vol. 14,4 823

5 Panda, Satchin. The Circadian Code. Harmony/Rodale.

6 Woodie, Lauren N et al. "The Circadian Regulation of Nutrient Metabolism in Diet-Induced Obesity and Metabolic Disease." Nutrients vol. 14,15 3136. 29 Jul. 2022

7 Jakubowicz D, Wainstein J, Tsameret S, Landau Z. Role of High Energy Breakfast "Big Breakfast Diet" in Clock Gene Regulation of Postprandial Hyperglycemia and Weight Loss in Type 2 Diabetes. Nutrients. 2021 May 5;13(5):1558

8 Wilkinson, Michael J et al. "Ten-Hour Time-Restricted Eating Reduces Weight, Blood Pressure, and Atherogenic Lipids in Patients with Metabolic Syndrome." Cell metabolism vol. 31,1 (2020): 92-104.e5

9 He, Mingqian et al. "Time-restricted eating with or without low-carbohydrate diet reduces visceral fat and improves metabolic syndrome: A randomized trial." Cell reports. Medicine vol. 3,10 (2022): 100777

10 He, Mingqian et al. "Time-restricted eating with or without low-carbohydrate diet reduces visceral fat and improves metabolic syndrome: A randomized trial." Cell reports. Medicine vol. 3,10 (2022): 100777

11 Jakubowicz D, Barnea M, Wainstein J, Froy O. High caloric intake at breakfast vs. dinner differentially influences weight loss of overweight and obese women. Obesity (Silver Spring). 2013 Dec;21(12):2504-12

12 Hadeel Ali Ghazzawi, Samar Mustafa; Effect of high-protein breakfast meal on within-day appetite hormones: Peptide YY, glucagon like peptide-1 in adults; Clin Nutr Experimental, vol 28, 2019. ISSN 2352-9393

13 Blom WA, Lluch A, Stafleu A, Vinoy S, Holst JJ, Schaafsma G, Hendriks HF. Effect of a high-protein breakfast on the postprandial ghrelin response. Am J Clin Nutr. 2006 Feb;83(2):211-20

14 https://www.valterlongo.com/the-fasting-mimicking-diet-as-opposed-to-the-more-traditional-water-fasting-results-in-a-decrease-in-intestinal-diseases-in-mice-and-in-systemic-inflammation-in-humans/

15 https://www.valterlongo.com/the-fasting-mimicking-diet-as-opposed-to-the-more-traditional-water-fasting-results-in-a-decrease-in-intestinal-diseases-in-mice-and-in-systemic-inflammation-in-humans/

16 https://www.newsweek.com/2021/12/17/americans-are-addicted-ultra-processed-foods-its-killing-us-1656977.html

17 https://www.healthyagingpoll.org/reports-more/report/addiction-highly-processed-food-among-older-adults

18 Fazzino TL, Rohde K, Sullivan DK. Hyper-Palatable Foods: Development of a Quantitative Definition and Application to the US Food System Database. Obesity (Silver Spring). 2019 Nov;27(11):1761-1768.

19 https://www.eurekalert.org/news-releases/1000520

20 Lane N. Power, Sex, Suicide: Mitochondria and the Meaning of Life. 2nd ed. Oxford University Press; Oxford, UK: 2018

21 Beal T, Ortenzi F. Priority Micronutrient Density in Foods. Front Nutr. 2022 Mar 7;9:806566

22 Beal Ty, Ortenzi F. Priority Micronutrient Density in Foods. Frontiers in Nutrition; 2022 March

23   Fuhrman, J., Sarter, B., Glaser, D. et al. Changing perceptions of hunger on a high nutrient density diet. Nutr J 9, 51 (2010)

24   Fuhrman, J., Sarter, B., Glaser, D. et al. Changing perceptions of hunger on a high nutrient density diet. Nutr J 9, 51 (2010)

25   Rhys Harrison, Vicki Warburton, Andrew Lux, et al. Blindness Caused by a Junk Food Diet. Ann Intern Med.2019;171:859-861. [Epub 30 September 2019]

26   Radulescu, Angela et al. "The effect on glucagon, glucagon-like peptide-1, total and acyl-ghrelin of dietary fats ingested with and without potato." The Journal of clinical endocrinology and metabolism vol. 95,7 (2010)

27   Rodgers, Diana; Wolf, Robb. Sacred Cow (p. 88). BenBella Books. Kindle Edition.

28   Arumugam, Madan Kumar et al. "Beneficial Effects of Betaine: A Comprehensive Review." Biology vol. 10,6 456. 22 May. 2021

29   Krok-Schoen JL, Archdeacon Price A, Luo M, Kelly OJ, Taylor CA. Low Dietary Protein Intakes and Associated Dietary Patterns and Functional Limitations in an Aging Population: A NHANES analysis. J Nutr Health Aging. 2019;23(4):338-347

30   Krok-Schoen JL, Archdeacon Price A, Luo M, Kelly OJ, Taylor CA. Low Dietary Protein Intakes and Associated Dietary Patterns and Functional Limitations in an Aging Population: A NHANES analysis. J Nutr Health Aging. 2019;23(4):338-347

31   Krok-Schoen JL, Archdeacon Price A, Luo M, Kelly OJ, Taylor CA. Low Dietary Protein Intakes and Associated Dietary Patterns and Functional Limitations in an Aging Population: A NHANES analysis. J Nutr Health Aging. 2019;23(4):338-347

32   Jean-François Lesgards. Benefits of Whey Proteins on Type 2 Diabetes Mellitus Parameters and Prevention of Cardiovascular Diseases; Nutrients 2023, 15(5), 1294

33   Frid AH, Nilsson M, Holst JJ, Björck IM. Effect of whey on blood glucose and insulin responses to composite breakfast and lunch meals in type 2 diabetic subjects. Am J Clin Nutr. 2005 Jul;82(1):69-75

34   Hadeel Ali Ghazzawi, Samar Mustafa, Effect of high-protein breakfast meal on within-day appetite hormones: Peptide YY, glucagon like peptide-1 in adults. Clinical Nutrition Experimental,
Volume 28; 2019,Pages 111-122, ISSN 2352-9393

35   Blom W. & Lluch A. et al. (2006). Effect of a high-protein breakfast on the postprandial ghrelin response. The American journal of clinical nutrition. 83. 211-20.

36   Stead, Eleanor R et al. Agephagy - Adapting Autophagy for Health During Aging. Frontiers in cell and developmental biology vol. 7 308. 28 Nov. 2019

37   Fascinating fact: fruits and vegetables respond favorably to cooking or freezing and canning, in most cases, unlocking even more nutrients due to the stress of the hot/cold temperatures.

38   Download the Nutrient Dense Food List at marisamoon.com/notsofast/resources

39   Epel E, Lapidus R, McEwen B, Brownell K. Stress may add bite to appetite in women: a laboratory study of stress-induced cortisol and eating behavior. Psychoneuroendocrinology. 2001 Jan;26(1):37-49

40   Exceptions may include person's with gastrointestinal issues, circadian disruption, and elderly people; all of whom can benefit from routine meal times.

41   Espelund U, Hansen T. K. et al. Fasting Unmasks a Strong Inverse Association between Ghrelin and Cortisol in Serum: Studies in Obese and Normal-Weight Subjects, The Journal of Clinical Endocrinology & Metabolism, Volume 90, Issue 2, 1 February 2005

42   Natalucci G, Riedl S, Gleiss A, Zidek T, Frisch H. Spontaneous 24-h ghrelin secretion pattern in fasting subjects: maintenance of a meal-related pattern. Eur J Endocrinol. 2005 Jun;152(6):845-50

43   van Anders SM, Steiger J, Goldey KL. Effects of gendered behavior on testosterone in women and men. Proc Natl Acad Sci U S A. 2015 Nov 10;112(45):13805-10. Epub 2015 Oct 26. PMID: 26504229; PMCID: PMC4653185

44   Testosterone is a precursor to estrogen, and women only need a small amount to make enough estrogen. When a woman's body makes excess testosterone, it can affect not only stress levels and anger management, but also cause irregular periods, increased body hair, balding, and acne. In some cases, this can develop into a hormonal disorder called Polycystic Ovary Syndrome (PCOS).

45   Marciniak Martyna et al., Effect of the one-day fasting on cortisol and DHEA daily rhythm regarding sex, chronotype, and age among obese adults, Frontiers in Nutrition 2023 Volume 10

46   Kim, Bo Hye et al. "Effects of Intermittent Fasting on the Circulating Levels and Circadian Rhythms of Hormones." Endocrinology and metabolism (Seoul, Korea) vol. 36,4 (2021): 745-756

47   Tasali, Esra et al. "Slow-wave sleep and the risk of type 2 diabetes in humans." Proceedings of the National Academy of Sciences of the United States of America vol. 105,3 (2008): 1044-9

Lemon-Cayenne Cleanse recipe

Daily batch:
60 oz of filtered water
6 tablespoons of raw honey, 100% pure dark maple syrup, or pure molasses (+ stevia to taste)
12 tablespoons of fresh squeezed lemon juice (approximately 8—12 lemons)
Optional 1/2 teaspoon cayenne pepper powder

Single serving:
10 oz purified water
2 tablespoons lemon juice (fresh squeezed from 1/2—1 lemon)
1 tablespoon of raw honey, 100% pure dark maple syrup, or pure molasses (+ stevia to taste)
Optional: pinch of cayenne

Printed in Great Britain
by Amazon